FIRST AID FOR THE

USMLE STEP 1

A STUDENT TO 2003 STUDENT GUIDE

VIKAS BHUSHAN, MD
University of California, San Francisco, Class of 1991
Diagnostic Radiologist

TAO LE, MD
University of California, San Francisco, Class of 1996
Johns Hopkins University, Fellow in Allergy and Immunology

CHIRAG AMIN, MD
University of Miami, Class of 1996

ANIL SHIVARAM
Yale University, Class of 2003

JOSHUA KLEIN
Yale University, Class of 2005

McGraw-Hill
Medical Publishing Division

New York   Chicago   San Francisco   Lisbon   London
Madrid   Mexico City   Milan   New Delhi   San Juan   Seoul
Singapore   Sydney   Toronto

This book was set in Goudy by Rainbow Graphics.
The editor was Catherine A. Johnson.
Project management was performed by Rainbow Graphics.
The production supervisor was Phil Galea.
The interior design is by Elizabeth Sanders.
Von Hoffman Graphics was printer and binder.

This book is printed on acid-free paper.

To the contributors to this and future editions, who took
time to share their knowledge, insight, and
humor for the benefit of students.

&

To our families, friends, and loved ones, who endured
and assisted in the task of assembling this guide.

Contributors

ZACHARY GOLDBERGER
Yale University,
Class of 2004

AIMEE LEE
Yale University,
Class of 2004

BRIAN NAHED
Yale University,
Class of 2004

MATTHEW WHITLEY
Yale University,
Class of 2004

KEVIN WANG
University of California, San Francisco,
Class of 2005

Faculty Reviewers

LINDA COSTANZO, PhD
Professor of Physiology
Medical College of Virginia
Virginia Commonwealth University

WILLIAM GANONG, MD
Lange Professor of Physiology Emeritus
University of California, San Francisco

BERTRAM KATZUNG, MD, PhD
Professor of Pharmacology
University of California, San Francisco

WILLIAM STEWART, PhD
Associate Professor of Surgery
Yale University School of Medicine

WARREN LEVINSON, MD, PhD
Professor of Microbiology and Immunology
University of California, San Francisco

STUART FLYNN, MD
Professor of Pathology
Yale University School of Medicine

Contents

Preface to the 2003 Edition

With the 2003 edition of *First Aid for the USMLE Step 1*, we continue our commitment to providing students with the most useful and up-to-date preparation guide for the USMLE Step 1. This edition represents a thorough revision in many ways and includes:

- A completely revised and updated exam preparation guide for the computerized USMLE Step 1. Includes detailed analysis as well as study and test-taking strategies for the computer-based testing (CBT) format.
- Revisions and new material based on student experience with the 2002 administrations of the computerized USMLE Step 1.
- Expanded USMLE advice for international medical graduates, osteopathic medical students, podiatry students, and students with disabilities.
- An updated collection of over 125 high-yield glossy photos similar to those appearing on the USMLE Step 1 exam.
- More than 900 frequently tested facts and useful mnemonics, including **hundreds of new or revised entries with many new diagrams and illustrations.**
- Useful reference links to prototypical clinical cases from the latest edition of the popular *Underground Clinical Vignette* (UCV) series (Blackwell Science/S2S Publishing).
- An updated listing of more than 100 high-yield clinical vignette topics that highlight key areas of basic science and clinical material recently emphasized on the USMLE Step 1.
- A completely revised, in-depth guide to over 300 basic science review and sample examination books, based on a random survey of third-year medical students across the country.

The 2003 edition would not have been possible without the help of the hundreds of students and faculty members who contributed their feedback and suggestions. We invite students and faculty to continue sharing their thoughts and ideas to help us improve *First Aid for the USMLE Step 1*. (See How to Contribute, p. xv, and User Survey, p. xxiii.)

Los Angeles	Vikas Bhushan
Baltimore	Tao Le
Miami	Chirag Amin
New Haven	Anil Shivaram
New Haven	Joshua Klein

November 2002

Foreword

The purpose of *First Aid for the USMLE Step 1: A Student-to-Student Guide* is to help medical students and international medical graduates review the basic medical sciences and prepare for the United States Medical Licensing Examination, Step 1 (USMLE Step 1). Preparing for this examination can be a stressful, difficult, and costly task. This book helps students make the most of their limited time, money, and energy. As is often the case in medical school, we found that the best advice a student can receive is from other medical students. We also recognized that certain basic science topics and details are "popular" and appear frequently on examinations. With this in mind, *First Aid for the USMLE Step 1* was started in 1989.

As we studied for the NBME Part I, we examined and evaluated scores of review books and thousands of sample questions. We kept track of useful study strategies, frequently tested facts, and helpful mnemonics through a simple computer database. The printed database was first distributed to the medical school class of 1992 at the University of California, San Francisco (UCSF). The next year, a revised edition was self-published under the name *High-Yield Basic Science Boards Review: A Student-to-Student Guide*. This guide was distributed to the UCSF class of 1993 and to numerous faculty and medical students at various institutions.

The title reflects the potential value of this book as the "first" one to get before buying others, and the fact that boards examinations are stressful and unpleasant experiences that students may "aid" each other in overcoming. We feel that this study guide provides a unique and pragmatic approach to the USMLE Step 1 and that it contains useful components not found in current boards review material. *First Aid for the USMLE Step 1* has three major sections:

Section I: Guide to Efficient Exam Preparation is a compilation of general student advice and study strategies for taking the computerized USMLE Step 1.

Section II: Database of High-Yield Facts contains short descriptions of frequently tested facts and concepts as well as mnemonics, diagrams, and high-quality photo illustrations to facilitate learning. It includes a unique summary of subject-by-subject examination emphases as estimated by students who have recently taken the examination.

Section III: Database of Basic Science Review Books is designed to save students time and money by identifying high-quality, reasonably priced review and sample examination books and software. The comments and ratings are based on our analyses and on an annual nationwide random sampling of third-year medical students.

First Aid for the USMLE Step 1 is not designed to be a comprehensive text or the sole study source for the USMLE Step 1; it is meant as a guide to one's preparation for the USMLE Step 1. The material in this book has been written to strengthen one's familiarity with a large number of topics in a short, fact-based review. The authors do not advocate blindly memorizing the lists of facts, and we hope medical students realize that memorization cannot replace an understanding of the concepts that underlie these key points.

Entries in *First Aid for the USMLE Step 1* originated from hundreds of students, international medical graduates, and faculty members, who synthesized the facts, notes, and mnemonics from a variety of textbooks, review books, lecture notes, and personal notes. We regret the inability to reference each individual fact or mnemonic owing to the diverse and often anecdotal sources. Although the material has been reviewed by faculty members and medical students, errors and omissions are inevitable. We urge readers to identify errors and suggest improvements. We regret that some students may find certain mnemonics trivializing or offensive. The mnemonics are meant solely as optional devices for learning.

The authors and McGraw-Hill intend to continue updating *First Aid for the USMLE Step 1* so that the book grows in quality and scope and continues to reflect the material covered on the USMLE Step 1. If you have any study strategies, high-yield facts with mnemonics, or book reviews for the next edition, please use the forms included to submit your contributions. (See How to Contribute, p xv.) Any student or faculty member who submits material subsequently used in the next edition of *First Aid for the USMLE Step 1* will receive personal acknowledgment in the next edition and a $10 gift certificate per complete entry.

Good luck in your studies!

Acknowledgments

This has been a collaborative project from the start. We gratefully acknowledge the thoughtful comments, corrections, and advice of the many hundreds of medical students, international medical graduates, and faculty who have supported the authors in the continuing development of *First Aid for the USMLE Step 1*.

Special thanks to Dr. Raoul Fresco for his generous contributions to the glossy photo section.

Thanks to Noam Maitless for the original book design, as well as Evenson Design Group, Ashley Pound, and Elizabeth Sanders for design revisions.

For support and encouragement throughout the process, we are grateful to Thao Pham and Jonathan Kirsch, Esq.

Thanks to our publisher, McGraw-Hill, for the valuable assistance of their staff. For enthusiasm, support, and commitment for this ongoing and ever-challenging project, thanks to our editor, Catherine Johnson. Thanks to Selina Bush for organizing and supporting the project. For editorial support, enormous thanks to Andrea Fellows. A special thanks to Jimmy and Bennie Sauls (Rainbow Graphics) for remarkable production work.

For submitting contributions and corrections for the 2003 edition, we thank Aileen Alviar, Lynn Marie Becker, Hind Bennani, Christina Checka, Carl Dragstedt, Ana Esteben, Alfred Fleming, Joseph Harburger, Pamela Herbert, Nancy Hernandez, Audrey Hong, John Ilgen, Jason Kuhl, Liza Le, Marci Levine, Vaishali Parikh, Mohamed Aiyub Patel, Naveen Pemmaraju, Elyse Pine, Sheldon Rockwood, Janelle Shin, Cynthia Soto, Marc Taylor, Emily Vail, Jaclyn van Nes, Nicholas Watson, Todd Wilkinson, Sarah Wiener, and Michael Shapiro.

For submitting book reviews, we thank Cristina Pacheco, Sujeet Achrya, Jocelyn Kim, Kristen McNamara, Melissa Brand, Rob Linden, Michael Tomblyn, Matthew Rrauen, Suzanne Emil, Amy Spizuoco, Una Ercegovac, Stephne Gamboa, Anjana Prasad, Nicholas Silvestri, Amil Patel, Tina Lin, Cheryl Clay, Kisa Seymore, Amousheh Sayah, Audrey Marcusen, Benjamin Snyder, Nancy Lares, Kerri Frank, Silvester Lim, Jennifer Turner, David Barrett, Kevin Pei, Heidi Lako-Adamson, Eva Hecht, Chirag Patel, Jennifer Gomez, Ken Park, Mike Mentari, Christopher Braushaw, Erica Pearson, Tara Kennedy, Matthew Belan, Tj Tanous, Nikola Ragusa, Hasan Syed, Jeremy Hogan, Alicia Chaves, John Acerra, Won Lee, Meena Nahata, Jill Thoman, Stephanie Kimberlain, Cheryl Quinn, Umesh Dave, Steven Lewis, Todd Anderson, Jennifer Thomas, Tara-Sharon Coyle, Karen Au, Brian Hess, Justin Maxhimer, Steve Leung, Jason Wilson, Andrew Louie, John Neilson, Amanda Barrett, Kris Jatana, Ajay Bhatia, Melinda Healy, Samir Thadani, Ryan Burri, Eric McGrath, Lien Huynh, Kristi Mizelle, David Herszenson, Erin Raci, Julie Gayle, Amanda Cooper, Kimberly Zuzak, Steven Conroy, Sheela Kadekar, Andrew

Chu, Michele Streeter, Carolyn Lex, Amanda Flint, Rupinder Tung, Derrick Chu, Michael Chu, Kirk Brown, and Christina Schwereb.

Special thanks to Navin Arora and Lisa Roy for their contributions to the Special Situations, Osteopathic Medicine, and Students with Disabilities sections.

Finally, thanks to Ted Hon, one of the founding authors of this book, for his vision in developing this guide on the computer.

Los Angeles	Vikas Bhushan
Baltimore	Tao Le
Miami	Chirag Amin
New Haven	Anil Shivaram
New Haven	Joshua Klein

How to Contribute

This version of *First Aid for the USMLE Step 1* incorporates hundreds of contributions and changes suggested by faculty and student reviewers. We invite you to participate in this process. We also offer **paid internships** in medical education and publishing ranging from three months to one year (see next page for details).

Please send us your suggestions for:

- Study and test-taking strategies for the new computerized USMLE Step 1
- New facts, mnemonics, diagrams, and illustrations
- High-yield topics that may reappear on future Step 1 exams
- Personal ratings and comments on review books that you have examined

For each entry incorporated into the next edition, you will receive a $10 gift certificate per entry from the author group, as well as personal acknowledgment in the next edition. Diagrams, tables, partial entries, updates, corrections, and study hints are also appreciated, and significant contributions will be compensated at the discretion of the authors. Also let us know about material in this edition that you feel is low yield and should be deleted.

The preferred way to submit entries, suggestions, or corrections is via electronic mail. Please include name, address, school affiliation, phone number, and e-mail address (if different from address of origin). Please send submissions to:

firstaidteam@yahoo.com

Otherwise, please send entries, neatly written or typed or on disk (Microsoft Word), to: **First Aid for the USMLE Step 1, 1015 Gayley Ave., #1113, Los Angeles, CA 90024, Attention: Contributions.** Please use the contribution and survey forms on the following pages. Each form constitutes an entry. (Attach additional pages as needed.)

Contributions received by July 15, 2003, receive priority consideration for the 2004 edition of *First Aid for the USMLE Step 1*.

Internship Opportunities

The author team of Bhushan and Le is pleased to offer part-time and full-time paid internships in medical education and publishing to motivated medical students and physicians. Internships may range from three months (e.g., a summer) up to a full year. Participants will have an opportunity to author, edit, and earn academic credit on a wide variety of projects, including the popular *First Aid* series.

English writing/editing experience, familiarity with Microsoft Word, and Internet access are required. For more information, e-mail a résumé or a short description of your experience along with a cover letter to Firstaidteam@yahoo.com. A sample of your work or a proposal of a specific project is helpful.

Note to Contributors

All contributions become property of the authors and are subject to editing and reviewing. Please verify all data and spellings carefully. In the event that similar or duplicate entries are received, only the first entry received will be used. Include a reference to a standard textbook to facilitate verification of the fact. Please follow the style, punctuation, and format of this edition if possible.

Contribution Form I

For entries, mnemonics, facts, strategies, corrections, diagrams, etc.

Contributor Name: ______________________

School/Affiliation: ______________________
(no acronyms please)

Address: ______________________

____

Telephone: ______________________

E-mail: ______________________

Topic:

Subject/Subsection:
Page number in '03 ed.:

Fact and Description:

Notes, Diagrams, and Mnemonics:

Reference:

Please return by July 15, 2003. You will receive personal acknowledgment and a $10 gift certificate for each entry that is used in future editions.

Please seal with tape only.
No staples or paper clips.

- - - - - - - - - - - - - (fold here) -

Place
Stamp
Here

FIRST AID FOR THE USMLE STEP 1
P.O. BOX 27
WOODSTOCK, MD   21163

- (fold here) -

Contribution Form II

For entries, mnemonics, facts,
strategies, corrections,
diagrams, etc.

Contributor Name: _____

School/Affiliation: _____
(no acronyms please)
Address: _____

_____

_____

Telephone: _____

E-mail: _____

Please place the subject heading (e.g., Anatomy) on the first line and the high-yield vignette or topic on the following two lines.

1. Subject: _____
    Vignette: _____
    _____

2. Subject: _____
    Vignette: _____
    _____

3. Subject: _____
    Vignette: _____
    _____

4. Subject: _____
    Vignette: _____
    _____

5. Subject: _____
    Vignette: _____
    _____

6. Subject: _____
    Vignette: _____
    _____

7. Subject: _____
    Vignette: _____
    _____

8. Subject: _____
    Vignette: _____
    _____

9. Subject: _____
    Vignette: _____
    _____

10. Subject: _____
    Vignette: _____
    _____

Please seal with tape only.
No staples or paper clips.

(fold here)

Place
Stamp
Here

FIRST AID FOR THE USMLE STEP 1
P.O. BOX 27
WOODSTOCK, MD   21163

(fold here)

Contribution Form III

For entries, mnemonics, facts, strategies, corrections, diagrams, etc.

Contributor Name: _____

School/Affiliation: _____
(no acronyms please)

Address: _____

_____

_____

Telephone: _____

E-mail: _____

We welcome additional comments on review resources rated in Section III as well as reviews of resources not rated in Section III. Please fill out each review entry as completely as possible. Please do not leave "Comments" blank. Rate texts using the letter grading scale provided on p. 404, taking into consideration current ratings of other books on that subject.

1. ***Title/Author:*** _____ Days needed to read: _____

   Publisher/Series: _____ ISBN Number: _____

   Rating: _____ ***Comments:*** _____

   _____

   _____

2. ***Title/Author:*** _____ Days needed to read: _____

   Publisher/Series: _____ ISBN Number: _____

   Rating: _____ ***Comments:*** _____

   _____

   _____

3. ***Title/Author:*** _____ Days needed to read: _____

   Publisher/Series: _____ ISBN Number: _____

   Rating: _____ ***Comments:*** _____

   _____

   _____

   _____

4. ***Title/Author:*** _____ Days needed to read: _____

   Publisher/Series: _____ ISBN Number: _____

   Rating: _____ ***Comments:*** _____

   _____

   _____

5. ***Title/Author:*** _____ Days needed to read: _____

   Publisher/Series: _____ ISBN Number: _____

   Rating: _____ ***Comments:*** _____

   _____

   _____

Please seal with tape only.
No staples or paper clips.

(fold here)

Place
Stamp
Here

FIRST AID FOR THE USMLE STEP 1
P.O. BOX 27
WOODSTOCK, MD   21163

(fold here)

User Survey

Contributor Name: _____

School/Affiliation: _____
(no acronyms please)
Address: _____

_____

_____

Telephone: _____

E-mail: _____

What student-to-student advice would you give someone preparing for the computerized USMLE Step 1? What on-line resources, if any, did you use for Step 1 prep?

What commercial review courses have you been enrolled in, and what were your overall assessments of the courses?

What would you change about the study and test-taking strategies listed in Section I: Guide to Efficient Exam Preparation?

Were there any high-yield facts, topics, or vignettes in Section II that you think were inaccurate or should be deleted? Which ones and why? What would you change or add? What high-yield images would you like to see?

What review resources for the USMLE Step 1 are not covered in Section III? Would you change the rating of any of the review resources in Section III? If so, which one(s) and why?

What other suggestions do you have for improving *First Aid for the USMLE Step 1*? Any other comments or suggestions? What did you dislike most about the book? What did you like most?

Please return by July 15, 2003. You will receive personal acknowledgment and a $10 gift certificate for each entry that is used in future editions.

Please seal with tape only.
No staples or paper clips.

--- (fold here) ---

FIRST AID FOR THE USMLE STEP 1
P.O. BOX 27
WOODSTOCK, MD   21163

--- (fold here) ---

How to Use This Book

Medical students who have used previous editions of this guide have given us feedback on how best to make use of the book.

It is recommended that you begin using this book as early as possible when learning the basic medical sciences. You can use Section III to select first-year course review books, internet resources, and then use those books for review while taking your medical school classes.

Use different parts of the book at different stages in your preparation for the USMLE Step 1. Before you begin to study for the USMLE Step 1, we suggest that you read Section I: Guide to Efficient Exam Preparation and Section III: Database of Basic Science Review Resources. **If you are an international medical graduate student, an osteopathic medical student, a podiatry student, or a student with a disability,** refer to the appropriate Section I supplement for additional advice. Devise a study plan and decide what resources to buy. We strongly recommend that you invest in at least one or two top-rated review books in each subject. *First Aid* is not a comprehensive review book, and it is not a panacea for not studying during the first two years of medical school. Scanning Section II will give you an initial idea of the diverse range of topics covered on the USMLE Step 1.

As you study each discipline, **use the corresponding high-yield-fact section in *First Aid for the USMLE Step 1* as a way of consolidating the material and testing yourself** to see if you have covered some of the frequently tested items. Use the UCV reference links to see corresponding clinical vignettes. Work with the book to integrate important facts into your fund of knowledge. Using *First Aid for the USMLE Step 1* as a review can serve as both a self-test of your knowledge and a repetition of important facts to learn. High-yield topics and vignettes are abstracted from recent exams to help guide your preparation.

Return to Section II frequently during your preparation and fill your short-term memory with remaining high-yield facts a few days before the USMLE Step 1. The book can serve as a useful way of retaining key associations and keeping high-yield facts fresh in your memory just prior to the examination.

Reviewing the book immediately after the exam is probably the best way to **help us improve the book in the next edition.** Decide what was truly high and low yield and **send in the contribution forms or your entire annotated book.**

First Aid Checklist for the USMLE Step 1

This is an example of how you might use the information in Section I to prepare for the USMLE Step 1. Refer to corresponding topics in Section I for more details.

Years Prior

☐ Select top-rated review books as study guides for first year medical school courses.

Months Prior

☐ Review computer test format and registration information.

☐ Register six months in advance. Carefully verify name and address printed on scheduling permit. Call Sylvan for test date ASAP.

☐ Define goals for the USMLE Step 1 (e.g., comfortably pass, beat the mean, ace the test).

☐ Set up a realistic timeline for study. Cover less crammable subjects first. Review subject-by-subject emphasis and clinical vignette format.

☐ Simulate the USMLE Step 1 to pinpoint strengths and weaknesses in knowledge and test-taking skills.

☐ Evaluate and choose study methods and materials (e.g., review books, practice tests, software).

☐ Ask advice from those who have recently taken the USMLE Step 1.

Weeks Prior

☐ Simulate the USMLE Step 1 again. Assess how close you are to your goal.

☐ Pinpoint remaining weaknesses. Stay healthy (exercise, sleep).

☐ Verify information on admission ticket (e.g., location, date).

One Week Prior

☐ Remember comfort measures (loose clothing, earplugs, etc.).

☐ Work out test site logistics such as location, transportation, parking, and lunch.

☐ Call Prometric and confirm your exam appointment.

One Day Prior

☐ Relax.

☐ Light review of short-term material if necessary. Skim high-yield facts.

☐ Get a good night's sleep.

☐ Make sure the name printed on your photo ID appears EXACTLY the same as the name printed on your scheduling permit. You will not be allowed to take the exam unless the names match EXACTLY.

Day of Exam

☐ Relax. Eat breakfast. Minimize bathroom breaks during exam by avoiding excessive morning caffeine.

☐ Analyze and make adjustments in test-taking technique. You are allowed to review notes/study material during breaks on exam day.

After the Exam

☐ Celebrate, regardless.

☐ Please fill out the contribution forms and receive $10 gift certificates. See p. xv for details.

Guide to Efficient Exam Preparation

Relax.

This section is intended to make your exam preparation easier, not harder. Our goal is to reduce your level of stress and help you make the most of your study effort by helping you understand more about the United States Medical Licensing Examination, Step 1 (USMLE Step 1)—especially what the new computer-based testing (CBT) is likely to mean to you. As a medical student, you are no doubt familiar with taking standardized examinations and quickly absorbing large amounts of material. When you first confront the USMLE Step 1, however, you may find it easy to become sidetracked and not achieve your goal of studying with maximum effectiveness. Common mistakes that students make when studying for the boards include the following:

- "Stressing out" owing to an inadequate understanding of new computer-based format
- Not understanding how scoring is performed or what your score means
- Starting *First Aid* too late
- Starting to study too late
- Using inefficient or inappropriate study methods
- Buying the wrong books or buying more books than you can ever use
- Buying only one publisher's review series for all subjects
- Not using practice examinations to maximum benefit
- Not using review books along with your classes
- Not analyzing and improving your test-taking strategies
- Getting bogged down by reviewing difficult topics excessively
- Studying material that is rarely tested on the USMLE Step 1
- Failing to master certain high-yield subjects owing to overconfidence
- Using *First Aid* as your sole study resource

In this section, we offer advice to help you avoid these pitfalls and be more productive in your studies. To begin, it is important for you to understand what the examination involves.

USMLE STEP 1—THE CBT BASICS

The USMLE assesses a physician's ability to apply knowledge, concepts, and principles that are important in health and disease and that constitute the basis of safe and effective patient care.[2]

Some degree of concern about your performance on the USMLE Step 1 examination is both expected and appropriate. All too often, however, medical students become unnecessarily anxious about the examination. It is therefore important to understand precisely what the USMLE Step 1 involves. As you become familiar with Step 1, you can translate your anxiety into more efficient preparation.

The USMLE Step 1 is the first of three examinations that you must pass in order to become a licensed physician in the United States.[1] The USMLE is a joint endeavor of the National Board of Medical Examiners (NBME) and the Federation of State Medical Boards (FSMB). In previous years, the examination was strictly organized around seven traditional disciplines: anatomy, behavioral science, biochemistry, microbiology, pathology, pharmacology, and physiology. In June 1991, the NBME began administering the "new" NBME Part I examination, which offered a more integrated and multidisciplinary format coupled with more clinically oriented questions.

In 1992, the USMLE replaced both the Federation Licensing Examination (FLEX) and the certifying examinations of the NBME.[3] The USMLE now serves as the single examination system for United States medical students and international medical graduates (IMGs) seeking medical licensure in the United States.

How Is the CBT Structured?

In 1999, the traditional two-day paper-and-pencil exam gave way to an eight-hour computer-based test. The exam, administered by Prometric, Inc®, a subsidiary of Thomson Learning™, is now offered year-round at hundreds of sites around the world.

The CBT format of Step 1 is simply a computerized version of the former paper exam.

The CBT Step 1 exam consists of seven question "blocks" of 50 questions each (Figure 1) for a total of 350 questions, timed at 60 minutes per block. A short 11-question survey follows the last question block. The computer begins the survey with a prompt to proceed to the next block of questions. Don't be fooled! "Block 8" is the NBME survey.

These blocks were designed to reduce eyestrain and fatigue during the exam. Once an examinee finishes a particular block, he or she must click on a screen icon to continue to the next block. Examinees will **not** be able to go back and change answers to questions from any previously completed block. Changing answers, however, is allowed **within** a block of questions as long as time permits.

Don't be fooled! After the last question block comes the NBME survey ("Block 8").

Prometric test centers offer Step 1 on a year-round basis, except for the first two weeks in January. The exam is given every day except Sunday at most centers. Some schools administer the exam on their own campuses.

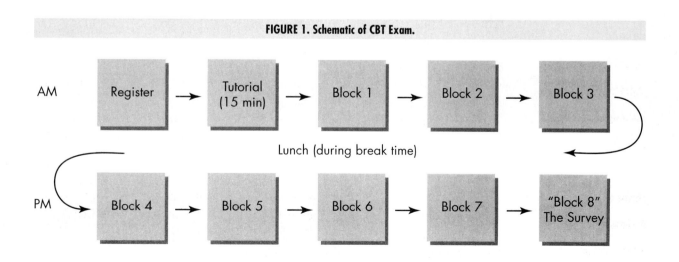

FIGURE 1. Schematic of CBT Exam.

AM: Register → Tutorial (15 min) → Block 1 → Block 2 → Block 3

Lunch (during break time)

PM: Block 4 → Block 5 → Block 6 → Block 7 → "Block 8" The Survey

What Is the CBT Like?

Skip the tutorial and add 15 minutes to your break time!

Because of the unique environment of the CBT, it's important that you be familiar ahead of time with what your test-day conditions will be like. Familiarizing yourself with the testing interface before the exam can add 15 minutes to your break time! This is because a 15-minute tutorial, offered on exam day, may be skipped if you are already familiar with the exam procedures and the testing interface (see description of CD-ROM below). The 15 minutes is added to your allotted break time (should you choose to skip the tutorial).

For security reasons, examinees are not allowed to bring any personal electronic equipment into the testing area. This includes digital watches, watches with computer communication and/or memory capability, cellular telephones, and electronic paging devices. Food and beverages are also prohibited. The testing centers are monitored by audio and video surveillance equipment.

The typical question screen (Figure 2) has a question followed by a number of choices on which an examinee can click, together with a number of navigational buttons at the bottom. There is also a button that allows the examinee to mark the question for review. There is a countdown timer in the upper right-hand corner of the screen as well. If the question happens to be longer than the screen (very rare), a scroll bar appears on the right, allowing the examinee to see the rest of the question. Regardless of whether the examinee clicks on an answer or leaves it blank, he or she must click the "Next" button to advance to the next question.

Some questions contain figures or color illustrations (Figure 3). These are typically situated to the right of the question. Although the contrast and bright-

FIGURE 2. Typical Question Screen.

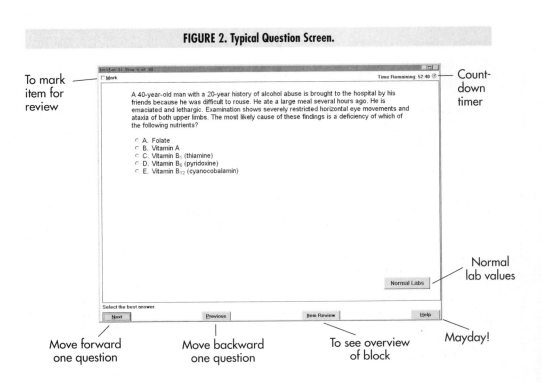

FIGURE 3. Question Screen with Illustration.

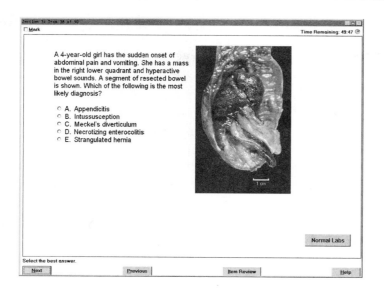

Test illustrations include:

- Gross photos
- Histology slides
- Radiographs
- EMs
- Line drawings

ness of the screen can be adjusted, there are no other ways to manipulate the picture (e.g., no zooming or panning).

The examinee can call up a window displaying normal lab values (Figure. 4). However, if he or she does not press "Tile" on the normal-values screen, the normal-values window may obscure the question. The examinee may have to scroll down searching for the needed laboratory values.

Clicking "Item Review" at the bottom of the screen brings up a screen showing an overview of the block (Figure 5). This screen allows the examinee to pinpoint questions marked for review as well as unanswered questions. This

FIGURE 4. Lab Values Screen—Floating and Tiled.

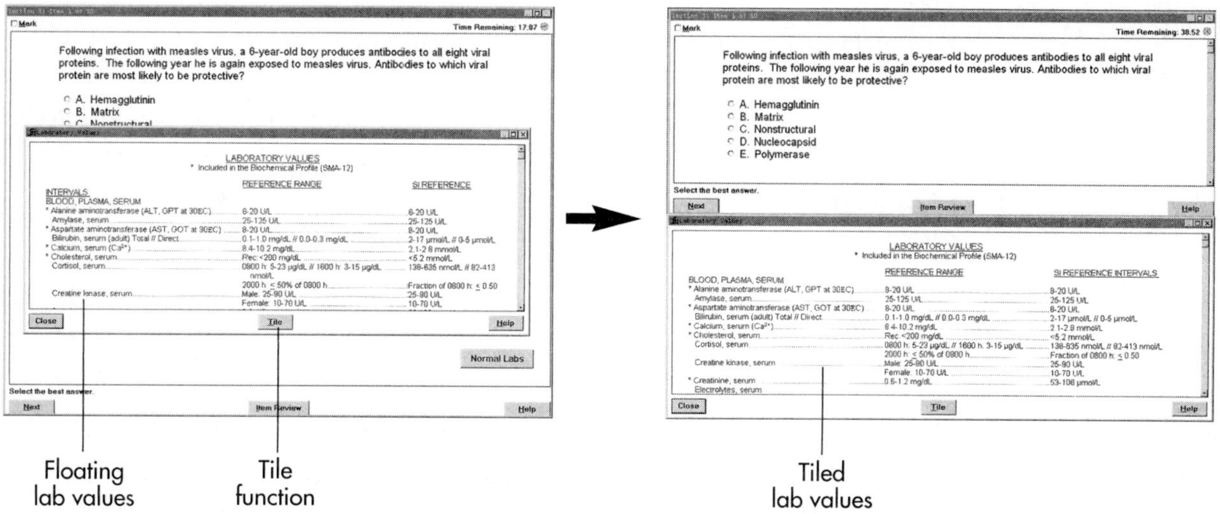

Floating lab values

Tile function

Tiled lab values

FIGURE 5. Item Review Screen.

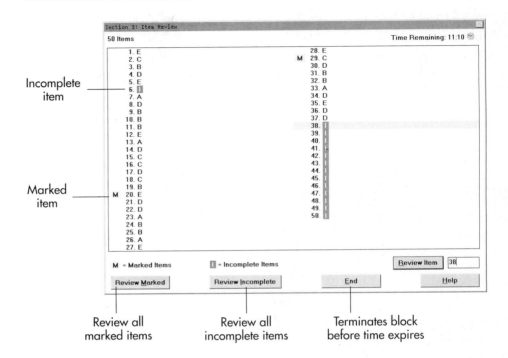

also serves as a quick way of navigating to any question in the block—even unmarked completed questions.

What Does the CBT Format Mean to Me?

The significance to you of the CBT depends on the requirements of your school and your level of computer knowledge. If you hate computers and freak out whenever you see one, you might want to face your fears as soon as possible. Spend some time playing with a Windows-based system and pointing and clicking icons or buttons with a mouse. These are the absolute basics, and you won't want to waste valuable exam time figuring them out on test day. Your test taking will proceed by pointing and clicking, essentially without the use of the keyboard. The free CD is an excellent way to become familiar with the test interface.

For those who feel they would benefit, the USMLE offers an opportunity to take a simulated test, or "CBT Practice Session at a Prometric center." Students are eligible to take the three-and-one-half-hour practice session after they have received their fluorescent orange scheduling permit (see below).

The same USMLE Step 1 sample test items (150 questions) available on the CD or USMLE Web site, www.usmle.org, are used at these sessions. *No new items will be presented.* The session is divided into three one-hour blocks of 50 test items each and costs about $42. The student receives a printed percent-correct score after completing the session. No explanations of questions are provided.

You may register for a practice session online at www.usmle.org.

How Do I Register to Take the Exam?

Starting with the 2001 USMLE application cycle, registration packets with printed materials are no longer provided to medical schools. Your medical school should have a supply of the 2003 CD, which contains electronic files of all of the printed materials, such as the *2003 USMLE Bulletin of Information*. Step 1 or Step 2 applications, which are not on the CD, may be printed from the USMLE Web site.

The preliminary registration process for the USMLE Step 1 is essentially unchanged, which is to say that students are required to complete registration forms and send exam fees to the NBME. The application allows applicants to select one of 12 overlapping three-month blocks in which to be tested (e.g., April–May–June, June–July–August). The application includes a photo ID form that must be certified by an official at your medical school to verify your enrollment. After the NBME processes your application, it will send you a fluorescent orange slip of paper called a scheduling permit.

The scheduling permit you receive from the NBME will contain your USMLE identification number, the eligibility period in which you may take the exam, and two unique numbers. One of these is known as your "scheduling number." You must have this number to make your exam appointment with Prometric. The other number is known as the "candidate identification number," or CIN. Examinees must enter their CINs at the Prometric workstation to access their exams. Prometric has no access to the codes. **Do not lose your permit!** You will not be allowed to take the boards unless you present this permit along with an unexpired, government-issued photo identification with your signature (such as a driver's license or passport). Make sure the name on your photo ID exactly matches the name appearing on your scheduling permit.

Once you receive your scheduling permit, you may call the Prometric toll-free number to arrange a time to take the exam. Although requests for taking the exam may be completed more than six months before the test date, examinees will not receive their scheduling permits earlier than six months before the eligibility period. The eligibility period is the three-month period you have chosen to take the exam. Most medical students choose the April–June or June–August period. Because exams are scheduled on a "first-come, first-served" basis, it is recommended that you telephone Prometric as soon as you have received your permit. After you've scheduled your exam, it's a good idea to confirm your exam appointment with Prometric at least one week prior to your test date. Prometric does not provide written confirmation of exam date, time, or location. Be sure to read the *2003 USMLE Bulletin of Information* for further details.

What If I Need to Reschedule the Exam?

You can change your date and/or center by contacting Prometric at 1-800-MED-EXAM (1-800-633-3926), www.prometric.com. Make sure to have your CIN when rescheduling. If you are rescheduling by phone, you must speak

Test scheduling is on a "first-come, first-served" basis. It's important to call and schedule an exam date as soon as you receive your scheduling permit.

Testing centers are closed on major holidays and during the first two weeks of January.

Register six months in advance for seating and scheduling preference.

with a Prometric representative; leaving a voice-mail message will not suffice. To avoid a rescheduling fee, you will need to request a change before noon EST at least five business days before your appointment. Please note that your rescheduled test date must fall within your assigned three-month eligibility period.

When Should I Register for the Exam?

Although there are no deadlines for registering for Step 1, you should plan to register at least six months ahead of your desired test date. This will guarantee that you will get either your test center of choice or one within a 50-mile radius of your first choice. For most U.S. medical students, the desired testing window is in June, since most medical school curricula for the second year end in May or June. Thus, U.S. medical students should plan to register before January for a June test date. The timing of the exam is more flexible for IMGs, as it is related only to when they finish exam preparation.

Choose your three-month eligibility period wisely. If you need to reschedule outside your initial three-month period, you must submit a new application along with another $405 application fee.

Where Can I Take the Exam?

Your testing location is arranged with Prometric when you call for your test date (after you receive your scheduling permit). For a list of Prometric locations nearest you, visit www.prometric.com.

How Long Will I Have to Wait Before I Get My Scores?

The USMLE reports scores three to six weeks after the examinee's test date. Scores are always released on a Wednesday. During peak times, score reports may take up to six weeks. Official information concerning the time required for score reporting is posted on the USMLE Web site.

What Did Other Students Like/Dislike About the CBT Format?

Feedback from students about the CBT format has been overwhelmingly positive. Students note that the testing environment was not as stressful as imagined and add that they enjoyed the test's point-and-click simplicity. "It's nice to be able to work at your own pace and take breaks whenever you want," commented one student.

Beware of the awkward lab-values screen, background noise, variable image quality, and eyestrain.

Of the complaints expressed, students were most concerned with image quality, eyestrain, temperature extremes (heat/cold), and background noise at the Prometric center. Students noted that the quality of some images made it difficult to answer certain questions and that they would like to be able to enlarge images. Eyestrain seemed to affect other test takers; taking a short break usually afforded relief. In addition, some students noted that the clicking of mice and keyboard chatter by other students bothered them. Earplugs helped but didn't completely block all such sounds.

What About Time?

Time is of special interest on the CBT exam. Here's a breakdown of the exam schedule:

15 minutes	Tutorial (skip if familiar)
7 hours	60-minute question blocks
45 minutes	Break time (includes time for lunch)

The computer will keep track of how much time has elapsed. However, the computer will show you only how much time you have remaining in a given block. Therefore, it is up to you to determine if you are pacing yourself properly (at a rate of approximately one question per 72 seconds).

The computer will **not** warn you if you are spending more than your allotted time for a break. Taking long breaks between question blocks or for lunch may result in your not being able to take breaks later. You should budget your time so that you can take a short break when you need it and have time to eat.

You must be especially careful not to spend too much time in between blocks (you should keep track of how much time elapses from when you finish a block of questions to when you start the next block). After you finish one question block, you'll need to click the mouse when you are ready to proceed to the next block of questions.

Forty-five minutes is the minimum break time for the day. You can gain extra break time (but not time for the question blocks) by skipping the tutorial or by finishing a block ahead of the allotted time.

For security reasons, digital watches are not allowed. This means that only analog watches are permitted. You should therefore get used to timing yourself with an analog watch so that you know exactly how much time you have left. Some analog watches come with a bevel that helps keep track of 60-minute periods. This may be useful for keeping track of break time.

If I Freak Out and Leave, What Happens to My Score?

Your scheduling permit shows a CIN that you will enter onto your computer screen to start your exam. Entering the CIN is the same as breaking the seal on a test book, and you are considered to have started the exam. However, no score will be reported if you do not complete the exam. In fact, if you leave at any time from the start of the test to the last block, no score will be reported. The fact that you started but did not complete the exam, however, will appear on your USMLE score transcript.

Be careful to watch the clock on your break time.

Gain extra break time by skipping the tutorial or finishing a block early.

If you have one unanswered question remaining during any block, the computer will allow you to answer it before you are closed out of the block. (Note: This will use up some of your break time.)

The exam ends when all blocks have been completed or their time has expired. As you leave the testing center, you receive a printed test-completion notice to document your completion of the exam.

To receive an official score, you must finish the entire exam. This means that you must start and either finish or run out of time for each block of the exam. Again, if you do not complete all blocks, your exam is documented as an incomplete attempt, and no score is reported.

What Types of Questions Are Asked?

Nearly three-fourths of the 2002 Step 1 questions began with a description of a patient.

Although numerous changes had to be made for the CBT format, the question types are the same as in previous years.

One-best-answer items have been the most commonly used multiple-choice format. Test takers report that every question was of this format. Most questions consist of a clinical scenario or a direct question followed by a list of five or more options. You are required to select the one best answer among the options. A number of options may be partially correct, in which case you must select the option that best answers the question or completes the statement. Additionally, keep in mind that experimental questions may appear on the exam (see Difficult Questions, p. 28).

How Is the Test Scored?

The mean Step 1 score for U.S. medical students rose from 200 in 1991 to 215 in 2000.

Each Step 1 examinee receives a score report that has the examinee's pass/fail status, two test scores, and a graphic depiction of the examinee's performance by discipline and organ system or subject area (Figures 6A and 6B). The actual organ-system profiles reported may depend on the statistical characteristics of a given administration of the examination.

For 1999, the NBME provided two overall test scores based on the total number of items answered correctly on the examination (Figure 7). The first score, the three-digit score, was reported as a scaled score in which the mean was 215 and the standard deviation was 20. The second score scale, the two-digit score, defines 75 as the minimum passing score (equivalent to a score of 179 on the first scale). A score of 82 is equivalent to a score of 200 on the first score scale. To avoid confusion, we refer to scores using the three-digit scale with a mean of 215 and a standard deviation of 20.

Passing the CBT Step 1 is estimated to correspond to answering 60 to 70% of the questions correctly.

Starting in 2001, a score of 182 or higher is required to pass Step 1. Passing the CBT Step 1 is estimated to correspond to answering 60 to 70% of questions correctly. In 2001, the pass rates for first-time test takers from accredited U.S. and Canadian medical schools were 93% and 91%, respectively (Table 1). These statistics prove it—you're much more likely to pass than fail. Although the NMBE may adjust the minimum passing score at any time, no further adjustment is expected for several years.

FIGURE 6A. Sample Score Report—Front Page

US·MLE
United States
Medical
Licensing
Examination

UNITED STATES MEDICAL LICENSING EXAMINATION™

USMLE Step 1 is administered to students and graduates of U.S. and Canadian medical schools by the
NATIONAL BOARD OF MEDICAL EXAMINERS® (NBME®)
3750 Market Street, Philadelphia, Pennsylvania 19104-3190.
Telephone: (215) 590-9700

STEP 1 SCORE REPORT

Schmoe, Joe T	USMLE ID: 1-234-567-8
Anytown, CA 12345	Test Date: June 2002

The USMLE is a single examination program for all applicants for medical licensure in the United States; it replaces the Federation Licensing Examination (FLEX) and the certifying examinations of the National Board of Medical Examiners (NBME Parts I, II and III). The program consists of three Steps designed to assess an examinee's understanding of and ability to apply concepts and principles that are important in health and disease and that constitute the basis of safe and effective patient care. Step 1 is designed to assess whether an examinee understands and can apply key concepts of the basic biomedical sciences, with an emphasis on principles and mechanisms of health, disease and modes of therapy. The inclusion of **Step 1** in the USMLE sequence is intended to ensure mastery of not only the basic medical sciences undergirding the safe and competent practice of medicine in the present, but also the scientific principles required for maintenance of competence through lifelong learning. Results of the examination are reported to medical licensing authorities in the United States and its territories for use in granting an initial license to practice medicine. The two numeric scores shown below are equivalent; each state or territory may use either score in making licensing decisions. These scores represent your results for the administration of Step 1 on the test date shown above.

PASS	This result is based on the minimum passing score set by USMLE for Step 1. Individual licensing authorities may accept the USMLE-recommended pass/fail result or may establish a different passing score for their own jurisdictions.
215	This score is determined by your overall performance on Step 1. For recent administrations, the mean and standard deviation for first-time examinees from U.S. and Canadian medical schools are approximately 215 and 20, respectively, with most scores falling between 175 and 255 A score of 179 is set by USMLE to pass Step 1. The standard error of measurement (SEM)‡ for this scale is four points.
85	This score is also determined by your overall performance on the examination. A score of 82 on this scale is equivalent to a score of 200 on the scale described above. A score of 75 on this scale, which is equivalent to a score of 182 on the scale described above, is set by USMLE to pass Step 1. The SEM‡ for this scale is one point.

‡Your score is influenced both by your general understanding of the basic biomedical sciences and the specific set of items selected for this Step 1 examination. The SEM provides an estimate of the range within which your scores might be expected to vary by chance if you were tested repeatedly using similar tests.

121JP452

NOTE: Original score report has copy-resistant watermark.

According to the USMLE, medical schools receive a listing of total scores and pass/fail results plus group summaries by discipline and organ system. Students can withhold their scores from their medical school if they wish. Official USMLE transcripts, which can be sent on request to residency programs, include only total scores, not performance profiles.

Consult the USMLE Web site or your medical school for the most current and accurate information regarding the examination.

What Does My Score Mean?

For students, the most important point with the Step 1 score is passing versus failing. Passing essentially means, "Hey, you're on your way to becoming a fully licensed doc."

FIGURE 6B. Sample Score Report—Back Page.

INFORMATION PROVIDED FOR EXAMINEE USE ONLY

The Performance Profile below is provided solely for the benefit of the examinee.
These profiles are developed as assessment tools for examinees only and will not be reported or verified to any third party.

USMLE STEP 1 PERFORMANCE PROFILES

	Lower Performance	Borderline Performance	Higher Performance
Behavioral Sciences			xxxxxxxxxxxxxx
Biochemistry			xxxxxxxxxxxx
Cardiovascular System			xxxxxxxxxxxxxx*
Gastrointestinal System			xxxxxxxxxxxxxxx
General Principles of Health & Disease			xxxxxxxxx
Genetics			xxxxxxxxxxxxxxx
Gross Anatomy & Embryology			xxxxxxxxxxxxx*
Hematopoietic & Lymphoreticular Systems		xxxxxxxxxxxxxx	
Histology & Cell Biology		xxxxxxxxxxxxxxx	
Microbiology & Immunology			xxxxxxxxxxx
Musculoskeletal, Skin & Connective Tissue		xxxxxxxxxxxxxxx	
Nervous System/Special Senses			xxxxxxxxxx
Pathology			xxxxxxxxx
Pharmacology			xxxxxxxx
Physiology			xxxxxxxx
Renal/Urinary System			xxxxxxxxxxxxxxxx
Reproductive & Endocrine Systems			xxxxxxxxxxxxx
Respiratory System			xxxxxxxxxxxxxxx

The above Performance Profile is provided to aid in self-assessment. The shaded area defines a borderline level of performance for each content area; borderline performance is comparable to a HIGH FAIL/LOW PASS on the total test.

Performance bands indicate areas of relative strength and weakness. Some bands are wider than others. The width of a performance band reflects the precision of measurement: narrower bands indicate greater precision. An asterisk indicates that your performance band extends beyond the displayed portion of the scale. Small differences in the location of bands should not be over interpreted. If two bands overlap, the performance in the associated areas should not be interpreted as significantly different.

This profile should not be compared to those from other Step 1 administrations.

Additional information concerning the topics covered in each content area can be found in the *USMLE Step 1 General Instructions, Content Description and Sample Items.*

452JP121

Beyond that, the main point of having a quantitative score is to give you a sense of how you've done beyond the fact that you've passed the exam. The two-digit or three-digit score gauges how you have done with respect to the content on the exam.

Since the content of the exam is what drives the score, the profile of the exam is what remains relatively constant over the years. That is to say that each exam profile includes a certain number of "very hard" questions along with "medium" and "easy" ones. The questions vary, but the profile of the exam doesn't change much. This ensures that someone who scored 200 on the boards yesterday achieved a level of knowledge similar to that of the person who scored 200 four years ago.

FIGURE 7. Scoring Scales for the USMLE Step 1.

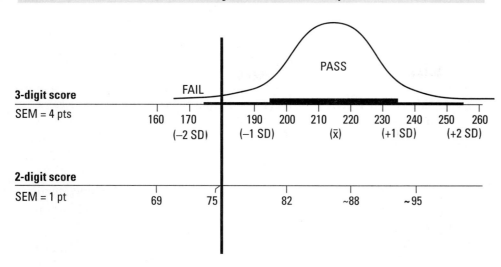

TABLE 1. Passing Rates for the 2000–2001 USMLE Step 1.[a]

	2000		2001	
	No. Tested	Passing (%)	No. Tested	Passing (%)
NBME-registered examinees (U.S./Canadian) Allopathic students First-time takers	16,412	93	16,368	91
Repeaters	1,855	58	2,012	58
Allopathic total	**18,267**	**90**	**18,380**	**88**
Osteopathic students First-time takers	785	77	723	72
Repeaters	38	40	51	31
Osteopathic total	**823**	**75**	**774**	**69**
Total (U.S./Canadian)	**19,090**	**89**	**19,154**	**87**
FMG examinees (ECFMG[b] registrants) First-time takers	8,767	65	9,835	66
Repeaters	4,688	36	4,259	35
FMG total	**13,455**	**55**	**14,094**	**56**
Total Step 1 examinees	**32,545**	**75**	**33,248**	**74**

[a]Reflects the most current data available at the time of publishing.

[b]Educational Commission for Foreign Medical Graduates.

Official NBME/USMLE Resources

We strongly encourage students to use the free materials provided by the testing agencies (see p. 32) and to study in detail the following NBME publications, all of which are available on CD-ROM or at the USMLE Web site www.usmle.org:

- *USMLE Step 1 2003 Computer-based Content and Sample Test Questions* (information given free to all examinees)
- *2003 USMLE Bulletin of Information* (information given free to all examinees)

The *USMLE Step 1 2003 Computer-based Content and Sample Test Questions* contains approximately 150 questions that are similar in format and content to the questions on the actual USMLE Step 1. This practice test offers one of the best methods for assessing your test-taking skills. However, it does not contain enough questions to simulate the full length of the examination, and its content represents a limited sampling of the basic science material that may be covered on Step 1. Most students felt that the questions on the actual 2002 exam were more challenging than those contained in these questions. Others report encountering a few near-duplicates of these questions on the actual Step 1. Presumably, these are "experimental" questions, but who knows! Bottom line: Know these questions!

The extremely detailed *Step 1 Content Outline* provided by the USMLE has not proved useful for students studying for the exam. The USMLE even states that ". . . the content outline is not intended as a guide for curriculum development or as a study guide."[4] We concur with this assessment.

The 2003 USMLE *Bulletin* of information is found on the CD-ROM. This publication contains detailed procedural and policy information regarding the CBT, including descriptions of all three Steps, scoring of the exams, reporting of scores to medical schools and residency programs, procedures for score rechecks and other inquiries, policies for irregular behavior, and test dates.

DEFINING YOUR GOAL

It is useful to define your own personal performance goal when approaching the USMLE Step 1. Your style and intensity of preparation can then be matched to your goal. Your goal may depend on your school's requirements, your specialty choice, your grades to date, and your personal assessment of the test's importance.

Fourth-year medical students have the best feel for how Step 1 scores factor into the residency application process.

Comfortably Pass

As mentioned earlier, the USMLE Step 1 is the first of three standardized examinations that you must pass in order to become a licensed physician in the United States. Also, at many medical schools, passing the USMLE Step 1 is required before you can continue with your clinical training. The NBME, however, feels that medical schools should not use Step 1 as the sole determinant of advancement to the third year.[5] If you are headed for a "non-competitive" residency program and you have consulted advisers and fourth-year medical students in your area of interest, you may feel comfortable with this approach. Obviously, however, aiming for a score of 182 is a risky way to "comfortably pass" the exam.

Beat the Mean

Although the NBME warns against the misuse of examination scores to evaluate student qualifications for residency positions, some residency program directors continue to use Step 1 scores to screen applicants. Thus, many students feel it is important to score higher than the national average.

Internship and residency programs vary greatly in their policy toward requesting scores. Some simply request your pass/fail status, whereas others ask for your total score. Some programs have even been known to request a photocopy of your score report to determine how well you performed on individual sections; however, this is unusual. It is unclear how continuing changes in USMLE Step 1 examination and score reporting will affect the application process for residency programs. The best sources of bottom-line information are fourth-year medical students who have recently completed the residency application process.

Some medical students may wish to "beat the mean" for their own personal satisfaction. For these students, there may be a psychological advantage to scoring higher than the national average.

Ace the Exam

Certain highly competitive residency programs, such as those in otolaryngology and orthopedic surgery, have acknowledged their use of Step 1 scores in the selection process. In such residency programs, greater emphasis may be placed on attaining a high score, so students who wish to enter these programs may wish to consider aiming for a very high score on the USMLE Step 1. However, use of the USMLE scores for residency selection has been criticized because neither Step 1 nor Step 2 was designed for this purpose.[6] In addition, only a subset of the basic science facts and concepts that are tested is important to functioning well on the wards. Alternatively, some students may wish to score well in order to feel a sense of mastery. High scores are particularly important for IMGs applying in all specialties.

Some competitive residency programs use Step 1 scores in their selection process.

TIMELINE FOR STUDY

Make a Schedule

After you have defined your goals, map out a study schedule that is consistent with your objectives, your vacation time, and the difficulty of your ongoing coursework (Figure 8). Determine whether you want to spread out your study time or concentrate it into 14-hour study days in the final weeks. Then factor in your own history in preparing for standardized examinations (e.g., SAT, MCAT).

Time management is key. Customize your schedule to your goals and available time following any final exams.

FIGURE 8. Typical Timeline for the USMLE Step 1.

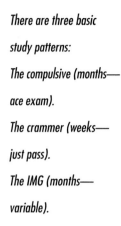

There are three basic
study patterns:
The compulsive (months—
ace exam).
The crammer (weeks—
just pass).
The IMG (months—
variable).

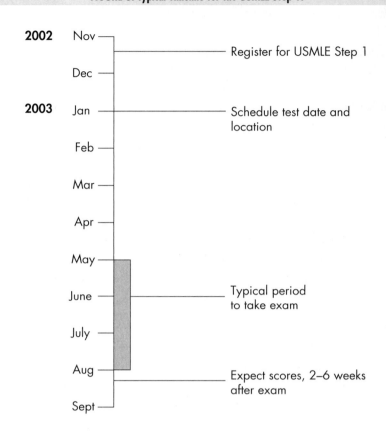

*"Crammable" subjects
should be covered later
and less crammable
subjects earlier.*

Another important consideration is when you will study each subject. Some subjects lend themselves to cramming, whereas others demand a substantial long-term commitment. The "crammable" subjects for Step 1 are those for which concise yet relatively complete review books are available. (See Section III for highly rated review and sample examination books.) Behavioral science and physiology are two subjects with concise review books. Three subjects with longer but quite complete review books are microbiology, pharmacology, and biochemistry. Thus, these subjects could be covered toward the end of your schedule, whereas other subjects (anatomy and pathology) require a longer time commitment and could be studied earlier. An increasing number of students report using a "systems-based" approach (e.g., GI, renal, cardiovascular) to integrate the material across basic science subjects.

*Allow time in your study
schedule for getting
sidetracked by personal
emergencies.*

Practically speaking, spending a given amount of time on a crammable or high-yield subject (particularly in the last few days before the test) generally produces more correct answers on the examination than spending the same amount of time on a low-yield subject. Student opinion indicates that knowing the crammable subjects extremely well probably results in a higher overall score than knowing all subjects moderately well.

If you are having difficulty deciding when to start your test preparation, you may find the reverse-calendar approach helpful. Start with the day of the test and plan backward, setting deadlines for objectives to be met. Where the planning ends on your calendar defines a possible starting point.

Make your schedule realistic, and set achievable goals. Many students make the mistake of studying at a level of detail that requires too much time for a comprehensive review—reading *Gray's Anatomy* in a couple of days is not a realistic goal! Revise your schedule regularly based on your actual progress. Be careful not to lose focus. Beware of feelings of inadequacy when comparing study schedules and progress with your peers. **Avoid students who stress you out.** Focus on a few top-rated books that suit your learning style—not on some obscure books your friends may pass down to you. Do not set yourself up for frustration. Accept the fact that you cannot learn it all. Maintain your sanity throughout the process.

Avoid burnout. Maintain proper diet, exercise, and sleep habits.

You will need time for uninterrupted and focused study. Plan your personal affairs to minimize crisis situations near the date of the test. Allot an adequate number of breaks in your study schedule to avoid burnout. Maintain a healthy lifestyle with proper diet, exercise, and sleep.

Year(s) Prior

The USMLE asserts that the best preparation for the USMLE Step 1 resides in "broadly based learning that establishes a strong general foundation of understanding of concepts and principles in basic sciences."[6] We agree. Although you may be tempted to rely solely on cramming in the weeks and months before the test, you should not have to do so. The knowledge you gained during your first two years of medical school and even during your undergraduate years should provide the groundwork on which to base your test preparation. The preponderance of your boards preparation should thus involve resurrecting dormant information that you have stored away during the basic science years.

Don't let the exam take over your life.

Some ways to help resurrect and integrate this information are as follows:

- Tutor first-year students during your second year.
- Review related first-year material in your second year. For example, review first-year cardiac physiology and histology while learning second-year cardiac pathology.
- At the end of each medical school course, compile and organize key tables, charts, and mnemonics into a "Step 1" binder. Then, when it comes time to study, you will have a head start with familiar high-yield material.
- Attend all "Introduction to Clinical Medicine" and "problem-based learning" classes and reviews to gain experience with clinical vignettes.
- Spend time using computer-based medical education software.

Buy review books early (first year) and use while studying for courses.

We also recommend that you buy highly rated review books early in your first year of medical school and use them as you study throughout the two years. When Step 1 comes along, the books will be familiar and personalized to the

Review first-year material in parallel with related second-year topics.

way in which you learn. It is risky and intimidating to use unfamiliar review books in the final two or three weeks.

You should talk with third- and fourth-year medical students to familiarize yourself with strengths and weaknesses in your school's curriculum. Identify subject areas in which you excel or with which you have difficulty. If you have any doubts concerning your reading speed, consider a speed-reading course. Content typically learned in the second year receives more coverage on Step 1 than do first-year topics owing to the emphasis placed on integration of basic science information across many courses.[7] Be aware of your school's testing format, and determine whether you have adequate exposure to multiple-choice and matching questions in the form of clinical vignettes.

Months Prior

Review test dates and the application procedure. In 2002, the testing for the USMLE Step 1 continues on a year-round basis (Table 2). Choose the most appropriate Prometric testing site for optimal performance. Many U.S. students simply take the exam at the closest site along with all their classmates. By contrast, a few students report a preference for traveling to more distant sites in the interest of privacy. Judge for yourself whether you find familiarity reassuring or stressful. If you have any disabilities or "special circumstances," contact the NBME as early as possible to discuss test accommodations (see p. 61, First Aid for the Student with a Disability).

Simulate the USMLE Step 1 under "real" conditions before beginning your studies.

Before you begin to study earnestly, simulate the USMLE Step 1 under "real" conditions (even down to the earplugs if you plan to use them during the real exam) to pinpoint strengths and weaknesses in your knowledge and test-taking skills. Be sure that you are well informed about the examination and that you have planned your strategy for studying. Consider what study methods you will use, the study materials you will need, and how you will obtain your materials. Some review books and software may not be available at your local bookstore, and you may have to order ahead of time to get copies (see the list of publisher contacts at the end of Section III). Plan ahead. Get advice from third- and fourth-year medical students who have recently taken the USMLE

		No. of Questions/	Test Schedule	Passing
Step	**Focus**	**No. of Blocks**	**Length of CBT Exam**	**Score**
Step 1	Basic mechanisms and principles	350/7	One day (eight hours)	182
Step 2	Clinical diagnosis and disease pathogenesis	400/8	One day (nine hours)	174
Step 3	Clinical management	500/10	Two days (16 hours)	182

TABLE 2. 2003 USMLE Schedule.

Step 1. There might be strengths and weaknesses in your school's curriculum that you should take into account in deciding where to focus your efforts. You might also choose to share books, notes, and study hints with classmates. That is how this book began.

Three Weeks Prior

Two to four weeks before the examination is a good time to resimulate the USMLE Step 1. You may want to do this earlier depending on the progress of your review, but do not do it later, when there will be little time to remedy defects in your knowledge or test-taking skills. Make use of remaining good-quality sample USMLE test questions, and try to simulate the computerized test conditions so that you get a fair assessment of your test performance. Recognize, too, that time pressure is increasing as more and more questions are framed as clinical vignettes. Most sample exam questions are shorter than the real thing. Focus on reviewing the high-yield facts, your own notes, picture books, and very short review books.

In the final two weeks, focus on review and endurance. Avoid unfamiliar material. Stay confident!

One Week Prior

Make sure you have your CIN (found on your scheduling permit) and other items necessary for the day of the examination, including a driver's license or other photo identification with signature (make sure your name on your ID *exactly* matches that on your scheduling permit), an analog watch, and possibly earplugs. Confirm the Prometric testing center location and test time. Work out how you will get to the testing center and what parking and traffic problems you might encounter. Visit the testing site (if possible) to get a better idea of the testing conditions. Determine what you will do for lunch. Make sure you have everything you need to ensure that you will be comfortable and alert at the test site. Prometric will provide earplugs on request. Assess your pre-exam living and sleeping arrangements. Take aggressive measures to ensure an environment fit for concentration and sufficient sleep. If you must travel a long distance to the test site, consider arriving the day before and staying overnight with a friend or at a nearby hotel (make early hotel reservations).

Confirm your testing date at least one week in advance.

One Day Prior

Try your best to relax and rest the night before the test. Double-check your admissions and test-taking materials as well as comfort measures as discussed earlier so you do not have to deal with such details the morning of the exam. Do not study any new material. If you feel compelled to study, then quickly review short-term-memory material (e.g., Section II: Database of High-Yield Facts) before going to sleep (the brain does a lot of information processing at night). However, do not quiz yourself, as you may risk becoming flustered and confused. Remember that regardless of how hard you studied, you cannot know everything. There will be things on the exam that you have never even seen before, so do not panic. Do not underestimate your abilities.

Ensure that you will be comfortable and alert. You must be able to think, not just regurgitate.

No notes, books, calculators, pagers, recording devices, or digital watches are allowed in the testing area.

Many students report difficulty sleeping the night prior to the exam. This is often exacerbated by going to bed much earlier than usual. Do whatever it takes to ensure a good night's sleep (e.g., massage, exercise, warm milk). Do not change your daily routine prior to the exam. Exam day is not the day for a caffeine-withdrawal headache.

Morning of the Exam

Wake up at your regular time and eat a normal breakfast. Drink coffee, tea, or soda in moderation, or you may end up wasting exam time on bathroom breaks. Make sure you have your scheduling permit admission ticket, test-taking materials, and comfort measures as discussed earlier. Wear loose, comfortable clothing. Plan for a variable temperature in the testing center. Remember that you will arrive early in the morning, when it may be cool, and that you will not leave until late in the afternoon, when it may be warmer. Arrive at the test site 30 minutes before the time designated on the admission ticket; however, do not come too early, as this may increase your anxiety. The proctor should give you a blue, laminated USMLE information sheet to read, which explains important things such as the use of break time. Seating may be assigned, but ask to be reseated if necessary; you need to be seated in an area that will allow you to remain comfortable and to concentrate. Get to know your testing station, especially if you have never been in a Prometric testing center before. Adjust your chair and the monitor. Test the mouse, keyboard, lamp, dry markers, and whiteboard to make sure everything is functioning properly before the exam starts. Listen to your proctors regarding any changes in instructions or testing procedures that may apply to your test site.

Arrive at the testing center 30 minutes before your scheduled exam time. If you arrive more than half an hour late you will not be allowed to take the test.

Remember that it is natural (and even beneficial) to be a little nervous. Focus on being mentally clear and alert. Avoid panic. Avoid panic. Avoid panic. When you are asked to begin the exam, take a deep breath, focus on the screen, and then begin. Keep an eye on the timer. Take advantage of breaks between blocks to stretch and relax for a moment.

Some students recommend reviewing certain "theme" topics that tend to recur throughout the exam.

The break for lunch is an excellent opportunity to relax, reorganize your thoughts, and regain composure if you are feeling overly stressed or panicked. Some students use the break to discuss questions with classmates or to look up information. Some even recommend reviewing theme topics during lunch. However, do what feels comfortable, as time will be short. If you decide to review the morning session, do not dwell on perceived mistakes.

After the Test

Have fun and relax regardless of how you may feel. Taking the test is an achievement in itself. Remember, you are much more likely to have passed than not. Enjoy the free time you have before your clerkships. Expect to experience some "reentry" phenomenon as you try to regain a real life. Once you have recovered sufficiently from the test (or from partying), we invite you to send us your feedback, corrections, and suggestions for entries, facts, mnemonics, strategies, book ratings, and so on (see p. xv, How to Contribute). Sharing your experience benefits fellow medical students and IMGs.

IF YOU THINK YOU FAILED

After the test, many examinees feel that they have failed, and most are at the very least unsure of their pass/fail status. There are several sensible steps you can take to plan for the future in the event that you do not achieve a passing score. First, save and organize all your study materials, including review books, practice tests, and notes. If you studied from borrowed materials, make sure you have immediate access to them. Review your school's policy regarding requirements for graduation and promotion to the third year. About one-half of the medical schools accredited by the Liaison Committee on Medical Education require passing Step 1 for promotion to the third year, and two-thirds require passing Step 1 as a requirement for graduation.[7] Familiarize yourself with the reapplication procedures for Step 1, including application deadlines and upcoming test dates. The CBT format allows an examinee who has failed the exam to retake it no earlier than the first day of the month after 60 days have elapsed since the last test date. Examinees will, however, be allowed to take the exam no more than three times within a 12-month period should they repeatedly fail.

If you pass Step 1, you are not allowed to retake the exam in an attempt to raise your score.

The performance profiles on the back of the USMLE Step 1 score report provide valuable feedback concerning your relative strengths and weaknesses (see Figure 6B). Study the performance profiles closely. Set up a study timeline to strengthen gaps in your knowledge as well as to maintain and improve what you already know. Do not neglect high-yield subjects. It is normal to feel somewhat anxious about retaking the test. If anxiety becomes a problem, however, seek appropriate counseling.

Fifty-two percent of the NBME-registered first-time takers who failed the June 1998 Step 1 repeated the exam in October 1998. The overall pass rate for that group in October was 60%. Eighty-five percent of those scoring near the old pass/fail mark of 176 (173–176) in June 1998 passed in October. However, 1999 pass rates varied widely depending on initial score (see Table 3, which reflects the most current data available at time of publishing).

Although the NBME allows an unlimited number of attempts to pass Step 1, both the NBME and the FSMB recommend that licensing authorities allow a minimum of three and a maximum of six attempts for each Step examination.[8] Again, review your school's policy regarding retakes.

TABLE 3. Pass Rates for USMLE Step 1 Repeaters 1999.[8]

Initial Score	% Pass
176–178	83
173–175	74
170–172	71
165–169	64
160–164	54
150–159	31
< 150	0
Overall	**67**

IF YOU FAILED

Even if you came out of the exam room feeling that you failed, seeing that failing grade can be traumatic, and it is natural to feel upset. Different people react in different ways: For some it is a stimulus to buckle down and study harder; for others it may "take the wind out of their sails" for a few days; and for still others it may lead to a reassessment of individual goals and abilities. In some instances, however, failure may trigger weeks or months of sadness, feelings of hopelessness, social withdrawal, and inability to concentrate—in other words, true clinical depression.

If you think you are depressed, seek help. Depression is a common yet potentially disabling, and at times even fatal, illness. Depression is also very treatable, so you must use the same resources that you plan to offer your patients. In other words, you must seek treatment, whether from a school counselor, a psychiatrist, or a psychologist. Do not "treat" yourself with alcohol, illicit drugs, or anything else; you need the same skilled help that anyone else with this problem warrants.

Near the failure threshold, each three-digit scale point is equivalent to about 1.5 questions answered correctly.[9]

As Table 3 shows, the majority of people who fail Step 1 the first time pass on their second attempt, especially if they were near the passing threshold. If you repeatedly fail the exam despite maximum preparation, you may need to reevaluate your goals. Seek testing and career counseling early.

STUDY METHODS

It is important to have a set of study methods for preparing for the USMLE Step 1. There is too much material to justify a studying plan that is built on random reading and memorization. Experiment with different ways of studying. You do not know how effective something might be until you try it. This is best done months before the test to determine what works and what you enjoy. Possible study options include:

- Studying review material in groups
- Creating personal mnemonics, diagrams, and tables
- Using *First Aid* as a framework on which to add notes
- Taking practice computer as well as pencil-and-paper tests (see Section III for reviews)
- Attending faculty review sessions
- Making or sharing flashcards
- Reviewing old syllabi and notes
- Making cassette tapes of review material to study during commuting time
- Playing Trivial Pursuit–style games with facts and questions
- Getting away from home for an extended period to avoid distractions and to immerse yourself in studying

Study Groups

A good study group has many advantages. It can relieve stress, organize your time, and allow people with different strengths to exchange information. Study groups also allow you to pool resources and spend less money on review books and sample tests.

There are, however, potential problems associated with study groups. Above all, it is difficult to study with people who have different goals and study paces. Avoid large, unwieldy groups. Otherwise, studying can be inefficient and time-consuming. Avoid study groups that tend to socialize more than study.

Balance individual and group study.

If you choose not to belong to a study group, it may be a good idea to find a support group or a study partner simply to keep pace with and share study ideas. It is beneficial to get different perspectives from other students in evaluating what is and is not important to learn. Do not become intimidated or discouraged by interactions with a few overly compulsive students; everyone studies and learns differently.

Mnemonics and Memorizing

Cramming is a viable way of memorizing short-term information just before a test, but after one or two days you will find that much of that knowledge has dissipated. For that reason, cramming and memorization by repetition ("brute force") in the weeks before the exam are not ideal techniques for long-term memorization of the overwhelming body of information covered in Step 1. Mnemonics are memory aids that work by linking isolated facts or abstract ideas to acronyms, pictures, patterns, rhymes, and stories—information that the mind tends to store well.[10] The best mnemonics are your own, and developing them takes work. The first step to creating a mnemonic is understanding the information to be memorized. Play around with the information and look for unique features that help you remember it. In addition, make the mnemonic as colorful, humorous, or outlandish as you can; such mnemonics are the most memorable. Effective mnemonics should link the topic with the facts in as specific and unambiguous a manner as possible. In memorizing the mnemonic, engage as many senses as possible by repeating the fact aloud or by writing or acting it out. Keep the information fresh by quizzing yourself periodically with flash cards, in study groups, and so on. Do not make the common mistake of simply rereading highlighted review material. The material may start to look familiar, but that does not mean you will be able to remember it in another context during the exam. Strive to gain an understanding rather than rote memorization.

Developing good mnemonics takes time and work. Quiz yourself periodically. Do not simply reread highlighted material.

Review Sessions

Faculty review sessions can also be helpful. Review sessions that are geared specifically toward the USMLE Step 1 tend to be more helpful than general review sessions. By contrast, open "question and answer" sessions tend to be inefficient and not worth the time. Focus on reviews given by faculty who are knowledgeable in the content and testing format of the USMLE Step 1.

Commercial Courses

Commercial preparation courses can be helpful for some students, but they are expensive and require significant time commitment. They are often effective in organizing study material for students preparing for Step 1 who feel over-whelmed by the sheer volume of material. Note, however, that multiple-week courses may be quite intense and may thus leave limited time for independent study. Note also that some commercial courses are designed for first-time test takers while others focus on students who are repeating the examination. Still other courses focus on IMGs, who must take all three Steps in a limited time period. See Section III for summarized data and excerpted information from several commercial review courses.

STUDY MATERIALS

Quality and Cost Considerations

Although an ever-increasing number of review books and software are now available on the market, the quality of such material is highly variable. Some common problems are as follows:

In 2002, many students felt that even the top-rated sample exams did not accurately reflect the clinical focus of the actual exam.

- Certain review books are too detailed for review in a reasonable amount of time or cover subtopics that are not emphasized on the exam (e.g., a 400-page histology book).
- Many sample question books were originally written years ago and have not been adequately updated to reflect trends on the revised USMLE Step 1.
- Many sample question books use poorly written questions or contain factual errors in their explanations.
- Explanations for sample questions range from nonexistent to overly detailed.
- The available review software is of highly variable quality, may be diffi-cult to install, and may be fraught with bugs.

Basic Science Review Books

Most review books are the products of considerable effort by experienced edu-cators. There are, however, many such books, so you must choose which ones to buy on the basis of their relative merits. Although recommendations from other medical students are useful, many students simply recommend whatever books they used without having compared them to other books on the same subject. Do not waste time with outdated "hand-me-down" review books. Some students blindly advocate one publisher's series without considering the broad range of quality encountered within most series. Weigh different opin-

If a given review book is not working for you, stop using it no matter how highly rated it may be or how much it costs.

ions against each other, read the reviews and ratings in Section III of this guide, examine the books closely in the bookstore, and choose review books carefully. You are investing not only money but also your limited study time. Do not worry about finding the "perfect" book, as many subjects simply do not have one, and different students prefer different styles.

There are two types of review books: books that are stand-alone titles and books that are part of a series. The books in a series generally have the same style, and you must decide if that style works for you. However, a given style is not optimal for every subject. For example, charts and diagrams may be the best approach for physiology and biochemistry, whereas tables and outlines may be preferable for microbiology.

You should also find out which books are up to date. Some new editions represent major improvements, whereas others contain only cursory changes. Take into consideration how a book reflects the format of the USMLE Step 1. Some of the books reviewed in Section III have not been updated adequately to reflect the clinical emphasis and question format of the current USMLE Step 1. Books that emphasize obscure facts and minute details tend to be less helpful for the current USMLE Step 1 because there are now fewer "picky" questions and more problem-solving questions.

Many students regret not having used the same books for medical school exam review and Step 1 review.

Practice Tests

Taking practice tests provides valuable information about potential strengths and weaknesses in your fund of knowledge and test-taking skills. Some students use practice examinations simply as a means of breaking up the monotony of studying and adding variety to their study schedule, whereas other students study almost solely from practice tests. There is, moreover, a wide range of quality in available practice material, and finding good practice exams is likely to become even more complicated with the advent of the computerized Step 1. Your best preview of the computerized exam can be found in the practice exams on the USMLE CD-ROM. Some students also recommend using computerized test simulation programs such as Kaplan's Qbank (see Section III for reviews). In addition, students report that many current practice-exam books have questions that are, on average, shorter and less clinically oriented than the current USMLE Step 1. Many Step 1 questions demand fast reading skills and application of basic science facts in a problem-solving format. Approach sample examinations and simulation software critically, and do not waste time with low-quality questions until you have exhausted better sources.

Most practice exams are shorter and less clinical than the real thing.

After taking a practice test, try to identify concepts and areas of weakness, not just the facts that you missed. Do not panic if you miss a lot of questions on a practice examination; instead, use the experience you have gained to motivate your study and prioritize those areas in which you need the most work. Use quality practice examinations to improve your test-taking skills. Analyze your ability to pace yourself so that you have enough time to complete each block of 50 questions comfortably. Practice examinations are also

Use practice tests to identify concepts and areas of weakness, not just facts that you missed.

a good means of training yourself to concentrate for long periods of time under appropriate time pressure. Consider taking practice tests with a friend or in a small group to increase motivation while simulating more accurately the format and schedule of the real examination. Analyze the pattern of your responses to questions to determine if you have made systematic errors in answering questions. Common mistakes are reading too much into the question, second-guessing your initial impression, and misinterpreting the question.

Clinical Review Books

Keep your eye out for more clinically oriented review books; purchase them early and begin to use them. A number of students are turning to Step 2 books, pathophysiology books, and case-based reviews to prepare for the clinical vignettes. Examples of such books include:

- *Blueprint* clinical series (Blackwell Science)
- *PreTest Physical Diagnosis* (McGraw-Hill)
- *Washington Manual* (Lippincott Williams & Wilkins)
- Various USMLE Step 2 review books

Texts, Syllabi, and Notes

Limit your use of texts and syllabi for Step 1 review. Many textbooks are too detailed for high-yield review and include material that is generally not tested on the USMLE Step 1 (e.g., drug dosages, complex chemical structures). Syllabi, although familiar, are inconsistent and frequently reflect the emphasis of individual faculty, which often does not correspond to that of the USMLE Step 1. Syllabi also tend to be less organized and to contain fewer diagrams and study questions than do top-rated review books. In our opinion, they are often a waste of time for the faculty to write and suboptimal for the student to read (when compared with the best review books). Make sure that your instructors are aware of the best books, and supplement your classes with case-based problem-solving curricula that reflect the current exam format. Your class notes have the advantage of presenting material in the way you learned it but suffer from the same disadvantages as syllabi.

When using texts or notes, engage in active learning by making tables, diagrams, new mnemonics, and conceptual associations whenever possible. Supplement unclear material with reference to other appropriate textbooks. Keep a good medical dictionary at hand to sort out definitions.

GENERAL STUDY STRATEGIES

The USMLE Step 1 was created according to an integrated outline that organizes basic science material in a multidisciplinary approach. Broad-based knowledge is now more important than it was in the exams of prior years. The exam is designed to test basic science material and its application to clinical situations. A little over half of the questions include clinical vignettes, although some are brief. Some useful studying guidelines are as follows:

- Be familiar with the CBT tutorial. This will give you 15 minutes of extra break time.
- Use computerized practice tests in addition to paper exams.
- Consider doing a simulated test at a Prometric center.
- Practice taking 50 questions in one-hour bursts.
- Be familiar with the Windows environment.
- Consider scheduling a light rotation for your first clinical block in case you get a test date later than you expected.

In spite of the change in the organization of the subject matter, the detailed Step 1 content outline provided by the USMLE has not proved useful for students. We feel that it is still best to approach the material along the lines of the seven traditional disciplines. In Section II, we provide suggestions on how to approach the material within each subject.

Practice questions that include case histories or descriptive vignettes are critical in preparing for the clinical slant of the USMLE Step 1. The normal lab values provided on the computerized test are difficult to use and access. For quick reference, see the table of high-yield laboratory values on the inside back cover.

Familiarize yourself with the commonly tested normal laboratory values.

Practice questions that include case histories or descriptive vignettes are critical for Step 1 preparation.

TEST-TAKING STRATEGIES

Your test performance will be influenced by both your fund of knowledge and your test-taking skills. You can increase your performance by considering each of these factors. Test-taking skills and strategies should be developed and perfected well in advance of the test date so that you can concentrate on the test itself. We suggest that you try the following strategies to see if they might work for you.

Practice and perfect test-taking skills and strategies well before the test date.

Pacing

You have seven hours to complete 350 questions (down from 720). Note that each one-hour block contains 50 questions. This works out to about 72 seconds per question. NBME officials note that time was not an issue for most takers of the CBT field test. However, pacing errors have in the past been detrimental to the performance of even highly prepared examinees. The bottom line is to keep one eye on the clock at all times! If you find yourself running out of time, fill in all remaining blanks with C or B or your favorite letter, but also click on the "mark" button for each so that you can come back to them from the item review screen.

Dealing with Each Question

There are several established techniques for efficiently approaching multiple-choice questions; see what works for you. One technique begins with identifying each question as easy, workable, or impossible. Your goal should be to answer all easy questions, work out all workable questions in a reasonable amount of time, and make quick and intelligent guesses on all impossible questions. Most students read the stem, think of the answer, and turn immediately to the choices. A second technique is to first skim the answer choices and the last sentence of the question and then read through the passage quickly, extracting only relevant information to answer the question. Try a variety of techniques on practice exams and see what works best for you.

In general, when you eliminate an incorrect choice on a question, avoid rereading it unnecessarily. Move on. If you are unsure about a choice, mark it for later review. When you think you have determined the best answer, click on it and move on.

Difficult Questions

Questions on the USMLE Step 1 require varying amounts of time to answer. Some problem-solving questions take longer than simple, fact-recall questions. Because of the exam's clinical emphasis, you may find that many of the questions appear workable but take more time than is available to you. It can be tempting to dwell on such a question for an excessive amount of time because you feel you are on the verge of "figuring it out," but resist this temptation and budget your time. Answer the question with your best guess, mark it for review, and come back to it if you have time after you have completed the rest of the questions in the block. This will keep you from inadvertently leaving any questions blank in your efforts to "beat the clock." Remember to save a few minutes at the end to make sure that all questions have been answered.

Inevitably, there will be some questions about which you will not have a clue (i.e., impossible questions). Do not be disturbed by these questions. Guess, mark them for later review, and move on. As a medical student, you are used to scoring well on standardized examinations (otherwise you would not be in medical school), so the USMLE Step 1 may be your first experience with facing lots of questions for which you do not know the answer. Prepare yourself for this. After narrowing down the answers as best you can, have a plan for guessing so that you do not waste time. Remember that you are not expected to know all the answers.

Another reason for not dwelling too long on any one question is that certain questions may be **experimental** or may be **incorrectly phrased.** Moreover, not all questions are scored. Some questions serve as "embedded pretest items" that do not count toward your overall score.[10] In fact, anywhere from 10 to 20% of exam questions have been designated as experimental on past exams.

Students have also noted several errors in past USMLE Step 1 examinations. The lesson here is that you should not waste too much time with ambiguous or "flawed" questions. The reason you are having difficulty with a question may lie in the question itself, not with you!

Guessing

There is **no penalty** for wrong answers. Thus, no test block should be left with unanswered questions. A hunch is probably better than a random guess. If you have to guess, we suggest selecting an answer you recognize over one that is totally unfamiliar. Go where the money is! If you have studied the subject and do not recognize a particular answer, then it is more likely a distractor than a correct answer.

Changing Your Answer

The conventional wisdom regarding "reconsidering" answers is not to change answers that you have already marked unless there is a convincing and logical reason to do so—in other words, go with your first hunch. You can test this strategy for yourself by keeping a running total of the questions on which you seriously considered changing your answer when taking practice exams. Experience eventually tells you how strongly to trust your first hunches. Remember, with the CBT format you can go back and change answers only within the question block you're working on. Once you move to the next block, you cannot return to questions in the previous block.

Fourth-Quarter Effect (Avoiding Burnout)

Pacing and endurance are important. Practice helps develop both. Fewer and fewer examinees are leaving the examination session early. Use any extra time you might have at the end of each block to return to marked questions or to recheck your answers; you cannot add the extra time to any remaining blocks of questions or to your break time. Do not be too casual in your review or you may overlook serious mistakes. A few students report that near the end of a section they suddenly remember facts that help answer questions they had guessed on earlier.

Do not terminate the block too early. Carefully review your answers if possible.

Remember your goals, and keep in mind the effort you have devoted to studying compared with the small additional effort to maintain focus and concentration throughout the examination.

Never give up. If you begin to feel frustrated, try taking a 30-second breather. Look away from the screen, breathe deeply, and slowly count to ten. Hopefully, you can return to the exam refreshed and clear. Every point you earn is to your advantage. The difference between passing and an average score is far fewer questions than you might think—about 25% of students who failed past exams were within 15 questions of passing.

CLINICAL VIGNETTE STRATEGIES

In recent years, the USMLE Step 1 has become increasingly clinically oriented. Students polled from 2002 exams report that nearly 80% of the questions were presented as clinical vignettes. This change mirrors the trend in medical education toward introducing students to clinical problem solving during the basic science years. The increasing clinical emphasis on Step 1 may be challenging to those students who attend schools with a more traditional curriculum.

The first step toward approaching the clinical vignette is not to panic. The same basic science concepts are often being tested in the guise of a clinical vignette.

What Is a Clinical Vignette?

Be prepared to read fast and think on your feet!

A clinical vignette is a short (usually paragraph-long) description of a patient, including demographics, presenting symptoms, signs, and other information concerning the patient. Sometimes this paragraph is followed by a brief listing of important physical findings and/or laboratory results. The task of assimilating all this information and answering the associated question in the span of one minute can be intimidating. Be prepared to read fast and think on your feet. Remember that the question is often indirectly asking something you already know.

Here are two examples of vignettes that appear complex but actually ask relatively straightforward questions.

Vignette #1

A 38-year-old African-American woman visits her physician. She explains that she has been experiencing palpitations, shortness of breath, and syncopal episodes for several months. In addition to a constant feeling of impending doom, she also has episodes of dizziness without nausea or vomiting. Her sleep pattern is normal. The physician's first course of action should be to:

    A) provide psychotherapy
    B) treat the patient with benzodiazepines
    C) perform a physical examination
    D) refer the patient to a psychiatrist
    E) teach the patient self-hypnosis

Answer: C. Regardless of whether a psychiatric or organic disorder is present, a history and physical examination should always be performed during the first visit. As the history is summarized in the vignette, the physical exam would be the first course of action before considering any of the other answer choices.

Vignette #2

J.B. is a seven-year-old white male who complains of a chronic, persistent cough. The cough is often elicited by physical activity or cold exposure. His mother says that she had an uncomplicated, full-term pregnancy and that the child has been healthy except for one episode of pneumonia when he was five years old. She also notes that his appetite is variable and that he frequently has light-colored and foul-smelling stool. On physical exam, his weight was 20.5 kg (25th percentile) and his height was 119.5 cm (25th percentile). His physician orders a sweat chloride test (Cook-Gibson method) and receives the following results:

Right arm   103 mEq/L
Left arm   108 mEq/L
Normal   < 70 mEq/L

What is the mode of inheritance of this disorder?

  A) autosomal dominant
  B) autosomal recessive
  C) mitochondrial
  D) X-linked recessive
  E) Y-linked

Answer: B.

Strategy

Remember that the Step 1 vignettes usually describe diseases or disorders in their most classic presentation. Look for buzzwords or cardinal signs (e.g., malar rash for SLE or nuchal rigidity for meningitis) in the narrative history. Be aware, however, that the question may contain classic signs and symptoms instead of mere buzzwords. Sometimes the data from labs and the physical exam will help you confirm or reject possible diagnoses, thereby helping you rule answer choices in or out. In some cases, they will be a dead giveaway for the diagnosis.

Step 1 vignettes usually describe diseases or disorders in their most classic presentation.

Making a diagnosis from the history and data is often not the final answer. Not infrequently, the diagnosis is divulged at the end of the vignette, after you have just struggled through the narrative to come up with a diagnosis of your own. The question instead asks about a related aspect of the diagnosed disease.

One strategy that many students suggest is to skim the questions and answer choices before reading a vignette, especially if the vignette is lengthy. This focuses your attention on the relevant information and reduces the time spent on that vignette. Sometimes you may not need much of the information in the vignette to answer the question.

Sometimes making a diagnosis is not necessary at all.

For vignette #2, consider the following approach:

- Take a look at the question and answer choices first. We see that a diagnosis of some inherited disease will likely have to be made to answer this question.
- As in many vignettes, the first sentence presents the patient's age, sex, and race. This information can help direct your diagnosis. For the case above, you are looking for a genetic disease in a young white male,

which may already tip you off to cystic fibrosis. If you are looking for an inherited anemia, sickle-cell disease would be more likely for an African-American patient. If, by contrast, the patient were Asian or Mediterranean, then thalassemia might be more likely.

- Next, look for the chief complaint, in this case "chronic, persistent cough."
- Even if the diagnosis of cystic fibrosis is not apparent at this point, fear not! The vignette further describes other classic symptoms of the disease (e.g., fat malabsorption due to pancreatic insufficiency, growth retardation, elevated sweat chloride levels).
- Instead of asking for the diagnosis, the question asks its mode of inheritance. Questions such as this require the test taker to go beyond the first stage in the reasoning process. **These "two-step questions" are appearing with increasing frequency on the Step 1 exam.**

"Two-step questions" are appearing with increasing frequency on the Step 1 exam.

TESTING AGENCIES

National Board of Medical Examiners (NBME)
Department of Licensing Examination Services
3750 Market Street
Philadelphia, PA 19104-3190
(215) 590-9700
Fax: (215) 590-9457
www.nbme.org

Educational Commission for Foreign Medical Graduates (ECFMG)
3624 Market Street, Fourth Floor
Philadelphia, PA 19104-2685
(215) 386-5900 or (215) 375-1913
Toll free within North America: (800) 500-8249
Fax: (215) 387-9963
www.ecfmg.org

Federation of State Medical Boards (FSMB)
400 Fuller Wiser Road, Suite 300
Euless, TX 76039-3855
(817) 868-4041
Fax: (817) 868-4099
www.fsmb.org

USMLE Secretariat
3750 Market Street
Philadelphia, PA 19104-3190
(215) 590-9700
www.usmle.org

REFERENCES

1. Bidese, Catherine M., *U.S. Medical Licensure Statistics and Current Licensure Requirements 1995*, Chicago, American Medical Association, 1995.

2. National Board of Medical Examiners, *2002 USMLE Bulletin of Information*, Philadelphia, 2001.

3. National Board of Medical Examiners, *Bulletin of Information and Description of National Board Examinations, 1991*, Philadelphia, 1990.

4. Federation of State Medical Boards and National Board of Medical Examiners, *USMLE: 1993 Step 1 General Instructions, Content Outline, and Sample Items*, Philadelphia, 1992.

5. Swanson, David B., Case, Susan M., Melnick, Donald E., et al., "Impact of the USMLE Step 1 on Teaching and Learning of the Basic Biomedical Sciences," *Academic Medicine*, September Supplement 1992, Vol. 67, No. 9, pp. 553–556.

6. Case, Susan M., and Swanson, David B., "Validity of NBME Part I and Part II Scores for Selection of Residents in Orthopaedic Surgery, Dermatology, and Preventive Medicine," *Academic Medicine*, February Supplement 1993, Vol. 68, No. 2, pp. S51–S56.

7. "Report on 1995 Examinations," *National Board Examiner*, Winter 1997, Vol. 44, No. 1, pp. 1–4.

8. "Report on 1996 Examinations," op. cit.

9. O'Donnell, M. J., Obenshain, S. Scott, and Erdmann, James B., "I: Background Essential to the Proper Use of Results of Step 1 and Step 2 of the USMLE," *Academic Medicine*, October 1993, Vol. 68, No. 10, pp. 734–739.

10. Robinson, Adam, *What Smart Students Know*, New York, Crown Publishers, 1993.

NOTES

Special Situations

"International medical graduate" (IMG) is the term now used to describe any student or graduate of a non-U.S., non-Canadian, non–Puerto Rican medical school, regardless of whether he or she is a U.S. citizen. The old term "foreign medical graduate" (FMG) was replaced because it was misleading when applied to U.S. citizens attending medical schools outside the United States.

The IMG's Steps to Licensure in the United States

If you are an IMG, you must go through the following steps (not necessarily in this order) to become licensed to practice in the United States. You must complete these steps even if you are already a practicing physician and have completed a residency program in your own country.

More detailed information can be found in the 2003 edition of the ECFMG Information Booklet, available at www.ecfmg.org/pubshome.html.

- Complete the basic sciences program of your medical school (equivalent to the first two years of U.S. medical school).
- Take the USMLE Step 1. You can do this while still in school or after graduating, but in either case your medical school must certify that you completed the basic sciences part of your school's curriculum before taking the USMLE Step 1.
- Complete the clinical clerkship program of your medical school (equivalent to the third and fourth years of U.S. medical school).
- Take the USMLE Step 2. If you are still in medical school, your school must certify that you are within one year of graduating for you to be allowed to take Step 2.
- Take the Test of English as a Foreign Language (TOEFL), recognized by the Educational Commission for Foreign Medical Graduates (ECFMG).
- Graduate with your medical degree.
- Then, send the ECFMG a copy of your degree, which they will verify with your medical school.
- Obtain an ECFMG certificate; to do this, candidates must accomplish the following:
    —Pass Step 1 and Step 2 within a seven-year period
    —Pass the TOEFL or the ECFMG English test
    —Pass the Clinical Skills Assessment (CSA) if the above three requirements were not met as of June 30, 1998
    —Have medical credentials verified by the ECFMG

Applicants may apply online for the USMLE Step 1 or Step 2, for the ECFMG Clinical Skills Assessment, or to request an extension of the USMLE eligibility period at iwa.ecfmg.org.

- The standard certificate is usually sent two weeks after all the above requirements have been fulfilled. You must have the certificate if you wish to obtain a position in an accredited residency program; some programs do not allow you to apply unless you already have a certificate.
- Apply for residency positions in your field of interest, either directly or through the National Residency Matching Program ("the Match"). To be entered into the Match, you need to have passed all the examinations necessary for ECFMG certification (i.e., Step 1, Step 2, the CSA, and the English test) by a certain deadline (January 31, 2003, for the next cycle). If you do not pass these exams by the deadline, you will be withdrawn from the Match.

- Obtain a visa that will allow you to enter and work in the United States if you are not already a U.S. citizen or a green-card holder (permanent resident).

- If required for IMGs by the state in which your residency is located, obtain an educational/training/limited medical license. Your residency program may assist you with this application. Note that medical licensing is the prerogative of each individual state, not of the federal government, and that states vary with respect to their laws about licensing (although all 50 states recognize the USMLE).

- Take the USMLE Step 3 during your residency, and then obtain a full medical license. Note that as an IMG you will not be able to take Step 3 and obtain an independent license until you have completed one, two, or three years of residency, depending on the state in which you live (except in the 11 states that allow IMGs to take Step 3 at the beginning of residency). However, if you live in a state that requires two or three years of residency as a prerequisite to taking Step 3, you can take Step 3 and then obtain a license in another state. Once you have a license in any state, you are permitted to practice in federal institutions such as VA hospitals and Indian Health Service facilities in any state. This can open the door to "moonlighting" opportunities and possibilities for an H1 visa application. For details on individual state rules, write to the licensing board in the state in question or contact the FSMB (see below).

- Complete your residency and then take the appropriate specialty board exams in order to become board certified (e.g., in internal medicine or surgery). If you already have a specialty certification in your home country (e.g., in surgery or cardiology), some specialty boards may grant you six months' or one year's credit toward your total residency time.

- Currently, many residency programs are accepting applications through the Electronic Residency Application Service (ERAS). For more information, see *First Aid for the Match* or contact:

  ECFMG/ERAS Program
  P.O. Box 11746
  Philadelphia, PA 19101-1746
  Phone: (215) 386-5900; Fax: (215) 222-5641
  www.ecfmg.org/eras
  email: eras_support@ecfmg.org

Timing of the USMLE

For an IMG, the timing of a complete application is critical. It is extremely important that you send in your application early if you are to garner the maximum number of interview calls. A rough guide would be to complete all exam requirements by August of the year in which you wish to apply. This would translate into sending both your score sheets and your ECFMG certificate, which is imperative for an interview call, by this date.

Many IMGs also benefit from taking the USMLE Step 1 before Step 2 because a sizable portion of the Step 2 exam tests fundamental concepts of basic sciences. It should be added, however, that it is up to each candidate to arrive at his or her own time frame and to avoid procrastinating about taking these crucial tests.

USMLE Step 1 and the IMG

Developing a good test-taking strategy is especially critical for the IMG.

The USMLE Step 1 is often the first—and, for most IMGs, the most challenging—hurdle to overcome. The USMLE is a standardized licensing system that gives IMGs a level playing field; it is the same exam series taken by U.S. graduates even though it is administered by the ECFMG rather than by the NBME. This means that pass marks for IMGs for both Step 1 and Step 2 are determined by a statistical process that is based on the scores of U.S. medical students in 1991. In general, to pass Step 1, you will probably have to score higher than the bottom 8 to 10% of U.S. and Canadian graduates. In 2001, however, only 66% of ECFMG candidates passed Step 1 on their first attempt, compared with 91% of U.S. and Canadian medical students and graduates.

Of note, 1994–1995 data showed that USFMGs (U.S. citizens attending non-U.S. medical schools) performed 0.4 SD lower than IMGs (non-U.S. citizens attending non-U.S. medical schools). Although their overall scores were lower, USFMGs performed better than IMGs on behavioral sciences.

A good Step 1 score is key to a strong IMG application.

In general, students from non-U.S. medical schools perform worst in behavioral science and biochemistry (1.9 and 1.5 SDs below U.S. students) and comparatively better in gross anatomy and pathology (0.7 and 0.9 SD below U.S. students). Although they are derived from 1994–1995, these data may help you focus your studying efforts.

As an IMG, it is imperative to do your best on Step 1. Few if any students feel totally prepared to take Step 1, but IMGs in particular require serious study and preparation to reach their full potential on this exam. A poor score on Step 1 is a distinct disadvantage when applying for most residencies. Remember that if you pass Step 1, you cannot retake it to try to improve your score. Your goal should thus be to beat the mean, because you can then assert confidently that you have done better than average for U.S. students. Good Step 1 scores will lend credibility to your residency application.

Do commercial review courses help improve your scores? Reports vary, and such courses can be expensive. Many IMGs decide to try the USMLE on their own and then consider a review course only if they fail. Just keep in mind that many states require that you pass the USMLE within three attempts. (For more information on review courses, see Section III.)

USMLE Step 2 and the IMG

In the past, the Step 2 examination had a reputation for being much easier than Step 1, but this no longer seems to be the case for IMGs or U.S. medical students. In 2000–2001, 75% of ECFMG candidates passed Step 2 on the first attempt, compared with 93% of U.S. and Canadian candidates. Also note that because this is a clinical sciences exam, cultural and geographic considerations play a greater role than is the case with Step 1. For example, if your medical education gave you a lot of exposure to malaria, brucellosis, and malnutrition but little to alcohol withdrawal, child abuse, and cholesterol screening, you must do some work to familiarize yourself with topics that are more heavily emphasized in U.S. medicine. You must also have a basic understanding of the legal and social aspects of U.S. medicine, because you will be asked questions about communicating with and advising patients.

There is a big difference between textbook learning of a language and actually being immersed in the culture that goes with it.

The English Language Test

If you did not pass the ECFMG English test by March 3, 1999, you will be required to pass the TOEFL to fulfill the English-language proficiency requirement for ECFMG certification. The administration date of a submitted TOEFL must be after March 3, 1999, to meet the requirement. A passing performance on the ECFMG English test taken prior to March 3, 1999, however, will continue to be accepted. For more information, check online at www.ecfmg.org/elpt/index.html or www.toefl.org.

Native English-speaking IMGs are also required to take the English-language test.

Clinical Skills Assessment

Starting in June 1998, the ECFMG introduced the CSA, an interactive test with role-playing "patients," in an effort to level the disparities that existed among the more than 1400 medical schools worldwide in both curricula and educational standards. The goal of the CSA is to ensure that IMGs can gather and interpret histories, perform physical examinations, and communicate in the English language at a level comparable to that of U.S. graduates.

The CSA simulates clinical encounters that are common in clinics, doctors' offices, and emergency departments. The test is standardized, which means that "standardized patients" (SPs)—i.e., laypeople who have been extensively trained to simulate various clinical problems—give the same responses to all candidates participating in the assessment. For quality assurance purposes, a videotape records all clinical encounters, but these are not used for scoring purposes. Eleven cases are presented to the IMG (ten of which are scored), with cases mixed in terms of age, sex, ethnicity, organ system, and discipline. The cases used in the CSA represent the types of patients who would typically be encountered during the core clerkships in the curricula of accredited U.S. medical schools. These include the following:

By 2004, the CSA will be mandatory for all applicants for licensure (including U.S. graduates).

- Internal medicine
- Surgery
- Obstetrics and gynecology
- Pediatrics
- Psychiatry
- Family medicine

Remember, candidates are scored on only 10 of the 11 patient encounters. The nonscored encounter is added for research purposes, with results applied to future administrations of the CSA.

Test Administration. Before entering a room to interact with an SP, you are given an opportunity to review preliminary information. This information, which is posted on the door of each room, includes the following:

- Patient characteristics (name, age, sex)
- Chief complaint and vitals (temperature, respiratory rate, pulse, BP)

After entering the room, you are given 15 minutes (with a warning bell sounded at 10 minutes) to perform the clinical encounter, which should include introducing yourself, obtaining an appropriate history, performing a focused clinical exam, formulating a differential diagnosis, and planning a diagnostic workup. You are expected to answer any questions the SP might ask as well as to discuss the diagnoses being considered and to advise the SP about follow-up plans. After you leave the room, you have 10 minutes to write a patient note (PN).

"Do's and Don'ts." Ground rules for the clinical encounter are as follows:

- Candidates are not permitted to perform rectal, pelvic/genital, or female breast exams. If a candidate feels that such examinations are warranted, he or she may suggest that they be conducted as part of the diagnostic workup.
- Candidates are not allowed to reenter a room once they have left it. It is therefore recommended that they obtain all the information they need before ending the clinical encounter.
- Time is not on the candidate's side, so it is advisable to "home in" on relevant problems and to conduct a focused clinical exam. For example, if a 40-year-old diabetic and smoker presents with chest pain, candidates should rule out problems of cardiopulmonary, gastrointestinal, and musculoskeletal origin to narrow the examination down to these systems. A CNS exam should therefore be the last one on the candidate's list in this particular example.

Scoring of the CSA. Your score will be based on the clinical encounter as a whole and on your overall communications skills.

ICE = DG + PN.

- **Integrated Clinical Encounter (ICE) score.** The skills you demonstrate in the clinical encounter will be evaluated as follows:
  1. Although SPs will not evaluate your performance, they will document your ability to gather data pertinent to the clinical encounter. Specifically, SPs will note on checklists whether you successfully obtained relevant information or correctly performed the physical exam. Your final data-gathering (DG) score represents an average of your performance with all ten SPs.

2. Health care professionals will score your PN according to predefined criteria, with your final PN score representing the average of your individual PN scores over all ten clinical encounters. Your ICE score will then represent the sum of your DG and PN scores.

- **Communication (COM) score.** In addition to assessing your data-gathering skills, SPs will evaluate your interpersonal skills (IPS) and your proficiency in spoken English. Your IPS will be assessed on four criteria: rapport, interviewing skills, personal manner, and counseling. Your overall COM score is the sum of your averaged IPS scores and your spoken English proficiency rating.

The grade you receive on the CSA is either a "pass" or a "fail." The "pass" grade indicates that you have met the standards set by experts for the ICE and COM. CSA scores, like those of all ECFMG tests, are mailed in four to six weeks. You can check the status of your CSA score report online using the ECFMG's OASIS Web site: oasis.ecfmg.org.

Applying for the CSA. Applicants seeking to take the CSA must complete the four-part application form (Form 706—pink form) in full and mail it to the ECFMG along with a $1200 registration fee. By calling (215) 386-5900 (Monday through Friday, 8 a.m. to 5:30 p.m. EST), you can have an operator help you schedule your test date. It is advisable to have several preferred dates in mind (all within one year of your notification of registration). The operator will formally schedule you on a mutually acceptable day, and your admissions permit will then be mailed to you. Alternatively, you can schedule your CSA date through the Internet via the ECFMG's Interactive Web Application (IWA) at iwa.ecfmg.org. There is no application deadline, since the CSA is administered throughout the year (except on major U.S. holidays).

After the ECFMG receives your fee and application form and determines that you are eligible to take the CSA, you must schedule your test date within four months and take the CSA within one year of the date indicated on your notification of registration.

Test Site Locations. The CSA is administered at the following locations:

ECFMG CSA Center—Philadelphia
3624 Market Street, Third Floor
Philadelphia, PA 19104-2685

ECFMG CSA Center—Atlanta
Two Crown Center
1745 Phoenix Boulevard, Suite 500
Atlanta, GA 30349-5585

If you are living outside the United States, you will need to apply for a visa that will allow you lawful entry into the United States in order to take the

41

CSA. A B2 visa may be issued by a consulate. Documents that are recommended to facilitate this process include:

- The CSA admission permit and a letter from the ECFMG (which explains why the applicant must enter the United States)
- Your medical diploma
- Transcripts from your medical school
- Your USMLE score sheets
- A sponsor letter or affidavit of support stating that you (if you are sponsoring yourself) or your sponsor will bear the expenses of your trip and that you have sufficient funds to meet that expense
- An alien status affidavit

Preparing for the CSA. You can prepare for the CSA by addressing common outpatient clinical issues. To improve doctor-patient communication skills, you can try "acting out" dialogue with friends or relatives. Since time will be a major factor, do not forget to time the encounter as if it were a real test by giving yourself 15 minutes for data gathering and 10 minutes for the patient note. The following volumes may also be of use to you in your preparation for the CSA:

- *Mastering the OSCE and CSA Examination: Second Edition*, Jo-Ann Reteguiz and Beverly Cornel-Avendaño (McGraw-Hill)
- NMS *Review for the Clinical Skills Assessment Exam*, Erich A. Arias (Lippincott Williams & Wilkins)
- *Bates' Guide to Physical Examination and History Taking*, Lynn S. Bickley, Barbara Bates, and Robert A. Hoekelman (Lippincott Williams & Wilkins)

Residencies and the IMG

It is becoming harder for IMGs to obtain residencies in the United States given the rising concerns about an oversupply of physicians in the United States. Official bodies such as the Council on Graduate Medical Education (COGME) have recommended that the total number of residency slots be reduced from the current 144% of the number of U.S. graduates to 110%. Furthermore, changes in immigration law are likely to make it much harder for noncitizens or legal residents of the United States to remain in the country after completing a residency.

In the residency Match, U.S.-citizen IMG applications decreased from 2169 in 2000 to 1999 in 2001, and the percentage of such IMGs accepted was 51% and 52%, an increase from 43.5% in 1997. For non-U.S.-citizen IMGs, applications fell from 7287 in 2000 to 5116 in 2001, while the percentage accepted rose to 38% and 45%, from 34.5% in 1997. The decrease in the total number of IMGs applying for the Match may be attributed to the decrease in the passing rate for the CSA to 80%. See Table 4.

TABLE 4. IMGs in the Match.			
IMG Applicants	1999	2000	2001
U.S. IMG citizens	1821	2169	1999
% U.S. IMGs accepted	47%	51%	52%
Non-U.S. citizens	7977	7287	5116
% Non-U.S. citizens accepted	32%	38%	45%

Visa Options for the IMG

As an IMG, you need a visa to work or train in the United States unless you are a U.S. citizen or a permanent resident (i.e, hold a green card). Two types of visas enable you to accept a residency appointment in the United States: J1 and H1B. Most sponsoring residency programs (SRPs) prefer a J1 visa. Above all, this is because SRPs are authorized by the U.S. Immigration and Naturalization Service (INS) to issue a Form IAP 66 directly to an IMG, whereas they have to go through considerable paperwork and an application to the Immigration and Labor Department to apply to the INS for an H1B visa on behalf of an IMG.

The J1 Visa. Also known as the Exchange Visitor Program, the J1 visa was introduced to give IMGs in diverse specialties the chance to use their training experience in the United States to improve conditions in their home countries. As mentioned above, the INS authorizes most SRPs to issue Form IAP 66 in the same manner that I20s are issued to regular international students in the United States.

To enable an SRP to issue an IAP 66, you must obtain a certificate from the ECFMG indicating that you are eligible to participate in a residency program in the United States. First, however, you must ask the Ministry of Health in your country to issue a statement indicating that your country needs physicians with the skills you propose to acquire by joining a U.S. residency program. This statement, which must bear the seal of your country's government and must be signed by a duly designated government official, is intended to satisfy the U.S. Secretary of Health and Human Services that there is such a need. The Health Ministry in your country should send this statement to the ECFMG (or they may allow you to mail it to the ECFMG).

How can you find out if the government of your country will issue such a statement? In many countries, the Ministry of Health maintains a list of medical specialties in which there is a need for further training abroad. You can also consult seniors in your medical school. A word of caution: If you are applying for a residency in internal medicine and internists are not in short supply in your country, it may help to indicate an intention to pursue a subspecialty after completing your residency training.

The text of your statement of need should read as follows:

> Name of applicant for visa: _____. There currently exists in _____ (your country) a need for qualified medical practitioners in the specialty of _____. (Name of applicant for visa) has filed a written assurance with the government of this country that he/she will return to _____ (your country) upon completion of training in the United States and intends to enter the practice of medicine in the specialty for which training is being sought.
>
> Stamp (or seal and signature) of issuing official of named country.
> Dated_____

To facilitate the issuing of such a statement by the Ministry of Health in your country, you should submit a certified copy of the agreement or contract from your SRP in the United States. The agreement or contract must be signed by you and the residency program official responsible for the training.

Armed with Form IAP 66, you should go to the U.S. consulate nearest to the residential address indicated in your passport. As for other nonimmigrant visas, you must show that you have a genuine nonimmigrant intent to return to your home country. You must also show that all your expenses will be paid.

When you enter the United States, bring your Form IAP 66 along with your visa. You are usually admitted to the United States for the length of the J1 program, designated as "D/S," or duration of status. The duration of your program is indicated on the IAP 66.

Duration of Participation. The duration of a resident's participation in a program of graduate medical education or training is limited to the time normally required to complete such a program. If you would like to get an idea of the typical training time for the various medical subspecialties, you may consult the *Directory of Medical Specialties,* published by Marquis Who's Who for the American Board of Medical Specialties. The authority charged with determining the duration of time required by an individual IMG is the State Department.

The maximum amount of time for participation in a training program is ordinarily limited to seven years unless the IMG has demonstrated to the satisfaction of the ECFMG and the State Department that his or her home country has an exceptional need for the specialty in which he or she will receive further training. An extension of stay may be granted in the event that an IMG needs to repeat a year of clinical medical training or needs time for training or education to take an exam required for board certification.

Requirements After Entry into the United States. Each year, all IMGs participating in a residency program on a J1 visa must furnish the Attorney General of the United States with an affidavit (Form I-644) attesting that they are in good standing in the program of graduate medical education or training in which they are participating and that they will return to their home countries upon completion of the education or training for which they came to the United States.

Restrictions Under the J1 Visa. Not later than two years after the date of entry into the United States, an IMG participating in a residency program on a J1 visa is allowed one opportunity to change his or her designated program of graduate medical education or training if his or her director approves that change.

The J1 visa includes a condition called the "two-year foreign residence requirement." The relevant section of the Immigration and Nationality Act states:

> Any exchange visitor physician coming to the United States on or after January 10, 1977, for the purpose of receiving graduate medical education or training is automatically subject to the two-year home-country physical presence requirement of section 212(e) of the Immigration and Nationality Act, as amended. Such physicians are not eligible to be considered for section 212(e) waivers on the basis of 'No Objection' statements issued by their governments.

The law thus requires that a J1 visa holder, upon completion of the training program, leave the United States and reside in his or her home country for a period of at least two years. Currently there is pressure from the American Medical Association to extend this period to five years.

An IMG on a J1 visa is ordinarily not allowed to change from J1 to most other types of visas or (in most cases) to change from J1 to permanent residence while in the United States until he or she has fulfilled the "foreign residence requirement." The purpose of the foreign residence requirement is to ensure that an IMG uses the training he or she obtained in the United States for the benefit of his or her home country. The U.S. government may, however, waive the two-year foreign residence requirement under the following circumstances:

- If you as an IMG can demonstrate a "well-founded fear of persecution" if forced to return to your country;
- If you as an IMG can prove that returning to your country would result in "exceptional hardship" to you or to members of your immediate family who are U.S. citizens or permanent residents; or
- If you are sponsored by an "interested governmental agency."

Applying for a J1 Visa Waiver. IMGs who have sought a waiver on the basis of the last alternative have found it beneficial to approach the following potentially "interested government agencies":

- **The Department of Health and Human Services (HHS).** HHS's considerations for a waiver have been as follows: (1) the program or activity in which the IMG is engaged is "of high priority and of national or international significance in an area of interest" to HHS (merely providing medical services in a medically underserved area would not be sufficient); (2) the IMG must be an "integral" part of the program or activity "so that the loss of his/her services would necessitate discontinuance of the program or a major phase of it"; and (3) the IMG "must possess outstanding qualifications, training, and experience well beyond the usually expected accomplishments at the graduate, postgraduate, and residency levels and must clearly demonstrate the capability to make original and significant contributions to the program."

In practice, HHS is more likely to recommend waivers for IMGs engaged in research than for those who treat patients. HHS waiver applications should be mailed to Joyce E. Jones, Executive Secretary, Exchange Visitor Review Board, Room 627-H, Hubert H. Humphrey Building, Department of Health and Human Services, 200 Independence Avenue, S.W., Washington, D.C. 20201.

- **The Veterans Administration.** With more than 170 health care facilities located in various parts of the United States, the VA is a major employer of physicians in this country. In addition, many VA hospitals are affiliated with university medical centers. Unlike HHS, the VA sponsors IMGs working not only in research but also in patient care (regardless of specialty) and in teaching. The waiver applicant may engage in teaching and research in conjunction with clinical duties. The VA's latest guidelines (issued on June 22, 1994) provide that it will act as an interested government agency only when the loss of the IMG's services would necessitate the discontinuance of a program or a major phase of it and when recruitment efforts have failed to locate a U.S. physician to fill the position.

  The procedure for obtaining a VA sponsorship for a J1 waiver is as follows: (1) the IMG should deal directly with the Human Resources Department at the local VA facility; and (2) the facility must request that the VA's chief medical director sponsor the IMG for a waiver. The waiver request should include the following documentation: (1) a letter from the director of the local facility describing the program, the IMG's immigration status, the health care needs of the facility, and the facility's recruitment efforts; (2) recruitment efforts, including copies of all job advertisements run within the preceding year; and (3) copies of the IMG's licenses, test results, board certifications, IAP 66 forms, etc.

  The VA contact person in Washington, D.C., should be contacted by the local medical facility rather than by IMGs or their attorneys.

- **The Appalachian Regional Commission (ARC).** The ARC sponsors physicians in certain places in the eastern and southern United States— namely, in Alabama, Georgia, Kentucky, Maryland, Mississippi, New York, North Carolina, Ohio, Pennsylvania, South Carolina, Tennessee, Virginia, and West Virginia. Since 1992, the ARC has sponsored approximately 200 primary care IMGs annually in counties within its jurisdiction that have been designated as Health Professional Shortage Areas (HPSAs) by HHS.

In accordance with its February 1994 revision of its J1 waiver policies, the ARC requires that waiver requests be initially submitted to the ARC contact person in the state of intended employment. If the state concurs, a letter from the state's governor recommending the waiver must be addressed to Jesse J. White, Jr., the federal co-chairman of the ARC. The waiver request should include the following: (1) a letter from the facility to Mr. White stating the proposed dates of employment, the IMG's medical specialty, the address of the practice location, an assertion that the IMG will practice primary care for at least 40 hours per week in the HPSA, and details as to why the facility needs the services of the IMG; (2) a J1 Visa Data Sheet; (3) the ARC federal co-chairman's J1 Visa Waiver Policy and the J1 Visa Waiver Policy Affidavit and Agreement with the notarized signature of the IMG; (4) a contract of at least two years' duration; (5) evidence of the IMG's qualifications, including a résumé, medical diplomas and licenses, and IAP 66 forms; and (6) evidence of recruitment efforts within the preceding six months. Copies of advertisements, copies of résumés received, and reasons for rejection must also be included. The ARC will not sponsor IMGs who have been out of status for six months or longer.

Requests for ARC waivers are processed in Washington, D.C., by Laura Dean Greathouse, ARC, 1666 Connecticut Avenue, N.W., Washington, D.C. 20235. ARC is usually able to forward a letter confirming that a waiver has been recommended to the United States Information Agency (USIA) to the requesting facility or attorney within 30 days of the request.

- **The Department of Agriculture (USDA).** The USDA sponsors physicians who practice in family medicine, general surgery, pediatrics, obstetrics and gynecology, emergency medicine, internal medicine, and general psychiatry in rural areas. The USDA does not sponsor physicians to practice in areas located within the jurisdiction of the ARC.

For an area to be deemed "rural," the county in which the health care facility is located must have a population of less then 20,000 according to the last census. Also, the facility must be located in an HPSA. The IMG must sign a contract with a health care facility for a minimum period of three years. An IMG whose immigration status has lapsed for six months or more will not be considered for sponsorship by the USDA.

Since August 1994, the USDA has required that each request for a waiver be supported by a letter of concurrence ("no objection") from the Department of Health in the state of intended employment. A few states (e.g., Georgia, Mississippi, New York, and Ohio) require that the USDA waiver request and accompanying documentation be submitted directly to them. If they concur with the request, they forward the entire packet together with a no-objection letter to the USDA.

USDA waiver requests should be mailed to Linda Seckel, Program Manager, J1 Visa Residency Waiver Program, Building 005, Room 320, BARC-West, 10300 Baltimore Boulevard, Beltsville, MD 20705-2350. The current processing time is approximately four months.

- **State Departments of Public Health.** There is no application form for a state-sponsored J1 waiver. However, USIA regulations specify that an application must include the following documents: (1) a letter from the State Department of Public Health identifying the physician and specifying that it would be in the public interest to grant him a J1 waiver; (2) an employment contract that is valid for a minimum of three years and that states the name and address of the facility that will employ the physician and the geographic areas in which he or she will practice medicine; (3) evidence that these geographic areas are located within HPSAs; (4) a statement by the physician agreeing to the contractual requirements; (5) copies of all IAP 66 forms; and (6) a completed USIA Data Sheet. Applications are numbered in the order in which they are received, since only 20 physicians per year may be granted waivers in a particular state. Individual states may choose to participate or not to participate in this program. Participating states include Alabama, Alaska, Arkansas, Arizona, Delaware, Florida, Georgia, Illinois, Indiana, Iowa, Kentucky, Maine, Massachusetts, Michigan, Minnesota, Mississippi, Missouri, Nebraska, Nevada, New Hampshire, New Mexico, New York, North Carolina, North Dakota, Ohio, Oklahoma, Pennsylvania, Rhode Island, South Carolina, Vermont, and Washington. Undecided states include California, Connecticut, New Jersey, Virginia, and Wyoming. Nonparticipating states include Hawaii, Idaho, Kansas, Louisiana, Montana, Oregon, South Dakota, Tennessee, Texas, and Utah.

The H1B Visa. Since 1991, the law has allowed medical residency programs to sponsor foreign-born medical residents for H1B visas. There are no restrictions to changing the H1B visa to any other kind of visa, including permanent resident status (green card), through employer sponsorship or through close relatives who are U.S. citizens or permanent residents. There was an overall ceiling of 65,000 H1B visas for professionals in all categories until mid-1998, when the number was raised to 95,000. It is advisable for SRPs to apply for H1B visas as soon as possible in the official year (beginning October 1) when the new quota officially opens up.

H1B visas are intended for "professionals" in a "specialty occupation." This means that an IMG intending to pursue a residency program in the United States with an H1B visa needs to clear all three USMLE Steps before becoming eligible for the H1B. The ECFMG administers Steps 1 and 2. Step 3 is conducted by the individual states. You will need to contact the FSMB or the medical board of the state where you intend to take the Step 3 for details.

USMLE Step 3 and the IMG

Basic eligibility requirements for the USMLE Step 3 are as follows:

- Obtain the MD degree (or its equivalent) or a DO degree by the application deadline.
- Pass both the USMLE Step 1 and Step 2 (or the equivalents). Applicants must receive notice of a passing score by the application deadline.
- Graduates of foreign medical schools should be ECFMG certified or should successfully complete a "fifth pathway" program (at a date no later than the application deadline).
- Apply to the following states, which do not have postgraduate training as an eligibility requirement:

    1. **California**
       Medical Board of California
       1426 Howe Avenue, #54
       Sacramento, CA 95825
       Phone: (916) 263-2382; Fax: (916) 263-2387
       Licensing inquiries: (916) 263-2499; (916) 263-2344
       www.medbd.ca.gov

    2. **Connecticut**
       Connecticut Medical Examining Board
       P.O. Box 340308
       Hartford, CT 06134-0308
       Phone: (860) 509-7648; Fax: (860) 509-7553
       Licensing inquiries: (860) 509-7563

    3. **Louisiana**
       Louisiana State Board of Medical Examiners
       P.O. Box 30250
       New Orleans, LA 70190-0250
       Phone: (504) 568-6820; Fax: (504) 599-0503
       www.lsbme.org

    4. **Maryland**
       Maryland Board of Physician Quality Assurance
       4201 Patterson Avenue
       Baltimore, MD 21215-0095
       Phone: (410) 764-4777; Fax: (410) 358-2252
       Step 3 inquiries: (800) 492-6836
       www.docboard.org

5. **Nebraska***

Nebraska Department of HHS Regulation and Licensure
P.O. Box 95007
Lincoln, NE 68509-5007
Phone: (402) 471-2133 Fax: (402) 471-3577
Step 3 inquiries: FSMB at (817) 571-2949
www.hhs.state.ne.us

6. **New York**

New York State Board for Medicine
Cultural Education Center, Room 3023
Empire State Plaza
Albany, NY 12230
Phone: (518) 474-3841; Fax: (518) 486-4846
www.op.nysed.gov/med.htm

7. **South Dakota**

South Dakota State Board of Medical and Osteopathic Examiners
1323 S. Minnesota Avenue
Sioux Falls, SD 57105
Phone: (605) 334-8343; Fax: (605) 336-0270
Step 3 inquiries: FSMB at (817) 571-2949

8. **Texas**

Texas State Board of Medical Examiners
P.O. Box 2018
Austin, TX 78768-2018
Phone: (512) 305-7010; Fax: (512) 305-7008
www.tsbme.state.tx.us

9. **Utah***

Utah Department of Commerce
Division of Occupational & Professional Licensure
160 East 300 South
Salt Lake City, UT 84114-6741
Phone: (801) 530-6628; Fax: (801) 530-6511
www.commerce.state.ut.us

10. **West Virginia**

West Virginia Board of Medicine
101 Dee Drive
Charleston, WV 25311
Phone: (304) 558-2921; Fax: (304) 558-2084
www.wvdhhr.org/wvbom

*Requires that IMGs obtain a "valid indefinitely" ECFMG certificate.

H1B Application. An application for an H1B visa is not filed by the IMG but by his or her employment sponsor—in your case, by the SRP in the United States. If an SRP is willing to do so, you will be told about it at the time of your interview for the residency program.

Before filing an H1B application with the INS, an SRP must file an application with the U.S. Department of Labor affirming that the SRP will pay at least the normal salary for your job that a U.S. professional would earn. After receiving approval from the Labor Department, your SRP should be ready to file the H1B application with the INS. The SRP's supporting letter is the most important part of the H1B application package; it must describe the job duties to make it clear that the physician is needed in a "specialty occupation" (resident) under the prevalent legal definition of that term.

Most SRPs prefer to issue an IAP 66 for a J1 visa rather than filing papers for an H1B visa because of the burden of paperwork and the attorney costs involved in securing approval of an H1B visa application. Even so, a sizable number of SRPs are willing to go through the trouble, particularly if an IMG is an excellent candidate or if the SRP concerned finds it difficult to fill all the available residency slots (although this is becoming rarer with continuing cuts in residency slots). If an SRP is unwilling to file for an H1B visa because of attorney costs, you could suggest that you would be willing to bear the burden of such costs. The entire process of getting an H1B visa can take anywhere from 10 to 20 weeks.

Although an H1B visa can be stamped by any U.S. consulate abroad, it is advisable to have it stamped at the U.S. consulate where you first applied for a visitor visa to travel to the United States for interviews.

Summary. Despite some significant obstacles, a number of viable methods are available to IMGs who seek to pursue a residency program or eventually practice medicine in the United States.

There is no doubt that the best alternative for IMGs is to obtain H1B visas to pursue their medical residencies. However, in cases where an IMG joins a residency program with a J1 visa, there are some possibilities for obtaining waivers of the two-year foreign residency requirement, particularly for those who are willing to make a commitment to perform primary care medicine in medically underserved areas.

Resources for the IMG

- ECFMG
  3624 Market Street, Fourth Floor
  Philadelphia, PA 19104-2685
  (215) 386-5900 or (202) 293-9320
  Fax: (215) 386-9196
  www.ecfmg.org

The ECFMG telephone number is answered only between 9:00 a.m. and 12:30 p.m. and between 1:30 p.m. and 5:00 p.m. Monday through Friday EST. The ECFMG often takes a long time to answer the phone, which is frequently busy at peak times of the year, and then gives you a long voice-mail message, so it is better to write or fax early than to rely on a last-minute phone call. Do not contact the NBME, as all IMG exam matters are conducted by the ECFMG. The ECFMG also publishes the *Information Booklet* on ECFMG certification and the USMLE program, which gives details on the dates and locations of forthcoming USMLE, CSA, and English tests for IMGs together with application forms. It is free of charge and is also available from the public affairs offices of U.S. embassies and consulates worldwide, as well as from Overseas Educational Advisory Centers. Single copies of the handbook may also be ordered by calling (215) 386-5900, preferably on weekends or between 6 p.m. and 6 a.m. Philadelphia time, or by faxing to (215) 387-9963. Requests for multiple copies must be made by fax or mail on organizational letterhead. The full text of the booklet is also available on the ECFMG's Web site at www.ecfmg.org.

- Federation of State Medical Boards
  P.O. Box 619850
  Dallas, TX 75261-9741
  (817) 868-4000
  Fax: (817) 868-4099
  www.fsmb.org

The FSMB publishes *The Exchange, Section I*, which gives detailed information on examination and licensing requirements in all U.S. jurisdictions. The 1999–2000 edition costs $30. (Texas residents must add 8.25% state sales tax.) To obtain publications, write to Federation Publications at the above address. All orders must be prepaid by a personal check drawn on a U.S. bank, a cashier's check, or a money order payable to the federation. Foreign orders must be accompanied by an international money order or the equivalent, payable in U.S. dollars through a U.S. bank or a U.S. affiliate of a foreign bank. For Step 3 inquiries, the telephone number is (817) 868-4041, and the fax number is (817) 868-4099. You may e-mail them at usmle@fsmb.org or write to the address above.

- United States Information Agency
  301 4th Street, S.W.
  Washington, D.C. 20547
  (202) 619-6531
  www.ecfmg.org

This Web site summarizes the agency's policy regarding various program administration issues arising from the pursuit of graduate medical education or training in the United States by foreign medical graduates under the aegis of the Exchange Visitor Program.

- The Internet newsgroups misc.education.medical and bit.listserv. medforum can be valuable forums through which to exchange information on licensing exams, residency applications, and the like.

- Immigration information for IMGs is available from the sites of Siskind, Susser, Haas & Devine, a firm of attorneys specializing in immigration law: www.visalaw.com/IMG/resources.html.

- Another source of immigration information can be found on the Web site of the law offices of Carl Shusterman, a Los Angeles lawyer specializing in medical immigration law: www.shusterman.com.

- International Medical Placement Ltd., a U.S. company specializing in recruiting foreign physicians to work in the United States, has a site at www.intlmedicalplacement.com. This site includes ordering information for several publications by FMSG, Inc., including USMLE study guides and residency matching information, as well as details on USMLE lecture courses offered by the author of these publications, Stanley Zaslau. The site also has information on seminars held by the company in foreign countries for physicians who are thinking of moving to the United States.

- *First Aid for the International Medical Graduate: Second Edition* by Keshav Chander (2002; 313 pages; ISBN 0071385320) is an excellent resource from a successful IMG. The book includes interviews of successful IMGs and students gearing up for the USMLE, plus complete "getting-settled" information for new residents. Various chapters provide a lot of useful advice on the U.S. curriculum, the health care delivery system, and ethical issues—and the differences IMGs should expect. Dr. Chander points out the weaknesses that are often found in IMG hopefuls and suggests ways of improving their performance on standardized tests as well as on academic and clinical evaluations. Also offered are tips on dealing with possible social and cultural transition difficulties. As an added bonus, the guide contains information on how to get good fellowships after residency.

Bottom line: A reassuring guide for IMGs to increase their confidence and proficiency. A great "first of its kind" that will empower IMGs with information that they need to succeed.

Other books that may be useful and of interest to IMGs are as follows:

- *International Medical Graduates in U.S. Hospitals: A Guide for Program Directors and Applicants*, by Faroque A. Khan and Lawrence G. Smith (1995; ISBN 094312641x).
- *Insider's Guide for the International Medical Graduate to Obtain a Medical Residency in the U.S.A.*, by Ahmad Hakemi (1999; ISBN 1929803001).

What Is the COMLEX Level 1?

In 1995, the National Board of Osteopathic Medicine Examiners (NBOME) introduced a new assessment tool called the Comprehensive Osteopathic Medical Licensing Examination, or COMLEX-USA. As with the former NBOME examination series, the COMLEX-USA is administered over three levels. In 1995, only Level 3 was administered, but by 1998 all three levels were implemented. The COMLEX-USA is now the only exam offered to osteopathic students. One goal of this changeover is to have all 50 states recognize this examination as equivalent to the USMLE. Currently, the COMLEX-USA exam sequence is accepted for licensure in all 50 states. Another stated goal of the COMLEX-USA Level 1 is to create a more primary care–oriented exam that integrates osteopathic principles into clinical situations.

To be eligible to take the COMLEX-USA Level 1, you must have satisfactorily completed at least one-half of your sophomore year in an American Osteopathic Association (AOA)–approved medical school. In addition, you must obtain verification that you are in good standing at your medical schol via approval of your dean.

For all three levels of the COMLEX-USA, raw scores are converted to a percentile score and a score ranging from 5 to 800. For Levels 1 and 2, a score of 400 is required to pass; for Level 3, a score of 350 is needed. COMLEX-USA scores are usually mailed six to eight weeks after the test date. The mean score on the June 2002 exam was 500 with a standard deviation of 79.

If you pass a COMLEX-USA examination, you are not allowed to retake it to improve your grade. If you fail, there is no specific limit to the number of times you can retake it in order to pass. Level 2 and 3 exams must be passed in sequential order within seven years of passing Level 1. Table 5 lists the upcoming examination dates for all levels of the COMLEX-USA in 2003.

What Is the Structure of the COMLEX Level 1?

The COMLEX-USA Level 1 is a multiple-choice examination that is administered over two days. The exam consists of four booklets, each of which must

TABLE 5. Test Dates for COMLEX-USA Exams in 2003.

Level 1	June 3–4
	October 7–8
Level 2	January 15–16
	August 26–27
Level 3	June 10–11
	December 9–10

be completed in four hours. In the 2002 exam, each booklet contained 200 questions for a two-day total of 800 questions. Since the number of questions may change, the best way to determine the number of questions to expect is to consult the most recent *Examination Guidelines and Sample Exam* (you can download this material from the Web site).

The COMLEX-USA Level 1 questions consist of one-best-answer questions, clinical vignettes, and matching sets. In the 2002 exam, approximately 50 to 60% of the questions were one-best-answer, 20 to 45% were clinical vignettes, and 3 to 5% were matching sets. There were no answer choices such as "all the above," "none of the above," negatively phrased best-answer questions, or K-type questions.

Each test booklet had a similar format. The 2002 COMLEX-USA exam consisted of 120 multiple-choice questions and 80 clinical vignette questions per test booklet. All four test booklets had approximately ten matching questions. Each multiple-choice question was preceded by a one- to two-sentence case.

The 2002 exam included only black-and-white (no color) photos with an accompanying brief clinical description, along with questions asking for the diagnosis. For example, there were photos of an eye movement deficit, an illustration of radical immunodiffusion, x-rays of upper and lower extremities, lung images showing lobar pneumonia, a blood smear showing megaloblastic anemia, ECGs, and an EEG. All photos appeared in the fourth book of the exam.

What Is the Difference Between the USMLE and the COMLEX-USA?

Although the COMLEX-USA and the USMLE are similar in scope, content, and emphasis, some differences are worth noting. For example, the COMLEX-USA Level 1 tests osteopathic principles in addition to basic science materials but does not emphasize lab techniques. In addition, although both exams often require that you apply and integrate knowledge over several areas of basic science to answer a given question, many students who took both tests in 2002 reported that the questions differed somewhat in style. Students reported, for example, that USMLE questions generally required that the test taker reason and draw from the information given (often a two-step process), whereas those on the COMLEX-USA exam tended to be more straightforward. Furthermore, USMLE questions were on average found to be considerably longer than those on the COMLEX-USA.

Students also commented that the COMLEX-USA utilized "buzzwords," although limited in their use (e.g., "rose spots" in typhoid fever), whereas the USMLE avoided buzzwords in favor of descriptions of clinical findings or symptoms (e.g., rose-colored papules on the abdomen rather than rose spots). Finally, the 2002 USMLE had many more photographs than did the COMLEX-USA. In general, the overall impression was that the USMLE was a more "thought-provoking" exam, while the COMLEX-USA was more of a "knowledge-based" exam.

Who Should Take Both the USMLE and the COMLEX-USA?

Aside from facing the COMLEX-USA Level 1, you must decide if you will also take the USMLE Step 1. We recommend that you consider taking both the USMLE and the COMLEX-USA under the following circumstances:

- **If you are applying to allopathic residencies.** Although there is growing acceptance of COMLEX-USA certification on the part of allopathic residencies, some allopathic programs prefer or even require passage of the USMLE Step 1. These include many academic programs, programs in competitive specialties (e.g., orthopedics, ophthalmology, or dermatology), and programs in competitive geographic areas (such as California). Fourth-year doctor of osteopathy (DO) students who have already matched may be a good source of information about which programs and specialties look for USMLE scores. It is also a good idea to contact program directors at the institutions you are interested in to ask about their policy regarding the COMLEX-USA versus the USMLE.
- **If you are unsure about your postgraduate training plans.** Successful passage of both the COMLEX-USA Level 1 and the USMLE Step 1 is certain to provide you with the greatest possible range of options when you are applying for internship and residency training.

The clinical coursework that some DO students receive during the summer of their third year (as opposed to their starting clerkships) is considered helpful in integrating basic science knowledge for the COMLEX-USA or the USMLE.

How Do I Prepare for the COMLEX-USA Level 1?

Student experience suggests that you should start studying for the COMLEX-USA four to six months before the test is given, as an early start will allow you to spend up to a month on each subject. The recommendations made in Section I regarding study and testing methods, strategies, and resources, as well as the books suggested in Section III for the USMLE Step 1, hold true for the COMLEX-USA as well.

Another important source of information is in the *Examination Guidelines and Sample Exam*, a booklet that discusses the breakdown of each subject while also providing sample questions. Many students, however, felt that this breakdown provided only a general guideline and was not representative of the level of difficulty of the actual COMLEX-USA. The sample questions did not provide examples of clinical vignettes, which made up approximately 25% of the exam. You will receive this publication with registration materials for the COMLEX-USA Level 1 exam, but you can also receive a copy and additional information by writing:

NBOME
8765 W. Higgins Road, Suite 200
Chicago, IL 60631-4101
Phone: (773) 714-0622; Fax: (773) 714-0631

or by visiting the NBOME Web page at www.nbome.org.

Level 1 Practice Items is a new feature offered by the NBOME. It contains about 200 COMLEX-USA Level 1 items and answers. It is important to note that items in this booklet have been used in previous exams. The booklet costs $15 and can be purchased via the NBOME Web site.

The 2002 COMLEX-USA exam consisted of 120 multiple-choice questions and 80 clinical vignette questions per test booklet. There were four test booklets, two of which had approximately ten matching questions. Each multiple-choice question accompanied a small case (about one to two sentences long).

In 2002, students reported an emphasis in certain areas. For example:

- There was an increased emphasis on lower limb anatomy.
- High-yield osteopathic manipulative technique (OMT) topics on the 2002 exam included basic craniosacral theory, sacral testing/diagnosis, lumbar mechanics, spinal motion and diagnosis, and an emphasis on the sympathetic and parasympathetic innervation of viscera.
- Specific topics were repeatedly tested on the exam. These included cardiovascular physiology and pathology, acid-base physiology, diabetes, benign prostatic hyperplasia, sexually transmitted diseases, measles, and rubella. Thyroid and adrenal function, neurology (head injury), specific drug treatments for bacterial infection, migraines/cluster headaches, and drug mechanisms also received heavy emphasis.
- Behavioral science questions were based on psychiatry.
- Since topics that were repeatedly tested appeared in all four booklets, students found it useful to review them in between the two test days. It is important to understand that the topics emphasized on the 2002 exam may not be stressed on the 2003 exam. However, some topics are heavily tested each year; it may be beneficial to have a solid foundation of the above-mentioned topics.

The National Board of Podiatric Medical Examiners (NBPME) tests are designed to assess whether a candidate possesses the knowledge required to practice as a minimally competent entry-level podiatrist. In all states that recognize them, the NBPME examinations are used as part of the licensing process governing the practice of podiatric medicine. Individual states use the examination scores differently; therefore, doctor of podiatric medicine (DPM) candidates should refer to the *NBPME Bulletin of Information: 2003 Examinations* (www.nbpme.info/PDFs/NBPME1and2Bull.pdf).

Candidates performing at extreme levels are passed or failed at 90 minutes.

The NBPME Part I is generally taken after the completion of the second year of podiatric medical education. Unlike the USMLE Step 1, there is no behavioral science section. The exam does sample the seven basic science disciplines: general anatomy; lower extremity anatomy; biochemistry; physiology; medical microbiology and immunology; pathology; and pharmacology. Questions covering these content areas are interspersed throughout the test.

Your NBPME Appointment

In early spring, your college registrar will have you fill out an application for the NBPME Part I. After your application and registration fees are received, you will be mailed the *NBPME Bulletin of Information: 2003 Examinations*. This bulletin gives you a list of Sylvan Learning Centers across the country that are administering the exam. You may then find the location nearest you and set up an appointment to take the exam. We suggest that you do this as soon as you receive your *NBPME Bulletin*, because reservation slots fill up quickly, especially in the home cities of the seven podiatric medical schools.

On the day of the exam, be sure to arrive at the testing center at least 30 minutes before your scheduled appointment. At that time, you will be registered, escorted to a computer terminal, and given a tutorial to acquaint you with the format of the examination. At the end of the examination, you will be asked to complete a survey regarding your computer-based testing experience.

Computer-Based Testing

The NBPME Part I is a Computerized Mastery Test (CMT) whose format is multiple choice. Each candidate is administered a base test of 90 questions. The maximum amount of time permitted for this base test is 90 minutes. Following the base test, candidates performing at either extreme (either high or low) are passed or failed immediately. By contrast, candidates with an intermediate level of performance are administered additional "testlets" (consisting of 15 questions each), permitting them additional opportunity to demonstrate minimal competence. The maximum time allowed for each additional testlet is 15 minutes. You should try your best on each question, marking any questions that you would like to review should time permit. There is no penalty for guessing. No more than 180 questions are administered to a candidate.

Interpreting Your Score

After you complete the NBPME Part I, a pass/fail decision is reported on the computer. You need a scaled score of at least 75 to pass. Eighty-five percent of first-time test takers pass the NBPME Part I. In computing the scaled score, the number of questions varies from candidate to candidate; however, this is taken into consideration along with the number of questions answered correctly. Approximately two weeks after the examination, you will receive your official score report by mail. Passing candidates receive a message of congratulations but no numerical score. Failing candidates receive a report with one score between 55 and 74 in addition to diagnostic messages intended to help identify strengths or weaknesses in particular content areas. If you fail the NBPME Part I, you must retake the entire examination at a later date. There is no limit to the number of times you can retake the exam.

Preparation for the NBPME Part I

Students suggest that you begin studying for the NBPME Part I at least three months prior to the test date. Each of the colleges of podiatric medicine conducts a series of board reviews. Ask a third-year student which review sessions are most informative. The suggestions made in Section I regarding study and testing methods for the USMLE Step 1 can be applied to the NBPME as well. This book should, however, be used as a supplement and not as the sole source of information.

Approximately 24% of the NBPME Part I focuses on lower extremity anatomy. In this area, students should rely on the notes and material that they received from their class. Remember, lower extremity anatomy is the podiatrist's specialty—so everything about it is important. Do not forget to study osteology. Keep your old tests and look through old lower extremity class exams, because each of the podiatric colleges submits questions from its own exams. This strategy will give you an understanding of the types of questions that may be asked.

Know everything about lower extremity anatomy.

The NBPME, like the USMLE, requires that you apply and integrate knowledge over several areas of basic science to answer the questions. Students report that many questions emphasize clinical presentations; however, the facts in this book are very useful in helping students recall the different diseases and organisms. DPM candidates should expand on the high-yield pharmacology section and study antifungal drugs and treatment protocols for *Pseudomonas*, candidiasis, erythrasma, and the like. The high-yield section focusing on pathology is very useful; however, additional emphasis on diabetes mellitus and all its secondary manifestations should not be overlooked. Students should also focus on classic podiatric dermatopathologies, gout, and arthritis.

A sample set of questions is found in the *NBPME Bulletin of Information: 2003 Examinations*. If you do not receive a *NBPME Bulletin* or if you have any questions regarding registration, fees, test centers, authorization forms, or score reports, please contact your college registrar or:

National Board of Podiatric Medical Examiners (NBPME)
P.O. Box 6516
Princeton, NJ 08541-6516
(877) 302-8952
www.nbpme.info

FIRST AID FOR THE STUDENT WITH A DISABILITY

The USMLE provides accommodations for students with documented disabilities. The basis for such accommodations is the Americans with Disabilities Act (ADA) of 1990. The ADA defines a disability as "a significant limitation in one or more major life activities." This includes both "observable/physical" disabilities (e.g., blindness, hearing loss, narcolepsy) and "hidden/mental disabilities" (e.g., attention deficit hyperactivity disorder, chronic fatigue syndrome, learning disabilities).

To provide appropriate support, the administrators of the USMLE must be informed of both the nature and the severity of an examinee's disability. Such documentation is required for an examinee to receive testing accommodations. Accommodations include extra time on tests, low-stimulation environments, extra or extended breaks, and zoom text.

Who Can Apply for Accommodations?

Students or graduates of a school in the United States or Canada that is accredited by the Liaison Committee for Medical Education (LCME) or the AOA may apply for test accommodations directly from the NBME. Requests are granted only if they meet the ADA definition of a disability. If you are a disabled student or a disabled graduate of a foreign medical school, you must contact the ECFMG (see below).

Who Is Not Eligible for Accommodations?

Individuals who do not meet the ADA definition of disabled are not eligible for test accommodations. Difficulties not eligible for test accommodations include test anxiety, slow reading without an identified underlying cognitive deficit, English as a second language, or learning difficulties that have not been diagnosed as a medically recognized disability.

Understanding the Need for Documentation

Although most learning-disabled medical students are all too familiar with the often exhausting process of providing documentation of their disability, you should realize that **applying for USMLE accommodation is different from these previous experiences.** This is because the NBME determines whether an individual is disabled solely on the basis of the guidelines set by the ADA.

Getting the Information

The first step in applying for USMLE special accommodations is to contact the NBME and obtain a guidelines and questionnaire booklet. This can be obtained by calling or writing to:

Testing Coordinator
Office of Test Accommodations
National Board of Medical Examiners
3750 Market Street
Philadelphia, PA 19104-3190
(215) 590-9500

Internet access to this information is also available at **www.nbme.org.** This information is also relevant for IMGs, since the information is the same as that sent by the ECFMG.

Foreign graduates should contact the ECFMG to obtain information on special accommodations by calling or writing to:

ECFMG
3624 Market Street, Fourth Floor
Philadelphia, PA 19104-2685
(215) 386-5900

When you get this information, take some time to read it carefully. The guidelines are clear and explicit about what you need to do to obtain accommodations.

Applying for Accommodations

Although the accommodation guidelines cited above are self-explanatory, here are some key points to keep in mind:

- **Produce a history.** Send the NBME extensive past records. Since almost all learning disabilities are present from birth, even the earliest records of your disability are invaluable in an assessment. Even if you were diagnosed at a late age, a "paper trail" of your learning disability should still be evident. Grade-school reports, tutoring letters, job reports, previous physician notes, report cards, teacher comments, medication history, and other documents will go a long way toward providing significant evidence of your learning disability.
- **Send your "official" documentation.** Most individuals who were diagnosed with a learning disability were tested with a specific battery of tests (an extensive list of these tests is given in the guidelines). Contact the physician who administered these tests and have the results sent to you. If you cannot locate that physician, obtain the documentation from the educational institutions you attended (college, high school, etc.). Verify that both the administering physician's clinical impressions and the results of your specific tests are included in your submitted material.

Reevaluating Your Disability

You might want to have your disability reevaluated for the USMLE. As stated previously, obtaining accommodations for the USMLE is different from any other process, as you are being evaluated solely on the basis of how well you meet the criteria specified by the ADA. Your evaluator should have this in mind when he or she performs the assessment. Sharing the information in the guidelines and questionnaire booklet with your evaluator will ensure that he or she is aware of this.

The purpose of a reevaluation is twofold. First, it is meant to produce further proof of the disability. Second, it is meant to determine the need for accommodation based on the level of current functioning.

Reevaluation is not for everyone. An evaluation represents a considerable time commitment and is difficult to schedule during the hectic second year. An evaluation is also expensive, usually costing anywhere from $500 to $2000. Furthermore, since such a reevaluation is not being ordered for a strictly "medical reason" and since it is investigating a "previous condition," your insurance company may not cover it.

If you do decide to get reevaluated, the following is highly recommended:

- **Choose an expert.** You're in medical school. Use it! Most of the leading experts on learning disabilities are associated with medical school faculty. Ask around for the leading expert on learning disabilities affiliated with your medical school, and use that physician as your evaluator. Make sure you stress to the evaluator that he or she is functioning as an independent evaluator and not as a school advocate. Using someone at your school is also desirable from a cost perspective; a faculty member may charge you a lower evaluation fee.
- **Undergo some testing.** If you have undergone previous cognitive testing, this step is probably not that important. However, you might want to undergo some basic tests that assess your current level of cognitive functioning. A purely clinical evaluation is commonly limited in both scope and ability. **If you have never undergone a full evaluation, a comprehensive diagnostic battery is essential.** Make sure that your evaluator is looking not just at one or two sessions or subtests but at the entire gestalt.
- **Share your previous history with the evaluator.** Even though the USMLE reviewer will examine your documentation, your evaluator should also have access to your medical history. In that way, he or she can highlight or emphasize certain aspects of your record.
- **Ask for a differential diagnosis.** Evaluators should offer a differential, not just a single diagnosis. Once the differential has been made, evidence for or against any alternative diagnosis should be presented.

Finally, it is highly advisable that you talk from the heart. Part of the application is an essay you write about your disability. This is your opportunity to shine. If you have problems with writing, just speak from your soul. No one else but you can truly describe your learning disability; view this as an opportunity to share your difficulties with a receptive audience.

The Accommodations

A wide variety of accommodations exist for the USMLE. Test accommodations include but are not limited to the following:

- Assistance with keyboard tasks
- Audio rendition
- Extended testing time
- Extra breaks
- Enlarged typeface

By far the most commonly requested and granted accommodation is for extra time. The ADA requires that individuals with a disability be provided with "equal access" to the testing program. Therefore, the purpose of accommodations is to "cancel" the effect of the disability, not to provide extra help in passing an examination.

Because the same types of impairments often vary in severity and frequently restrict different people to different degrees or in different ways, each request is considered individually to determine the effect of the impairment on the life of the applicant and whether a particular accommodation is even appropriate for that person.

The following additional material is excerpted from the NBME Web site (www.nbme.org) and is copyright 1996–2002 by the NBME.

If I am requesting an accommodation from the NBME on Step 1 or Step 2, when should I send in my request and documentation?

Mail your request and supporting documentation for test accommodations directly to the NBME Office of Test Accommodations at the *same time* you submit your Step 1 application. Don't submit your test accommodations request with your application.

Can my evaluator or my medical school send in my request for test accommodations?

No. A request for accommodations, by law, must be initiated by the person with a disability. Also, to protect your confidentiality, the NBME does not provide information concerning your request to third parties.

How does the NBME determine what is an appropriate accommodation for USMLE?

As part of the documentation, the examinee's evaluator should recommend appropriate accommodations to ease the impact of the impairment on the testing activity. Professional consultants in learning disabilities, attention deficit hyperactivity disorder (ADHD), and various other psychiatric and physical conditions review the documentation and recommendations of evaluators to help match the type of assistance with the demonstrated need. The NBME consults with the examinee to determine what accommodations have been effectively used in the past.

If I apply for test accommodations on USMLE, does my disability evaluation have to be up to date?

For someone with a continuing history of accommodation, which would likely include high school and college as well as medical school, current testing is usually not necessary if objective documentation of the past accommodations is provided. However, the impact of the disability may change over time, and new testing may be necessary to demonstrate the current level of impairment and resulting need for accommodation. You will be advised if updated testing is needed.

What are some reasons my request for accommodations might not be approved?

- Insufficient documentation of a need for accommodation. Conditions such as learning disabilities and ADHD are permanent and lifelong. A diagnosis requires an objective history of chronic symptoms from childhood to adulthood as well as evidence of significant impairment currently.
- Lack of presence of a moderate to severe level of impairment attributable to the disorder.
- The identified difficulty is not considered to be a disability under the law, i.e., slow reading without evidence of an underlying language-processing disorder; language difficulties as a result of English as a second language.

Approximately 75% of the total number of requests for all Steps are approved.

Once my request for accommodations has been approved, do I need to arrange for accommodations the next time I register for a Step?

An examinee with a disability must request accommodations at the time of registration. NBME examinees must send a letter requesting accommodations to the Office of Test Accommodations. A repeated request must state whether any change in the accommodations is required, and if so, documentation of the needed change must be provided.

Accommodations are not granted automatically even if they were approved for previous Step administrations.

Miscellaneous Suggestions

- **Get your information to the USMLE early.** The earlier your information is received, the more time the USMLE will have for evaluating and considering your case. They will also have time to ask you for additional material should this prove necessary.

- **Use your winter holiday.** It is a lot easier to get this material ready for the USMLE when you are not in school. It is also immeasurably easier to be evaluated when you are not facing the pressures of the second year.

Database of High-Yield Facts

"There comes a time when for every addition of knowledge you forget something that you knew before. It is of the highest importance, therefore, not to have useless facts elbowing out the useful ones."
—Arthur Conan Doyle, *A Study in Scarlet*

"Never regard study as a duty, but as the enviable opportunity to learn."
—Albert Einstein

"Live as if you were to die tomorrow. Learn as if you were to live forever."
—Gandhi

Anatomy
Behavioral Science
Biochemistry
Microbiology
Pathology
Pharmacology
Physiology
Rapid Review

The 2003 edition of *First Aid for the USMLE Step 1* contains a revised and expanded database of basic science material that student authors and faculty have identified as high yield for board reviews. The facts are loosely organized according to the seven traditional basic medical science disciplines (anatomy, behavioral science, biochemistry, microbiology, pathology, pharmacology, and physiology). Each discipline is then divided into smaller subsections of related facts. Individual facts are generally presented in a three-column format, with the **Title** of the fact in the first column, the **Description** of the fact in the second column, and the **Mnemonic** or **Special Note** in the third column. Some facts do not have a mnemonic and are presented in a two-column format. Others are presented in list or tabular form in order to emphasize key associations.

The database structure is useful for reviewing material already learned. This section is not ideal for learning complex or highly conceptual material for the first time. At the beginning of each basic science section we list supplementary high-yield clinical vignettes and topics that have appeared on recent exams in order to help focus your review.

Selected facts have embedded references to the **third edition** of the *Underground Clinical Vignettes (UCV) Basic Science—Step 1* series (Blackwell Science). These annotations link the high-yield fact to a corresponding vignette, illustrating how that fact may appear in a Step 1 clinical scenario. The following annotation, for example, refers to cases 23 and 45 from *UCV Anatomy:* **UCV** *Anat.23, 45*

UCV REFERENCE LEGEND	
UCV Title	**Abbreviation**
Anatomy	Anat
Behavioral Science	BehSci
Biochemistry	Bio
Microbiology, Vol. 1	Micro1
Microbiology, Vol. 2	Micro2
Pathophysiology, Vol. 1	Path1
Pathophysiology, Vol. 2	Path2
Pathophysiology, Vol. 3	Path3
Pharmacology	Pharm

The Database of High-Yield Facts is not comprehensive. Use it to complement your core study material and not as your primary study source. The facts and notes have been condensed and edited to emphasize the essential material, and as a result each entry is "incomplete." Work with the material, add your own notes and mnemonics, and recognize that not all memory techniques work for all students.

We update Section II annually to keep current with new trends in boards content as well as to expand our database of high-yield information. However, we must note that inevitably many other very high yield entries and topics are not yet included in our database.

We actively encourage medical students and faculty to submit entries and mnemonics so that we may enhance the database for future students. We also solicit recommendations of alternate tools for study that may be useful in preparing for the examination, such as diagrams, charts, and computer-based tutorials (see How to Contribute, p. xv).

Disclaimer

The entries in this section reflect student opinions of what is high yield. Owing to the diverse sources of material, no attempt has been made to trace or reference the origins of entries individually. We have regarded mnemonics as essentially in the public domain. All errors and omissions will gladly be corrected if brought to the attention of the authors, either through the publisher or directly by e-mail.

Anatomy

"Dispel from your mind the thought that an understanding of the human body in every aspect of its structure can be given in words ..."
—Leonardo da Vinci

Several topics fall under this heading, including embryology, gross anatomy, histology, and neuroanatomy. Do not memorize all the small details; however, do not ignore anatomy altogether. Review what you have already learned and what you wish you had learned. Many questions require two steps. The first step is to identify a structure on anatomic cross-section, electron micrograph, or photomicrograph. The second step may require an understanding of the clinical significance of the structure.

When studying, stress clinically important material. For example, be familiar with gross anatomy related to specific diseases (e.g., Pancoast's tumor, Horner's syndrome), traumatic injuries (e.g., fractures, sensory and motor nerve deficits), procedures (e.g., lumbar puncture), and common surgeries (e.g., cholecystectomy). There are also many questions on the exam involving x-rays, CT scans, and neuro MRI scans. Many students suggest browsing through a general radiology atlas, pathology atlas, and histology atlas. Focus on learning basic anatomy at key levels in the body (e.g., sagittal brain MRI; axial CT of midthorax, abdomen, and pelvis). Basic neuroanatomy (especially pathways, blood supply, and functional anatomy) also has good yield. Use this as an opportunity to learn associated neuropathology and neurophysiology. Basic embryology (especially congenital malformations) is worth reviewing.

High-Yield Clinical Vignettes
High-Yield Images
High-Yield Topics
Cell Type
Embryology
Gross Anatomy
Histology
Neuroanatomy

These abstracted case vignettes are designed to demonstrate the thought processes necessary to answer multistep clinical reasoning questions.

Vignette	Question	Answer
■ Baby vomits milk when fed and has a gastric air bubble.	What kind of fistula is present?	Blind esophagus with lower segment of esophagus attached to trachea.
■ 20-year-old dancer reports decreased plantar flexion and decreased sensation over the back of her thigh, calf, and lateral half of her foot.	What spinal nerve is involved?	Tibial (L4 to S3).
■ Patient presents with decreased pain and temperature sensation over the lateral aspects of both arms.	What is the lesion?	Syringomyelia.
■ Penlight in patient's right eye produces bilateral pupillary constriction. When moved to the left eye, there is paradoxical bilateral pupillary dilatation.	What is the defect?	Atrophy of the left optic nerve.
■ Patient describes decreased prick sensation on the lateral aspect of her leg and foot.	A deficit in what muscular action can also be expected?	Dorsiflexion and eversion of foot (common peroneal nerve).
■ Elderly woman presents with arthritis and tingling over the lateral digits of her right hand.	What is the diagnosis?	Carpal tunnel syndrome, median nerve compression.
■ Woman involved in motor vehicle accident cannot turn head to the left and has right shoulder droop.	What structure is damaged?	Right CN XI (runs through jugular foramen with CN IX and X), innervating sternocleidomastoid and trapezius muscles.
■ Man presents with one wild, flailing arm.	Where is the lesion?	Contralateral subthalamic nucleus (hemiballismus).
■ Pregnant woman in 3rd trimester has normal blood pressure when standing and sitting. When supine, blood pressure drops to 90/50.	What is the diagnosis?	Compression of the inferior vena cava.
■ Soccer player who was kicked in the leg suffered a damaged medial meniscus.	What else is likely to have been damaged?	Anterior cruciate ligament (remember the "unhappy triad").

Vignette	Question	Answer
■ Gymnast dislocates her shoulder anteriorly.	What nerve is most likely to have been damaged?	Axillary nerve (C5, C6).
■ Patient with cortical lesion does not know that he has a disease.	Where is the lesion?	Right parietal lobe.
■ Child presents with cleft lip.	Which embryologic process failed?	Fusion of maxillary and medial nasal processes.
■ Patient cannot protrude tongue toward left side and has a right-sided spastic paralysis.	Where is the lesion?	Left medulla, CN XII.
■ Teen falls while rollerblading and hurts his elbow. He can't feel the medial part of his palm.	Which nerve and what injury?	Ulnar nerve due to broken medial condyle.
■ 24-year-old male develops testicular cancer.	Metastatic spread occurs by what route?	Para-aortic lymph nodes (recall descent of testes during development).
■ Field hockey player presents to the ER after falling on her arm during practice. X-ray shows midshaft break of humerus.	Which nerve and which artery are most likely damaged?	Radial nerve and deep brachial artery, which run together.

The high-yield images referenced below may not all appear in this chapter or in the high-yield glossy photo insert; however, they are still worthy of consideration.

- Carotid angiography → identify the anterior cerebral artery → occlusion of this artery will produce a deficit where? → contralateral leg.
- H&E of normal liver → identify the central vein, portal triad, bile canaliculi, etc.
- X-ray of fractured humerus → what nerve is most likely damaged? → radial nerve.
- X-ray of hip joint → what part undergoes avascular necrosis with fracture at the neck of the femur? → femoral head.
- Abdominal CT cross-section → obstruction of what structure results in enlarged kidneys? → inferior vena cava.
- Intravenous pyelogram with right ureter dilated → where is the obstruction and what is the likely cause? → ureterovesicular junction; stone.
- Illustration of fetal head → medial maxillary eminence gives rise to what? → primary palate.
- Abdominal MRI cross-section → locate the splenic artery, portal vein, etc.
- EM of cell → lysosomes (digestion of macromolecules), RER (protein synthesis), SER (steroid synthesis).
- Coronal MRI section of the head at the level of the eye → find the medial rectus muscle → what is its function? → medial gaze.
- Optic nerve path → defect that would cause diminished pupillary reflex in right eye? Defect that would cause right homonymous hemianopsia? → right optic nerve; left optic tract.
- Aortogram → identify adrenal artery, renal arteries, SMA, etc.
- Chest x-ray showing pleural effusion with layering → where is the fluid located? → costodiaphragmatic recess.
- MRI abdominal cross-section → what structure is derivative of the common cardinal veins? → inferior vena cava.
- Sagittal MRI of brain of patient with hyperphagia, increased CSF pressure, and visual problems → where is the lesion? → hypothalamus.

Embryology

1. Development of the heart, lung, liver, kidney (i.e., what are the embryologic structures that give rise to these organs?).
2. Etiology and clinical presentation of important congenital malformations (e.g., neural tube defects, cleft palate, tetralogy of Fallot, tracheoesophageal fistula, horseshoe kidney).
3. Development of the central nervous system (e.g., telencephalon, diencephalon, mesencephalon).
4. Derivatives of the foregut, midgut, and hindgut as well as their vascular supply.
5. Derivatives of the somites, and malformations associated with defects in somite migration.
6. Changes in the circulatory/respiratory system on the first breath of a newborn.
7. Development of the embryonic plate in weeks 2 and 3.

Gross Anatomy

1. Anatomic landmarks in relation to medical procedures (e.g., direct and indirect hernia repair, lumbar puncture, pericardiocentesis).
2. Anatomic landmarks in relation to major organs (e.g., lungs, heart, kidneys).
3. Common injuries of the knee (including clinical examination), hip, shoulder, and clavicle, paying attention to the clinical deficits caused by these injuries (e.g., shoulder separation, hip fracture).
4. Clinical features and anatomic correlations of specific brachial plexus lesions (e.g., waiter's tip, wrist drop, claw hand, scapular winging).
5. Clinical features of common peripheral nerve injuries (e.g., common vs. deep peroneal nerve palsy, radial nerve palsy).
6. Etiology and clinical features of common diseases affecting the hands (e.g., carpal tunnel syndrome, Dupuytren's contracture).
7. Major blood vessels and collateral circulatory pathways of the gastrointestinal tract (e.g., collaterals between the superior and inferior mesenteric arteries).
8. Bone structures (metaphysis, epiphysis, diaphysis), including histologic features; linear (epiphysis) and annular (diaphysis) bone growth.

Histology

1. Histology of the respiratory tract (i.e., differentiate between the bronchi, terminal bronchioles, respiratory bronchioles, and alveoli).
2. Structure, function, and electron microscopic (EM) appearance of major cellular organelles and structures (e.g., lysosomes, peroxisomes, glycogen, mitochondria, ER, Golgi apparatus, nucleus, nucleolus).
3. Structure, function, and EM appearance of cell-cell junctional structures (e.g., tight junctions, gap junctions, desmosomes).
4. Histology of lymphoid organs (e.g., lymph nodes, spleen).

HIGH-YIELD FACTS

Anatomy

5. Resident phagocytic cells of different organisms (e.g., Langerhans' cells, Kupffer cells, alveolar macrophages, microglia).
6. Histology of muscle fibers and changes seen with muscle contraction (sarcomere structure, different bands, rigor mortis).
7. Cellular basis for the blood-testis barrier.

Neuroanatomy

1. Etiology and clinical features of important brain, cranial nerve, and spinal cord lesions (e.g., brain stem lesions and "crossed signs," dorsal root lesions, effects of schwannoma, Weber and Parinaud syndromes).
2. Production, circulation, and composition of cerebrospinal fluid.
3. Neuroanatomy of hearing (central and peripheral hearing loss).
4. Extraocular muscles (which muscle abducts, adducts, etc.) and their innervation.
5. Structure and function of a chemical synapse (e.g., neuromuscular junction).
6. Major neurotransmitters, receptors, second messengers, and effects.
7. Blood supply of the brain (anterior, middle, posterior cerebral arterial areas, "watershed" areas) and neurologic deficits corresponding to various vascular occlusions.
8. Functional anatomy of the basal ganglia (e.g., globus pallidus, caudate, putamen).
9. Anatomic landmarks near the pituitary gland.
10. Brain MRI/CT, including morphologic changes in disease states (e.g., Huntington's chorea, MS, aging).
11. Clinical exam of pupillary light reflex: pathway tested, important anatomic lesions, swinging light test.

Radiology

1. X-rays; plain films.
   a. Fractures (skull, humerus, etc.) and associated clinical findings.
   b. PA and lateral chest films, including important landmarks (costodiaphragmatic recess, major blood vessels, cardiac chambers, and abnormalities seen with different diseases [consolidation, pneumothorax, mitral stenosis, cardiomyopathy]).
   c. Abdominal films, including vasculature (locate important vessels in contrast films) and other important structures.
   d. Joint films (e.g., shoulder, wrist, knee, hip, spine), including important injuries/diseases (e.g., osteoarthritis, herniated disk).
2. CT/MRI studies.
   a. Brain cross-section (e.g., hematomas, brain lesions, extraocular muscles).
   b. Chest cross-section (e.g., superior vena cava, aortic arch, heart).
   c. Abdominal cross-section (e.g., liver, kidney, pancreas, aorta, inferior vena cava, rectus abdominis muscle, splenic artery).

Blood cell differentiation

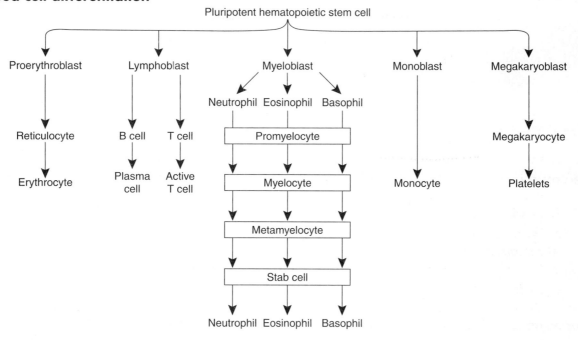

Pluripotent hematopoietic stem cell

Proerythroblast → Reticulocyte → Erythrocyte

Lymphoblast → B cell → Plasma cell; T cell → Active T cell

Myeloblast → Neutrophil Eosinophil Basophil → Promyelocyte → Myelocyte → Metamyelocyte → Stab cell → Neutrophil Eosinophil Basophil

Monoblast → Monocyte

Megakaryoblast → Megakaryocyte → Platelets

Erythrocyte 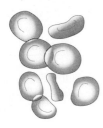	Anucleate, biconcave → large surface area: volume ratio → easy gas exchange (O_2 and CO_2). Source of energy—glucose (90% anaerobically degraded to lactate, 10% by HMP shunt). Survival time—120 days. Membrane contains the chloride-bicarbonate antiport important in the "physiologic chloride shift," which allows the RBC to transport CO_2 from the periphery to the lungs for elimination.	*Eryth* = red; *cyte* = cell. Erythrocytosis = polycythemia = ↑ number of red cells. Anisocytosis = varying sizes. Poikilocytosis = varying shapes. Reticulocyte = baby erythrocyte.
Leukocyte	Types: granulocytes (basophils, eosinophils, neutrophils) and mononuclear cells (lymphocytes, monocytes). Responsible for defense against infections. Normally 4,000–10,000 per microliter.	*Leuk* = white; *cyte* = cell.
Basophil	Mediates allergic reaction. < 1% of all leukocytes. Bilobate nucleus. Densely basophilic granules containing heparin (anticoagulant), histamine (vasodilator) and other vasoactive amines, and SRS-A.	*Basophilic*—staining readily with *basic* stains.
Mast cell 	Mediates allergic reaction. Degranulation—release of histamine, heparin, and eosinophil chemotactic factors. Can bind IgE to membrane. Mast cells resemble basophils structurally and functionally but are not the same cell type.	Involved in type I hypersensitivity reactions. Cromolyn sodium prevents mast cell degranulation.

Eosinophil

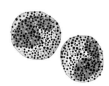

1–6% of all leukocytes. Bilobate nucleus. Packed with large eosinophilic granules of uniform size. Defends against helminthic and protozoan infections (major basic protein). Highly phagocytic for antigen-antibody complexes.

Produces histaminase and arylsulfatase.

Eosin = a dye; *philic* = loving.
Causes of eosinophilia =
 NAACP:
  Neoplastic
  Asthma
  Allergic processes
  Collagen vascular
   diseases
  Parasites

Neutrophil

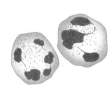

Acute inflammatory response cell. 40–75% WBCs. Phagocytic. Multilobed nucleus. Large, spherical, azurophilic 1° granules (called lysosomes) contain hydrolytic enzymes, lysozyme, myeloperoxidase, and lactoferrin.

Hypersegmented polys are seen in vitamin B_{12}/ folate deficiency.

Monocyte

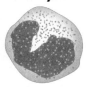

2–10% of leukocytes. Large. Kidney-shaped nucleus. Extensive "frosted glass" cytoplasm. Differentiates into macrophages in tissues.

Mono = one, single; *cyte* = cell.

Lymphocyte

Small. Round, densely staining nucleus. Small amount of pale cytoplasm. B lymphocytes produce antibodies. T lymphocytes manifest the cellular immune response as well as regulate B lymphocytes and macrophages.

B lymphocyte

Part of humoral immune response. Arises from stem cells in bone marrow. Matures in marrow. Migrates to peripheral lymphoid tissue (follicles of lymph nodes, white pulp of spleen, unencapsulated lymphoid tissue). When antigen is encountered, B cells differentiate into plasma cells and produce antibodies. Has memory. Can function as antigen-presenting cell (APC) via MHC class II.

B = **B**one marrow.

Plasma cell

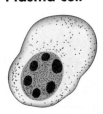

Off-center nucleus, clock-face chromatin distribution, abundant RER and well-developed Golgi apparatus. B cells differentiate into plasma cells, which can produce large amounts of antibody specific to a particular antigen.

Multiple myeloma is a plasma cell neoplasm.

T lymphocyte	Mediates cellular immune response. Originates from stem cells in the bone marrow, but matures in the thymus. T cells differentiate into cytotoxic T cells (MHC I, CD8), helper T cells (MHC II, CD4), suppressor T cells, and delayed hypersensitivity T cells.	**T** is for **T**hymus. **CD** is for **C**luster of **D**ifferentiation. $\mathbf{MHC \times CD = 8}$ (e.g., MHC 2 × CD4 = 8).
Macrophage 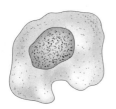	Phagocytizes bacteria, cell debris, and senescent red cells and scavenges damaged cells and tissues. Long life in tissues. Macrophages differentiate from circulating blood monocytes. Activated by γ-IFN. Can function as APC.	*Macro* = large; *phage* = eater.
Airway cells	Ciliated cells extend to the respiratory bronchioles; goblet cells extend only to the terminal bronchioles. Type I cells (97% of alveolar surfaces) line the alveoli. Type II cells (3%) secrete pulmonary surfactant (dipalmitoylphosphatidylcholine), which ↓ the alveolar surface tension. Also serve as precursors to type I cells and other type II cells.	All the mucus secreted can be swept orally (ciliated cells run deeper). A lecithin:sphingomyelin ratio of > 2.0 in amniotic fluid is indicative of fetal lung maturity.
Microglia 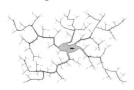	CNS phagocytes. Mesodermal origin. Not readily discernible in Nissl stains. Have small irregular nuclei and relatively little cytoplasm. In response to tissue damage, transform into large ameboid phagocytic cells.	HIV-infected microglia fuse to form multinucleated giant cells in the CNS.
Oligodendroglia 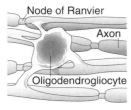 Node of Ranvier — Axon — Oligodendrogliocyte	Function to myelinate multiple CNS axons. In Nissl stains, they appear as small nuclei with dark chromatin and little cytoplasm. Predominant type of glial cell in white matter.	These cells are destroyed in multiple sclerosis.
Schwann cells	Function to myelinate PNS axons. Unlike oligodendroglia, a single Schwann cell myelinates only 1 PNS axon. Schwann cells promote axonal regeneration.	Acoustic neuroma is an example of a schwannoma. Location commonly associated with internal acoustic meatus (CN VII, VIII).

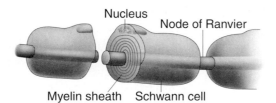

Nucleus
Node of Ranvier
Myelin sheath   Schwann cell

Gas exchange barrier

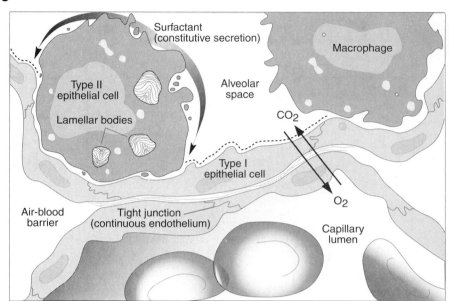

Surfactant (constitutive secretion)

Macrophage

Type II epithelial cell

Alveolar space

Lamellar bodies

CO_2

Type I epithelial cell

O_2

Air-blood barrier

Tight junction (continuous endothelium)

Capillary lumen

Type II epithelial cells also serve as progenitor for type I cells

Fetal landmarks

Within week 1	Implantation (as a blastocyst).
Within week 2	Bilaminar disk.
Within week 3	Gastrulation.
Within week 3	Primitive streak and neural plate begin to form.
Weeks 3–8	Organogenesis; susceptible to teratogens.
Week 4	Heart begins to beat; upper and lower limb buds begin to form.
Week 10	Genitalia have male/female characteristics.

Teratogens

Most susceptible in 3rd–8th week (organogenesis) of pregnancy.

Examples	Effects on fetus
ACE inhibitors	Renal damage
Cocaine	Abnormal fetal development and fetal addiction
DES	Vaginal clear cell adenocarcinoma
Iodide	Congenital goiter or hypothyroidism
13-cis-retinoic acid	Extremely high risk for birth defects
Thalidomide	Limb defects ("flipper" limbs)
Warfarin, x-rays	Multiple anomalies

Fetal infections can also cause congenital malformations. (Other medications contraindicated in pregnancy are shown in the pharmacology section.)

HIGH-YIELD FACTS

Anatomy

Umbilical cord

Contains 2 umbilical arteries, which return deoxygenated blood from the fetus, and 1 umbilical vein, which supplies oxygenated blood from the placenta to the fetus.

Single umbilical artery is associated with congenital and chromosomal anomalies.

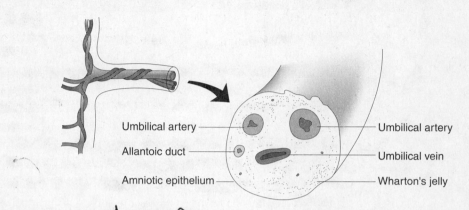

Umbilical artery
Allantoic duct
Amniotic epithelium

Umbilical artery
Umbilical vein
Wharton's jelly

Embryologic derivatives

Anterior pituitary

Ectoderm

Surface ectoderm	Adenohypophysis, lens of eye, epithelial linings, epidermis.
Neuroectoderm	Neurohypophysis, CNS neurons, oligodendrocytes, astrocytes, pineal gland.
Neural crest	ANS, dorsal root ganglia, melanocytes, chromaffin cells of adrenal medulla, enterochromaffin cells, pia, celiac ganglion, Schwann cells, odontoblasts, parafollicular (C) cells of thyroid.

Mesoderm — Dura connective tissue, muscle, bone, cardiovascular structures, lymphatics, blood, urogenital structures, and serous linings of body cavities (e.g., peritoneal), spleen, adrenal cortex.

Endoderm — Gut tube epithelium and derivatives (e.g., lungs, liver, pancreas, thymus, thyroid, parathyroid).

Notochord — Induces ectoderm to form neuroectoderm (neural plate). Its postnatal derivative is the nucleus pulposus of the intervertebral disk.

Early development

Rule of 2's for 2nd week	2 germ layers (bilaminar disk): epiblast, hypoblast. 2 cavities: amniotic cavity, yolk sac. 2 components to placenta: cytotrophoblast, syncytiotrophoblast.	The epiblast (precursor to ectoderm) invaginates to form primitive streak. Cells from the primitive streak give rise to both intraembryonic mesoderm and endoderm.
Rule of 3's for 3rd week	3 germ layers (gastrula): ectoderm, mesoderm, endoderm.	

Fetal erythropoiesis

Fetal erythropoiesis occurs in:
1. Yolk sac (3–8 wk)
2. Liver (6–30 wk)
3. Spleen (9–28 wk)
4. Bone marrow (28 wk onward)

Young Liver Synthesizes Blood.

Heart embryology

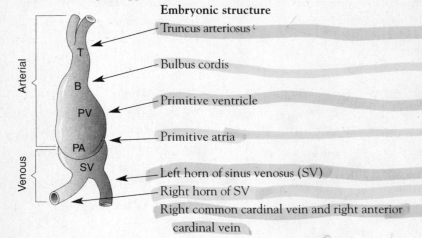

Embryonic structure	Gives rise to
Truncus arteriosus	Ascending aorta and pulmonary trunk
Bulbus cordis	Smooth parts of left and right ventricle
Primitive ventricle	Trabeculated parts of left and right ventricle
Primitive atria	Trabeculated left and right atrium
Left horn of sinus venosus (SV)	Coronary sinus
Right horn of SV	Smooth part of right atrium
Right common cardinal vein and right anterior cardinal vein	Superior vena cava

Twinning

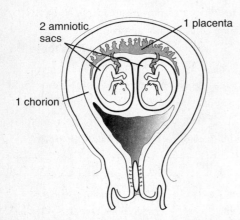

Monozygotic

2 amniotic sacs

1 placenta

1 chorion

1 zygote splits evenly to develop 2 amniotic sacs with a single common chorion and placenta.

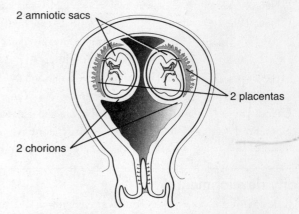

Dizygotic (fraternal) or monozygotic

2 amniotic sacs

2 placentas

2 chorions

Dizygotes develop individual placentas, chorions, and amniotic sacs.

Monozygotes develop 2 placentas (separate/fused), chorions, and amniotic sacs.

Fetal circulation

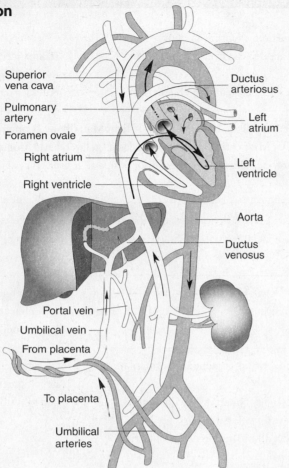

Superior vena cava

Pulmonary artery

Foramen ovale

Right atrium

Right ventricle

Ductus arteriosus

Left atrium

Left ventricle

Aorta

Ductus venosus

Portal vein

Umbilical vein

From placenta

To placenta

Umbilical arteries

Blood in umbilical vein is ≈ 80% saturated with O_2.

Most oxygenated blood reaching the heart via the IVC is diverted through the foramen ovale and pumped out the aorta to the head.

Deoxygenated blood from the SVC is expelled into the pulmonary artery and ductus arteriosus to the lower body of the fetus.

At birth, infant takes a breath; ↓ resistance in pulmonary vasculature causes ↑ left atrial pressure vs. right atrial pressure; foramen ovale closes; ↑ in oxygen leads to ↓ in prostaglandins, causing closure of ductus arteriosus.

Indomethacin closes the foramen ovale.

UCV *Anat.6*   (Adapted, with permission, from Ganong WF. *Review of Medical Physiology,* 19th ed. Stamford, CT: Appleton & Lange, 1999:600.)

Fetal-postnatal derivatives

1. Umbilical vein—ligamentum teres hepatis
2. Umbilical arteries—**medial** umbilical ligaments
3. Ductus arteriosus—ligamentum arteriosum
4. Ductus venosus—ligamentum venosum
5. Foramen ovale—fossa ovalis
6. Allantois—urachus—**median** umbilical ligament
7. Notochord—nucleus pulposus

Urachal cyst or sinus is a remnant of the allantois (urine drainage from bladder).

Aortic arch derivatives

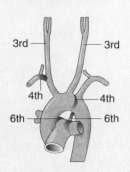

3rd   3rd

4th   4th

6th   6th

1st—part of **MAX**illary artery.
2nd—Stapedial artery and hyoid artery.
3rd—common **C**arotid artery and proximal part of internal carotid artery.
4th—on left, aortic arch; on right, proximal part of right subclavian artery.
6th—proximal part of pulmonary arteries and (on left only) ductus arteriosus.

1st arch is **MAX**imal.
Second = Stapedial.
C is 3rd letter of alphabet.

4th arch (4 limbs) = systemic.

6th arch = pulmonary and the pulmonary-to-systemic shunt (ductus arteriosus).

HIGH-YIELD FACTS

Anatomy

Branchial apparatus	Branchial clefts are derived from ectoderm. Branchial arches are derived from mesoderm and neural crests. Branchial pouches are derived from endoderm.	**CAP** covers outside from inside (**C**lefts = ectoderm, **A**rches = mesoderm, **P**ouches = endoderm).
Branchial arch 1 derivatives	Meckel's cartilage: **M**andible, **M**alleus, incus, spheno**M**andibular ligament. Muscles: Muscles of **M**astication (temporalis, **M**asseter, lateral and **M**edial pterygoids), **M**ylohyoid, anterior belly of digastric, tensor tympani, tensor veli palatini. Nerve: CN V_3.	
Branchial arch 2 derivatives	Reichert's cartilage: **S**tapes, **S**tyloid process, lesser horn of hyoid, **S**tylohyoid ligament. Muscles: muscles of facial expression, **S**tapedius, **S**tylohyoid, posterior belly of digastric. Nerve: CN VII.	
Branchial arch 3 derivatives	Cartilage: greater horn of hyoid. Muscle: stylopharyngeus. Nerve: CN IX.	Think of pharynx: stylo**pharyngeus** innervated by glosso**pharyngeal** nerve.
Branchial arches 4 to 6 derivatives	Cartilages: thyroid, cricoid, arytenoids, corniculate, cuneiform. Muscles (4th arch): most pharyngeal constrictors, cricothyroid, levator veli palatini. Muscles (6th arch): all intrinsic muscles of larynx **except cricothyroid.** Nerve: 4th arch—CN X; 6th arch—CN X (recurrent laryngeal branch).	Arch 5 makes no major developmental contributions.
Branchial arch innervation	Arch 1 derivatives supplied by CN V_2 and V_3. Arch 2 derivatives supplied by CN VII. Arch 3 derivatives supplied by CN IX. Arch 4 and 6 derivatives supplied by CN X.	
Branchial cleft derivatives	1st cleft develops into external auditory meatus. 2nd through 4th clefts form temporary cervical sinuses, which are obliterated by proliferation of 2nd arch mesenchyme.	Persistent cervical sinus can lead to a branchial cyst in the neck.

Ear development

Bones	Muscles	Miscellaneous
Incus/malleus—1st arch	Tensor tympani (V_3)—1st arch	External auditory meatus—1st cleft
Stapes—2nd arch	Stapedius (VII)—2nd arch	Eardrum, eustachian tube—1st pharyngeal membrane

Branchial pouch derivatives	1st pouch develops into middle ear cavity, eustachian tube, mastoid air cells.	1st pouch contributes to endoderm-lined structures of ear.
	2nd pouch develops into epithelial lining of palatine tonsil.	3rd pouch contributes to 3 structures (thymus, L and R inferior parathyroids).
	3rd pouch (dorsal wings) develops into **inferior** parathyroids.	Aberrant development of 3rd and 4th pouches → DiGeorge syndrome → leads to T-cell deficiency (thymic hypoplasia) and hypocalcemia (parathyroid glands).
	3rd pouch (ventral wings) develops into thymus.	
	4th pouch develops into **superior** parathyroids.	

Thymus	Site of T-cell maturation. Encapsulated. From epithelium of 3rd branchial pouches. Lymphocytes of mesenchymal origin. Cortex is dense with immature T cells; medulla is pale with mature T cells and epithelial reticular cells and contains Hassall's corpuscles. Positive and negative selection occurs at the corticomedullary junction.	Think of the **T**hymus as "finishing school" for **T** cells. They arrive immature and "dense" in the cortex; they are mature in the medulla.

Thyroid development	Thyroid diverticulum arises from floor of primitive pharynx, descends into neck. Connected to tongue by thyroglossal duct, which normally disappears but may persist as pyramidal lobe of thyroid. Foramen cecum is normal remnant of thyroglossal duct. Most common ectopic thyroid tissue site is the tongue.

Tongue development	1st branchial arch forms anterior $^2/_3$ (thus pain via CN V_3, taste via CN VII).	Taste is CN VII, IX, X (solitary nucleus); pain is CN V_3, IX, X; motor is CN XII.
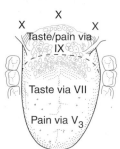	3rd and 4th arches form posterior $^1/_3$ (thus pain and taste mainly via CN IX, extreme posterior via CN X).	
	Motor innervation is via CN XII.	

Cleft lip and cleft palate	Cleft lip—failure of fusion of the maxillary and medial nasal processes.	
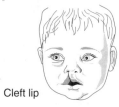	Cleft palate—failure of fusion of the lateral palatine processes, the nasal septum, and/or the median palatine process.	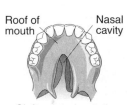
Cleft lip		Cleft palate (partial)

Diaphragm embryology

Diaphragm is derived from:

1. **S**eptum transversum
2. **P**leuroperitoneal folds
3. **B**ody wall
4. **D**orsal mesentery of esophagus

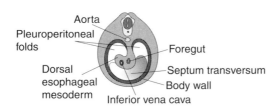

Aorta
Pleuroperitoneal folds
Foregut
Dorsal esophageal mesoderm
Septum transversum
Body wall
Inferior vena cava

Several **P**arts **B**uild **D**iaphragm.

Diaphragm descends during development but maintains innervation from above C3–C5.

Abdominal contents may herniate into the thorax due to incomplete development (hiatal hernia).

UCV *Anat.44*

Bone formation

Intramembranous
Endochondral

Spontaneous bone formation without preexisting cartilage.
Ossification of cartilaginous molds. Long bones form by this type of ossification at 1° and 2° centers.

Meckel's diverticulum

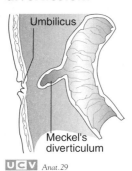

Umbilicus

Meckel's diverticulum

UCV *Anat.29*

Persistence of the vitelline duct or yolk stalk. May contain ectopic acid–secreting gastric mucosa and/or pancreatic tissue. Most common congenital anomaly of the GI tract. Can cause bleeding or obstruction near the terminal ileum. Contrast with omphalomesenteric cyst = cystic dilatation of vitelline duct.

Associated with intussusception and volvulus.

The five **2**'s:

2 inches long.

2 feet from the ileocecal valve.

2% of population.

Commonly presents in first **2** years of life.

May have **2** types of epithelia.

Pancreas and spleen embryology

Pancreas is derived from the foregut. Ventral pancreatic bud becomes pancreatic head, uncinate process (lower half of head), and main pancreatic duct. Dorsal pancreatic bud becomes everything else (body, tail, isthmus, and accessory pancreatic duct).

Spleen arises from dorsal mesentery but is supplied by artery of foregut.

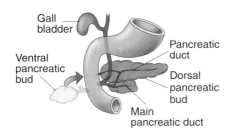

Gall bladder
Pancreatic duct
Ventral pancreatic bud
Dorsal pancreatic bud
Main pancreatic duct

HIGH-YIELD FACTS

Anatomy

Genital ducts

Mesonephric (wolffian) duct

Paramesonephric (müllerian) duct

Develops into **S**eminal vesicles, **E**pididymis, **E**jaculatory duct, and **D**uctus deferens.

Develops into fallopian tube, uterus, and part of . vagina.

Müllerian inhibiting substance secreted by testes suppresses development of paramesonephric ducts in males.

SEED.

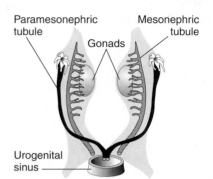

Paramesonephric tubule

Mesonephric tubule

Gonads

Urogenital sinus

Bicornuate uterus

Results from incomplete fusion of the paramesonephric ducts. Associated with urinary tract abnormalities and infertility.

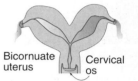

Bicornuate uterus

Cervical os

Male/female genital homologues

Male	Female
Corpus spongiosum	Vestibular bulbs
Bulbourethral glands (of Cowper)	Greater vestibular glands (of Bartholin)
Prostate gland	Urethral and paraurethral glands (of Skene)
Glans penis	Glans clitoris
Ventral shaft of the penis (from genital tubercle)	Labia minora
Scrotum	Labia majora

Congenital penile abnormalities

Hypospadias

Epispadias

Abnormal opening of penile urethra on inferior (ventral) side of penis due to failure of urethral folds to close.

Abnormal opening of penile urethra on superior (dorsal) side of penis due to faulty positioning of genital tubercle.

Hypospadias is more common than epispadias.

Exstrophy of the bladder is associated with epispadias.

Sperm development

Spermatogenesis begins with spermatogonia (type A and type B). Full development takes 2 months. Spermatogenesis occurs in Seminiferous tubules. Type A forms both type A and type B spermatogonia.

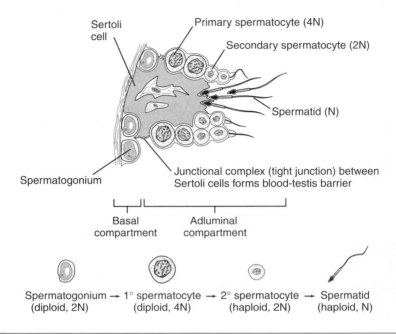

Derivation of sperm parts

Acrosome is derived from the Golgi apparatus and flagellum (tail) from one of the centrioles. **M**iddle piece (neck) has **M**itochondria. Sperm food supply is fructose.

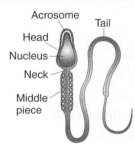

Meiosis and ovulation

1° oocytes begin meiosis I during fetal life and complete meiosis I just prior to ovulation.

Meiosis I is arrested in pr**O**phase for years until **O**vulation.

Meiosis II is arrested in **MET**aphase until fertilization.

An egg **MET** a sperm.

Amniotic fluid abnormalities

Polyhydramnios	> 1.5–2 L of amniotic fluid; associated with esophageal/duodenal atresia, causing inability to swallow amniotic fluid, and with anencephaly.
Oligohydramnios	< 0.5 L of amniotic fluid; associated with bilateral renal agenesis or posterior urethral valves (in males) and resultant inability to excrete urine.

| **Potter's syndrome** | Bilateral renal agenesis → oligohydramnios → limb deformities, facial deformities, pulmonary hypoplasia. | Babies with **Potter's** can't "**Pee**" in utero. |

| **Horseshoe kidney** | Inferior poles of both kidneys fuse. As they ascend from pelvis during fetal development, horseshoe kidneys get trapped under inferior mesenteric artery and remain low in the abdomen. | 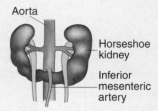 |

| **Landmark dermatomes** | C2 is a posterior half of a skull "cap."
 C3 is a high turtleneck shirt.
 C4 is a low-collar shirt.
 T4 is at the nipple.
 T7 is at the xiphoid process.
 T10 is at the umbilicus (important for early appendicitis pain referral).
 L1 is at the inguinal ligament.
 L4 includes the kneecaps.
 S2, S3, S4 erection and sensation of penile and anal zones. | Gallbladder pain referred to the right shoulder via the phrenic nerve.
 T4 at the **teat pore.**

 T10 at the belly but**TEN.**

 L1 is **IL** (Inguinal Ligament).
 Down on **L4s (all fours).**
 "**S2, 3, 4** keep the penis off the floor." |

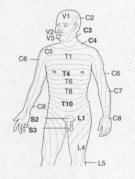

| **Rotator cuff muscles** | Shoulder muscles that form the rotator cuff: **S**upraspinatus, **I**nfraspinatus, **t**eres minor, **S**ubscapularis. | **S I t S** (small t is for teres minor). |

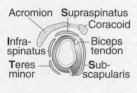

| **Thenar-hypothenar muscles** | Thenar—**O**pponens pollicis, **A**bductor pollicis brevis, **F**lexor pollicis brevis.
 Hypothenar—**O**pponens digiti minimi, **A**bductor digiti minimi, **F**lexor digiti minimi. | Both groups perform the same functions: **O**ppose, **A**bduct, and **F**lex **(OAF).** |

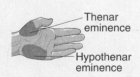

Unhappy triad/ knee injury

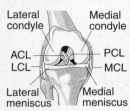

UCV *Anat.89*

This common football injury (caused by clipping from the lateral side) consists of damage to medial collateral ligament (MCL), medial meniscus, and anterior cruciate ligament (ACL).

PCL = posterior cruciate ligament. LCL = lateral collateral ligament.

"Anterior" and "posterior" in ACL and PCL refer to sites of **tibial** attachment.

Positive anterior drawer sign indicates tearing of the ACL.

Abnormal passive abduction indicates a torn MCL.

Recurrent laryngeal nerve

Supplies all intrinsic muscles of the larynx **except the cricothyroid muscle.** Left recurrent laryngeal nerve wraps around the arch of the aorta and the ligamentum arteriosum. Right recurrent laryngeal nerve wraps around right subclavian artery. Damage results in hoarseness. Complication of thyroid surgery.

Branch of CN X.

View from posterior

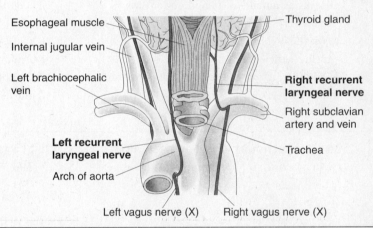

UCV *Anat.70*

Scalp and meninges: layers

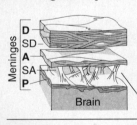

Skin
Connective tissue
Aponeurosis
Loose connective tissue (vascular layer)
Pericranium (skull)
Dura mater, subdural (SD) space, Arachnoid, subarachnoid (SA) space, Pia mater, brain

SCALP–skull–DAP.

Mastication muscles

3 muscles close jaw: Masseter, teMporalis, Medial pterygoid. 1 opens: lateral pterygoid. All are innervated by the trigeminal nerve (V₃).

M's Munch.
Lateral Lowers (when speaking of pterygoids with respect to jaw motion).

Muscles with *glossus*

All muscles with root *glossus* in their names (**except palatoglossus**, innervated by vagus nerve) are innervated by hypo*glossal* nerve.

Palat: vagus nerve.
Glossus: hypo*glossal* nerve.

Muscles with *palat*	All muscles with root *palat* in their names (**except tensor veli palatini**, innervated by mandibular branch of CN V) are innervated by vagus nerve.	Palat: vagus nerve (except **TENS**or, who was too **TENSE**).
Carotid sheath	3 structures inside: 1. Internal jugular **V**ein (lateral) 2. Common carotid **A**rtery (medial) 3. Vagus **N**erve (posterior)	**VAN.**

Diaphragm structures

Structures perforating diaphragm:
At T8: IVC.
At T10: esophagus, vagus (two trunks).
At T12: aorta (red), thoracic duct (white), azygous vein (blue).

Diaphragm is innervated by **C3, 4,** and **5** (phrenic nerve). Pain from the diaphragm can be referred to the shoulder.

I 8 10 EGGs AT 12:
I = IVC @ **8th** vertebra; **EG** = **E**sopha**G**us; **G** = va**G**us @ **10th** vertebra; **A** = **A**orta, **A**zygous; **T** = **T**horacic duct @ **12th** vertebra.
"**C3, 4,** and **5** keeps the diaphragm alive."

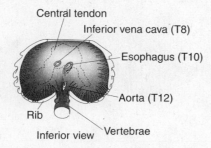

Central tendon
Inferior vena cava (T8)
Esophagus (T10)
Aorta (T12)
Rib
Inferior view   Vertebrae

Coronary artery anatomy

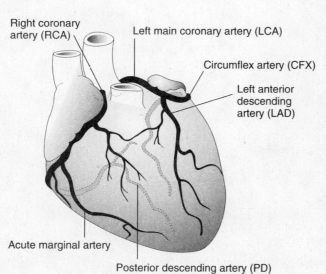

Right coronary artery (RCA)
Left main coronary artery (LCA)
Circumflex artery (CFX)
Left anterior descending artery (LAD)
Acute marginal artery
Posterior descending artery (PD)

(Adapted, with permission, from Ganong WF. *Review of Medical Physiology*, 19th ed. Stamford, CT: Appleton & Lange, 1999:592.)

In the majority of cases, the SA and AV nodes are supplied by the RCA. 80% of the time, the RCA supplies the inferior portion of the left ventricle via the PD artery (= right dominant).
Coronary artery occlusion occurs most commonly in the LAD, which supplies the anterior interventricular septum.
Coronary arteries fill during diastole.

Bronchopulmonary segments

Each bronchopulmonary segment has a 3° (segmental) bronchus and 2 arteries (bronchial and pulmonary) in the center; veins and lymphatics drain along the borders.

Arteries run with Airways.

Lung relations

Right lung has 3 lobes; Left has 2 lobes and Lingula (homologue of right middle lobe). Right lung is more common site for inhaled foreign body owing to less acute angle of right main stem bronchus.

Instead of a middle lobe, the left lung has a space occupied by the heart. The relation of the pulmonary artery to the bronchus at each lung hilus is described by **RALS**—Right Anterior; Left Superior.

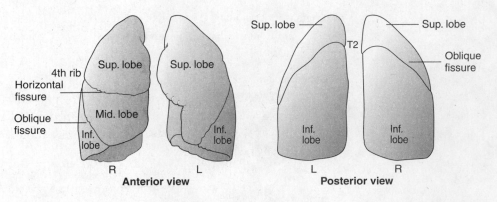

Femoral triangle

Femoral sheath contains femoral artery, femoral vein, and femoral canal (containing deep inguinal lymph nodes). Femoral nerve lies outside femoral sheath.

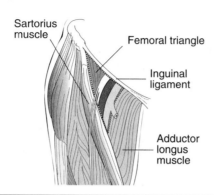

Lateral to medial: **N–(AVEL)** = **Nerve–(A**rtery–**V**ein–**E**mpty space–**L**ymphatics).

Femoral hernia is entrance of abdominal contents through the femoral canal.

The femoral triangle contains the femoral **V**ein, femoral **A**rtery, and femoral **N**erve.

Femoral hernia protrudes below and lateral to the pubic tubercle.

Abdominal hernias

Hernias are protrusions of peritoneum through an opening, usually sites of weakness.

Diaphragmatic hernia — Abdominal retroperitoneal structures enter the thorax; may occur in infants as a result of defective development of pleuroperitoneal membrane. Most commonly a hiatal hernia, in which stomach herniates upward through the esophageal hiatus of the diaphragm. *Anat.18*

Direct hernia — Protrudes through the inguinal (Hesselbach's) triangle (bounded by inguinal ligament, inferior epigastric artery, and lateral border of rectus abdominis). Direct hernia bulges directly through abdominal wall medial to inferior epigastric artery. Goes through the external inguinal ring only. Usually in older men. *Anat.27*

Indirect hernia — **IN**direct hernia goes through the internal (deep) inguinal ring and external (superficial) inguinal ring and **IN**to the scrotum. Indirect hernia enters internal inguinal ring lateral to inferior epigastric artery. **IN**direct hernias occur in **IN**fants owing to failure of processus vaginalis to close. *Anat.28*

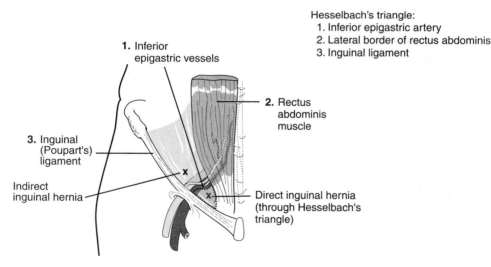

Hesselbach's triangle:
1. Inferior epigastric artery
2. Lateral border of rectus abdominis
3. Inguinal ligament

Arterial supply of stomach

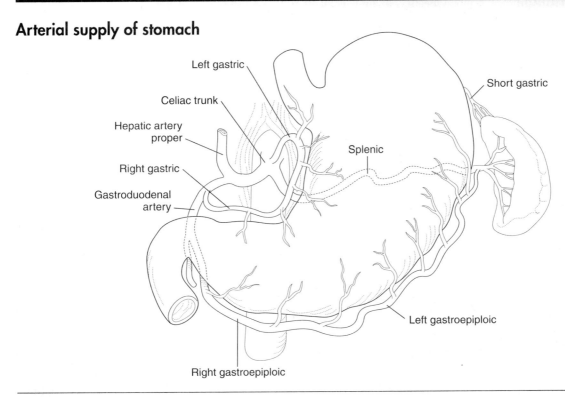

Portal-systemic anastomoses

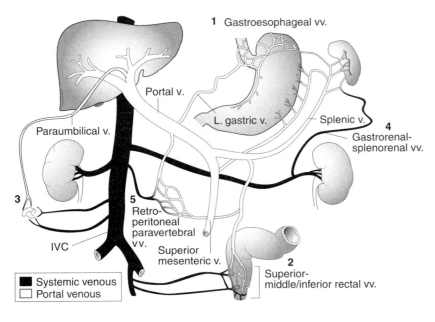

1. Left gastric–azygos → **esophageal varices.**
2. Superior–middle/inferior rectal → **hemorrhoids.**
3. Paraumbilical–inferior epigastric → **caput medusae** (navel).
4. Retroperitoneal → renal.
5. Retroperitoneal → paravertebral.

Gut, butt, and caput, the anastomoses 3. Commonly seen in alcoholic cirrhosis.

UCV *Anat.22*

Pectinate line

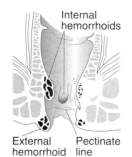

Internal hemorrhoids

External hemorrhoid

Pectinate line

Formed where hindgut meets ectoderm.

Above pectinate line—internal hemorrhoids (not painful), adenocarcinoma. **V**isceral innervation. Arterial supply is from the superior rectal artery (branch of IMA). Venous drainage is to superior rectal vein → inferior mesenteric vein → portal system.

Below pectinate line—external hemorrhoids (painful), squamous cell carcinoma. Somatic innervation. Arterial blood supply is from the inferior rectal artery (branch of internal pudendal artery). Venous drainage is to inferior rectal vein → internal pudendal vein → internal iliac vein → IVC.

Internal hemorrhoids receive visceral innervation.

External hemorrhoids receive somatic innervation and are therefore painful.

Retroperitoneal structures

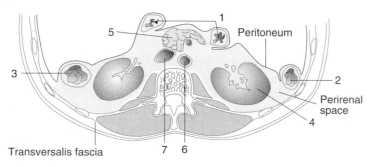

5

1

Peritoneum

3

2

Perirenal space

4

Transversalis fascia   7 6

1. Duodenum (2nd, 3rd, 4th parts)
2. Descending colon
3. Ascending colon
4. Kidney and ureters
5. Pancreas (except tail)
6. Aorta
7. Inferior vena cava

Adrenal glands and rectum (not shown in diagram)

Digestive tract anatomy

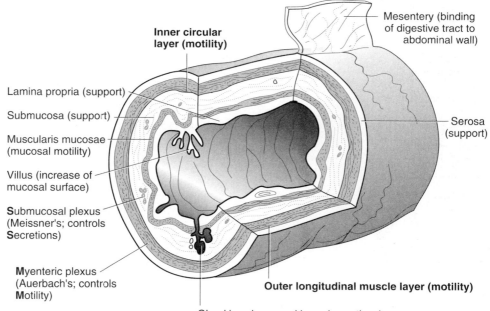

Inner circular layer (motility)

Mesentery (binding of digestive tract to abdominal wall)

Lamina propria (support)

Submucosa (support)

Muscularis mucosae (mucosal motility)

Villus (increase of mucosal surface)

Submucosal plexus (Meissner's; controls **S**ecretions)

Myenteric plexus (Auerbach's; controls **M**otility)

Serosa (support)

Outer longitudinal muscle layer (motility)

Gland in submucosal layer (secretions)

(Adapted, with permission, from McPhee S et al. *Pathophysiology of Disease: An Introduction to Clinical Medicine*, 3rd ed. New York: McGraw-Hill, 2000:296.)

Enteric plexuses

Myenteric	Coordinates **M**otility along entire gut wall. Also known as Auerbach's plexus. Contains cell bodies of some parasympathetic terminal effector neurons. Located between inner and outer layers (longitudinal and circular) of smooth muscle in GI tract wall.
Submucosal	Regulates local **S**ecretions, blood flow, and absorption. Also known as Meissner's plexus. Contains cell bodies of some parasympathetic terminal effector neurons. Located between mucosa and inner layer of smooth muscle in GI tract wall.

GI blood supply

Artery	Gut region	Structures supplied
Celiac	Foregut	Stomach to duodenum; liver, gallbladder, pancreas
SMA	Midgut	Duodenum to proximal $2/3$ of transverse colon
IMA	Hindgut	Distal $1/3$ of transverse colon to upper portion of rectum

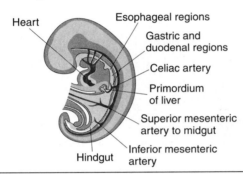

Heart
Esophageal regions
Gastric and duodenal regions
Celiac artery
Primordium of liver
Superior mesenteric artery to midgut
Inferior mesenteric artery
Hindgut

Kidney anatomy and glomerular structure

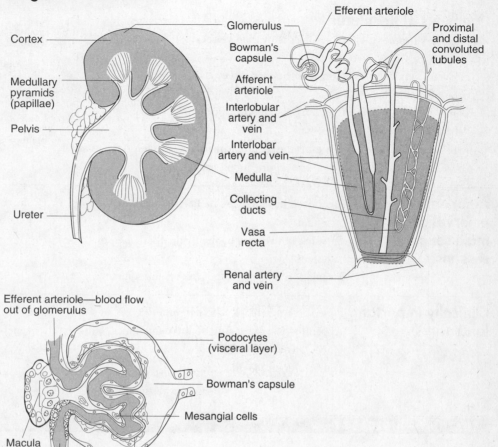

(Adapted, with permission, from McPhee S et al. *Pathophysiology of Disease: An Introduction to Clinical Medicine,* 3rd ed. New York: McGraw-Hill, 2000:384.)

Juxtaglomerular apparatus (JGA)	JGA—JG cells (modified smooth muscle of afferent arteriole) and macula densa (Na$^+$ sensor, part of the distal convoluted tubule). JG cells secrete renin (leading to ↑ angiotensin II and aldosterone levels) in response to ↓ renal blood pressure, ↓ Na$^+$ delivery to distal tubule, and ↑ sympathetic tone. JG cells also secrete erythropoietin.	JGA defends glomerular filtration rate via the renin-angiotensin system. *Juxta* = close by.
Ureters: course	Ureters pass **under** uterine artery and **under** ductus deferens (retroperitoneal).	Water (ureters) **under** the bridge (artery, ductus deferens).

Ligaments of the uterus

Suspensory ligament of ovaries	Contains the ovarian vessels.
Transverse cervical (cardinal) ligament	Contains the uterine vessels.
Round ligament of uterus	Contains no important structures.
Broad ligament	Contains the round ligaments of the uterus and ovaries and the uterine tubules and vessels.

Autonomic innervation of the male sexual response

Erection is mediated by the **P**arasympathetic nervous system.

Emission is mediated by the **S**ympathetic nervous system.

Ejaculation is mediated by visceral and somatic nerves.

Point and Shoot.

Clinically important landmarks

Pudendal nerve block—ischial spine.

Appendix—$^2/_3$ of the way from the umbilicus to the anterior superior iliac spine (McBurney's point).

Lumbar puncture—iliac crest.

Peripheral nerve layers

Endoneurium invests single nerve fiber.

Perineurium (permeability barrier) surrounds a fascicle of nerve fibers.

Epineurium (dense connective tissue) surrounds entire nerve (fascicles and blood vessels).

Perineurium—Permeability barrier; must be rejoined in microsurgery for limb reattachment.

Endo = inner.

Peri = around.

Epi = outer.

Corpuscles

Meissner's	Small, encapsulated sensory receptors found in dermis of palm, soles, and digits of skin. Involved in light discriminatory touch of glabrous (hairless) skin.
Pacinian	Large, encapsulated sensory receptors found in deeper layers of skin at ligaments, joint capsules, serous membranes, mesenteries. Involved in pressure, coarse touch, vibration, and tension.

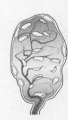
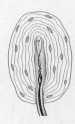

HIGH-YIELD FACTS

Anatomy

Inner ear

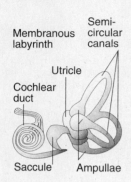

Membranous labyrinth
Semi-circular canals
Utricle
Cochlear duct
Saccule
Ampullae

The bony labyrinth is filled with perilymph (Na^+ rich: similar to ECF) and includes the cochlea (hearing), the vestibule (linear acceleration), and the semicircular canals (angular acceleration).

The membranous labyrinth is filled with endolymph (K^+ rich: similar to ICF) and contains the cochlear duct, utricle, saccule, and semicircular canals. Hair cells are the sensory elements in both the cochlear and vestibular apparatus.

The base of the cochlea picks up high-frequency sound; the apex, low frequency.

Peri—think outside of cell (Na^+).
Endo—think inside of cell (K^+).
Endolymph is made by the stria vascularis.
Utricle and saccule contain maculae—for linear acceleration.
Semicircular canals contain **ampullae**—for **angular** acceleration.

Collagen types

Collagen is the most abundant protein in the human body.

Type I (90%)—bone, tendon, skin, dentin, fascia, cornea, late wound repair.

Type II—cartilage (including hyaline), vitreous body, nucleus pulposus.

Type III (reticulin)—skin, blood vessels, uterus, fetal tissue, granulation tissue.

Type IV—basement membrane or basal lamina.

Type X—epiphyseal plate.

Type **I**: BONE.

Type **II**: car**TWO**lage.

Type **IV**: Under the **floor** (basement membrane).

Epidermis layers

From surface to base: stratum Corneum, stratum Lucidum, stratum Granulosum, stratum Spinosum, stratum Basalis.

Californians Like Girls in String Bikinis.

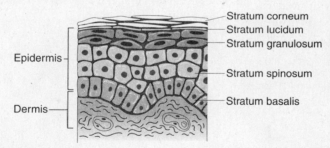

Epidermis
Dermis
Stratum corneum
Stratum lucidum
Stratum granulosum
Stratum spinosum
Stratum basalis

Epithelial cell junctions

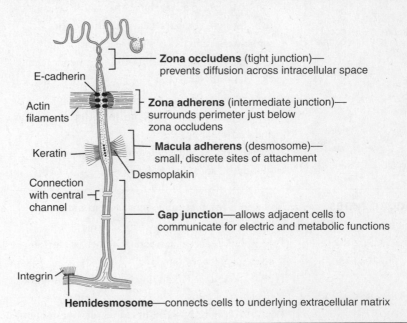

E-cadherin

Actin filaments

Keratin

Connection with central channel

Integrin

Zona occludens (tight junction)— prevents diffusion across intracellular space

Zona adherens (intermediate junction)— surrounds perimeter just below zona occludens

Macula adherens (desmosome)— small, discrete sites of attachment

Desmoplakin

Gap junction—allows adjacent cells to communicate for electric and metabolic functions

Hemidesmosome—connects cells to underlying extracellular matrix

Glomerular basement membrane	Formed from fused endothelial and podocyte basement membranes and coated with negatively charged heparan sulfate. Responsible for actual filtration of plasma according to net charge and size.	In **N**ephrotic syndrome, **N**egative charge is lost (and plasma protein is lost in urine as a consequence).
Cilia structure	9 + 2 arrangement of microtubules. Dynein is an ATPase that links peripheral 9 doublets and causes bending of cilium by differential sliding of doublets.	Kartagener's syndrome is due to a dynein arm defect, resulting in immotile cilia.

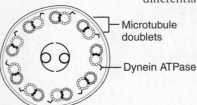

Microtubule doublets

Dynein ATPase

UCV *Bio.59*

Nissl bodies	Nissl bodies (in neurons)—rough ER; not found in axon or axon hillock. Synthesize enzymes (e.g., ChAT) and peptide neurotransmitters.

Functions of Golgi apparatus	1. Distribution center of proteins and lipids from ER to the plasma membrane, lysosomes, and secretory vesicles 2. Modifies N-oligosaccharides on asparagine. 3. Adds O-oligosaccharides to serine and threonine residues 4. Proteoglycan assembly from proteoglycan core proteins 5. Sulfation of sugars in proteoglycans and of selected tyrosine on proteins 6. Addition of mannose-6-phosphate to specific lysosomal proteins, which targets the protein to the lysosome	**I-cell disease** is caused by the failure of addition of mannose-6-phosphate to lysosome proteins, causing these enzymes to be secreted outside the cell instead of being targeted to the lysosome.
Rough endoplasmic reticulum (RER)	RER is the site of synthesis of secretory (exported) proteins and of N-linked oligosaccharide addition to many proteins.	Mucus-secreting goblet cells of the small intestine and antibody-secreting plasma cells are rich in RER.
Smooth endoplasmic reticulum (SER)	SER is the site of steroid synthesis and detoxification of drugs and poisons.	Liver hepatocytes and steroid hormone–producing cells of the adrenal cortex are rich in SER.
Sinusoids of liver	Irregular "capillaries" with round pores 100–200 nm in diameter. No basement membrane. Allows macromolecules of plasma full access to surface of liver cells through space of Disse.	
Sinusoids of spleen	Long, vascular channels in red pulp with fenestrated "barrel hoop" basement membrane. Macrophages found nearby.	T cells are found in the PALS and the red pulp of the spleen. B cells are found in follicles within the white pulp of the spleen.

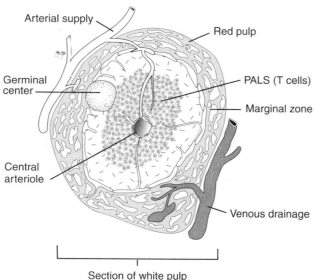

Arterial supply

Red pulp

Germinal center

PALS (T cells)

Marginal zone

Central arteriole

Venous drainage

Section of white pulp

(Adapted, with permission, from Janeway CA, Travers P, Walport M, Capra JD. *Immunobiology: The Immune System in Health and Disease*, 4th ed. New York: Garland, 1999.)

Pancreas endocrine cell types   Islets of Langerhans are collections of endocrine cells (most numerous in tail of pancreas). α = glucagon; β = insulin; δ = somatostatin. Islets arise from pancreatic buds.

Adrenal cortex and medulla

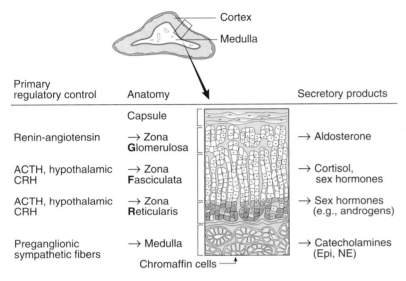

Primary regulatory control	Anatomy	Secretory products
	Capsule	
Renin-angiotensin	→ Zona **G**lomerulosa	→ Aldosterone
ACTH, hypothalamic CRH	→ Zona **F**asciculata	→ Cortisol, sex hormones
ACTH, hypothalamic CRH	→ Zona **R**eticularis	→ Sex hormones (e.g., androgens)
Preganglionic sympathetic fibers	→ Medulla	→ Catecholamines (Epi, NE)

Chromaffin cells

GFR corresponds with **salt** (Na^+), **sugar** (glucocorticoids), and **sex** (androgens).

"The deeper you go, the sweeter it gets."

Pheochromocytoma—most common tumor of the adrenal medulla in adults. *Bio.26*

Neuroblastoma—most common in children. *Path3.26*

Pheochromocytoma causes episodic hypertension; neuroblastoma does not.

UCV

Brunner's glands

Secrete alkaline mucus. Located in submucosa of duodenum (the only GI submucosal glands). Duodenal ulcers cause hypertrophy of Brunner's glands.

Lymph node

A 2° lymphoid organ that has many afferents, 1 or more efferents. Encapsulated, with trabeculae. Functions are nonspecific filtration by macrophages, storage/proliferation of B and T cells, Ab production.

Follicle
: Site of B-cell localization and proliferation. In outer cortex. 1° follicles are dense and dormant. 2° follicles have pale central germinal centers and are active.

Medulla
: Consists of medullary cords (closely packed lymphocytes and plasma cells) and medullary sinuses. Medullary sinuses communicate with efferent lymphatics and contain reticular cells and macrophages.

Paracortex
: Houses T cells. Region of cortex between follicles and medulla. Contains high endothelial venules through which T and B cells enter from blood. In an extreme cellular immune response, paracortex becomes greatly enlarged. Not well developed in patients with DiGeorge's syndrome.

Paracortex enlarges in an extreme cellular immune response (i.e., viral).

Subcapsular sinus
Capsule
Capillary supply
Postcapillary (high endothelial) venules
Afferent lymphatic
Medullary sinus (macrophages)
Medullary cords (plasma cells)
Trabecula
Efferent lymphatic
Follicle of cortex (B cells)
Paracortex (T cells)
Artery Vein

| Peyer's patch | Unencapsulated lymphoid tissue found in lamina propria and submucosa of small intestine. Covered by single layer of cuboidal enterocytes (no goblet cells) with specialized M cells interspersed. M cells take up antigen. Stimulated B cells leave Peyer's patch and travel through lymph and blood to lamina propria of intestine, where they differentiate to IgA-secreting plasma cells. IgA receives protective secretory component and is then transported across epithelium to gut to deal with intraluminal Ag. | Think of **IgA,** the **I**ntra-gut **A**ntibody. And always say, "secretory IgA." |

ANATOMY — NEUROANATOMY

Lumbar puncture

Cauda equina — Spinous process

L3

L4

L4/5 disk

L5

Needle in subarachnoid space

CSF obtained from lumbar subarachnoid space between L4 and L5 (at the level of iliac crests). Structures pierced as follows:

1. Skin/superficial fascia
2. Ligaments (supraspinous, interspinous, ligamentum flavum)
3. Epidural space
4. Dura mater
5. Subdural space
6. Arachnoid
7. Subarachnoid space—CSF

Pia is not pierced.

Lower extremity nerve injury

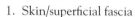

Nerve	Deficit in motion	
Common peroneal (L4–S2)	Loss of dorsiflexion (→ foot drop) *Anat.56*	**PED** = **P**eroneal **E**verts and **D**orsiflexes.
Tibial (L4–S3)	Loss of plantar flexion	**TIP** = **T**ibial **I**nverts and **P**lantarflexes; if injured, can't stand on **TIP**toes.
Femoral (L2–L4)	Loss of knee jerk *Anat.61*	
Obturator (L2–L4)	Loss of hip adduction	

UCV

| Spinal cord lower extent | In adults, spinal cord extends to lower border of L1–L2; subarachnoid space extends to lower border of S2. Lumbar puncture is usually performed in L3–L4 or L4–L5 interspaces, at level of cauda equina. | To keep the cord alive, keep the spinal needle between L3 and L5. |
| Spinal nerves | There are 31 spinal nerves altogether: 8 cervical, 12 thoracic, 5 lumbar, 5 sacral, 1 coccygeal. | 31, just like 31 flavors! Vertebral disk herniation usually occurs between L5 and S1. |

HIGH-YIELD FACTS

Anatomy

CNS/PNS supportive cells

Astrocytes—physical support, repair, K^+ metabolism.
Microglia—phagocytosis.
Oligodendroglia—central myelin production.
Schwann cells—peripheral myelin production.
Ependymal cells—inner lining of ventricles.

Blood-brain barrier

Formed by 3 structures:
1. **C**horoid plexus epithelium
2. **I**ntracerebral capillary endothelium
3. **A**rachnoid

Glucose and amino acids cross by carrier-mediated transport mechanism.

Nonpolar/lipid-soluble substances cross more readily than polar/water-soluble ones.

L-dopa, rather than dopamine, is used to treat parkinsonism because dopamine does not cross the blood-brain barrier.

Blood-brain barrier guarded by **CIA.**
Other barriers include:
1. Blood-gas barrier
2. Blood-testis barrier

Hypothalamus: functions

Thirst and water balance (supraoptic nucleus).
Adenohypophysis control via releasing factors.
Neurohypophysis releases hormones synthesized in hypothalamic nuclei.

Hunger (lateral nucleus) and satiety (ventromedial nucleus).

Autonomic regulation (anterior hypothalamus regulates parasympathetic activity), circadian rhythms (suprachiasmatic nucleus).

Temperature regulation (posterior hypothalamus regulates heat conservation and production when cold; Anterior hypothalamus coordinates Cooling when hot).

Sexual urges and emotions (Septate nucleus).

The hypothalamus wears **TAN HATS.**

If you zap your **ventromedial** nucleus, you grow **vent**rally and **medial**ly (hyperphagia and obesity).

If you zap your **P**osterior hypothalamus, you become a **P**oikilotherm (cold-blooded snake).
A/C = anterior cooling.

[handwritten annotations: "Posterior is used when you fee Cold!" and "Anterior → when you feel hot."]

Posterior pituitary (neurohypophysis)

Receives hypothalamic axonal projections from supraoptic (ADH) and paraventricular (oxytocin) nuclei.

Oxytocin: *oxys* = quick; *tocos* = birth.

Functions of thalamic nuclei	Lateral geniculate nucleus—visual.	Lateral to Look.
	Medial geniculate nucleus—auditory.	Medial for Music.

Ventral posterior nucleus, lateral part—body senses (proprioception, pressure, pain, touch vibration).

Ventral posterior nucleus, medial part—facial sensation, including pain.

Ventral anterior/lateral nuclei—motor.

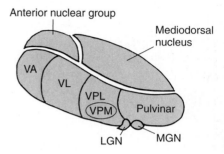

Limbic system: functions

Responsible for **F**eeding, **F**ighting, **F**eeling, **F**light, and sex.

The famous **5 F's.**

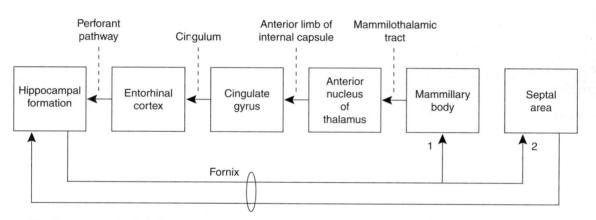

The hippocampus projects to:
1. Subiculum (projecting to mammillary nuclei)
2. Septal area

Basal ganglia   Important in mitigating voluntary movements and making postural adjustments.

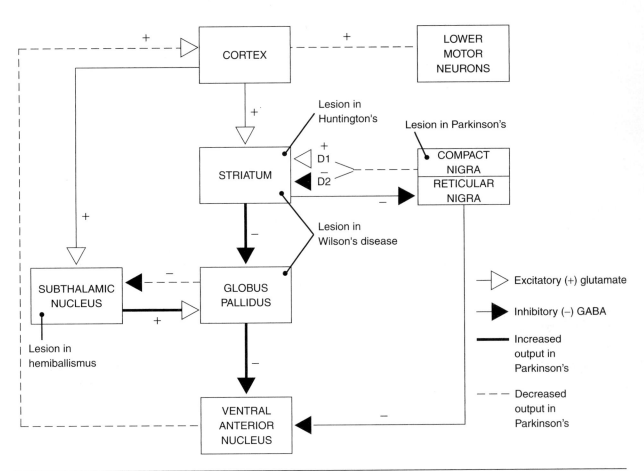

Chorea	Sudden, jerky, purposeless movements. Characteristic of basal ganglia lesion (e.g., Huntington's disease).	*Chorea* = dancing (Greek). Think choral dancing or choreography.
Athetosis	Slow, writhing movements, especially of fingers. Characteristic of basal ganglia lesion.	*Athetos* = not fixed (Greek). Think snakelike.
Hemiballismus	Sudden, wild flailing of 1 arm. Characteristic of contralateral subthalamic nucleus lesion.	Half ballistic (as in throwing a baseball).

Cerebral cortex functions

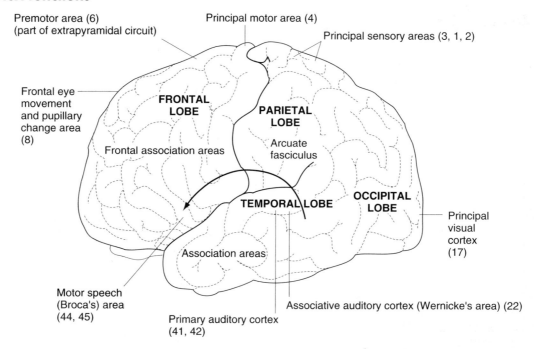

Premotor area (6)
(part of extrapyramidal circuit)

Principal motor area (4)

Principal sensory areas (3, 1, 2)

Frontal eye
movement
and pupillary
change area
(8)

**FRONTAL
LOBE**

**PARIETAL
LOBE**

Arcuate
fasciculus

Frontal association areas

TEMPORAL LOBE

**OCCIPITAL
LOBE**

Principal
visual
cortex
(17)

Association areas

Motor speech
(Broca's) area
(44, 45)

Primary auditory cortex
(41, 42)

Associative auditory cortex (Wernicke's area) (22)

Brain lesions

Area of lesion	Consequence	
Broca's area	Motor (expressive) aphasia with good comprehension *Path3.2*	BROca's is BROken speech. Wernicke's is Wordy but makes no sense.
Wernicke's area	Sensory (fluent/receptive) aphasia with poor comprehension *Anat.51*	
Arcuate fasciculus	Conduction aphasia; poor repetition with good comprehension, fluent speech.	Connects Wernicke's to Broca's area.
Amygdala (bilateral)	Klüver-Bucy syndrome (hyperorality, hypersexuality, disinhibited behavior) *Path3.17*	
Frontal lobe	Frontal release signs (e.g., personality changes and deficits in concentration, orientation, judgment)	
Right parietal lobe	Spatial neglect syndrome (agnosia of the contralateral side of the world)	
Reticular activating system	Coma	
Mammillary bodies (bilateral)	Wernicke-Korsakoff's encephalopathy (confabulations, anterograde amnesia) *Bio.86*	

UCV

Cavernous sinus

CN III, IV, V_1, V_2, and VI and postganglionic sympathetic fibers en route to the orbit all pass through the cavernous sinus. Only CN VI is "free-floating." Cavernous portion of internal carotid artery is also here.

The nerves that control extraocular muscles (plus V_1 and V_2) pass through the cavernous sinus.

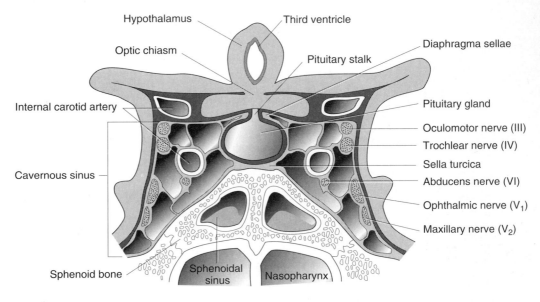

Hypothalamus — Third ventricle
Optic chiasm — Pituitary stalk — Diaphragma sellae
Internal carotid artery — Pituitary gland
— Oculomotor nerve (III)
— Trochlear nerve (IV)
— Sella turcica
Cavernous sinus — Abducens nerve (VI)
— Ophthalmic nerve (V_1)
— Maxillary nerve (V_2)
Sphenoid bone — Sphenoidal sinus — Nasopharynx

(Adapted, with permission, from Stobo J et al. *The Principles and Practice of Medicine*, 23rd ed. Stamford, CT: Appleton & Lange, 1996:277.)

UCV *Anat.55*

Foramina: middle cranial fossa (CN II–VI)

1. Optic canal (CN II, ophthalmic artery, central retinal vein)
2. **S**uperior orbital fissure (CN III, IV, V_1, VI, ophthalmic vein)
3. Foramen **R**otundum (CN V_2)
4. Foramen **O**vale (CN V_3)
5. Foramen spinosum (middle meningeal artery)

All structures pass through sphenoid bone. Divisions of CN V exit owing to **S**tanding **R**oom **O**nly (**S**uperior orbital fissure, foramen **R**otundum, foramen **O**vale).

Foramina: posterior cranial fossa (CN VII–XII)

1. Internal auditory meatus (CN VII, VIII)
2. Jugular foramen (CN IX, X, XI, jugular vein)
3. Hypoglossal canal (CN XII)
4. Foramen magnum (spinal roots of CN XI, brain stem, vertebral arteries)

All structures pass through temporal or occipital bones.

Extraocular muscles and nerves

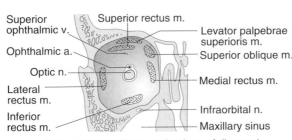

Superior ophthalmic v. — Superior rectus m.
Ophthalmic a. — Levator palpebrae superioris m.
Optic n. — Superior oblique m.
Lateral rectus m. — Medial rectus m.
Inferior rectus m. — Infraorbital n.
— Maxillary sinus

(Note: inferior oblique not in plane of diagram)

Lateral **R**ectus is CN VI, **S**uperior **O**blique is CN IV, the **R**est are CN III. The "chemical formula" $LR_6SO_4R_3$. The superior oblique **a**bducts, **i**ntroverts, **d**epresses.

Pupillary light reflex

Light in either retina sends a signal to pretectal nuclei (dashed lines) in midbrain that activate bilateral Edinger-Westphal nuclei; pupils contract bilaterally (consensual reflex). Note that the illumination of 1 eye results in bilateral pupillary constriction.

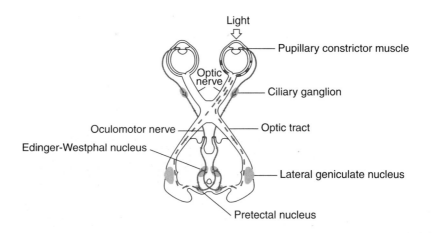

(Adapted, with permission, from Simon RP et al. *Clinical Neurology*, 3rd ed. Stamford, CT: Appleton & Lange, 1996.)

Internuclear ophthalmoplegia

Lesion in the medial longitudinal fasciculus (MLF). Results in medial rectus palsy on attempted lateral gaze. Nystagmus in abducting eye. Convergence is normal. MLF syndrome is seen in many patients with multiple sclerosis.

MLF = MS.

When looking left, the nucleus of CN VI fires, which contracts the left lateral rectus and stimulates the contralateral nucleus of CN III via the MLF to contract the medial rectus.

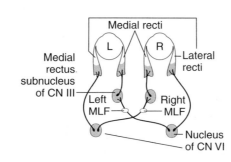

Visual field defects

1. Right anopsia
2. Bitemporal hemianopsia
3. Left homonymous hemianopsia
4. Left upper quadrantic-anopsia (right temporal lesion)
5. Left lower quadrantic-anopsia (right parietal lesion)
6. Left hemianopsia with macular sparing

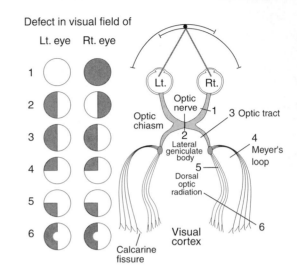

Cranial nerves

Nerve	CN	Function	Type	Mnemonic
Olfactory	I	Smell	Sensory	Some
Optic	II	Sight	Sensory	Say
Oculomotor	III	Eye movement, pupil constriction, accommodation, eyelid opening	Motor	Marry
Trochlear	IV	Eye movement	Motor	Money
Trigeminal	V	Mastication, facial sensation	Both	But
Abducens	VI	Eye movement	Motor	My
Facial	VII	Facial movement, anterior $^2/_3$ taste, lacrimation, salivation (submaxillary and submandibular salivary glands)	Both	Brother
Vestibulocochlear	VIII	Hearing, balance	Sensory	Says
Glossopharyngeal	IX	Posterior $^1/_3$ taste, swallowing, salivation (parotid gland), monitoring carotid body and sinus	Both	Big
Vagus	X	Taste, swallowing, palate elevation, talking, thoracoabdominal viscera	Both	Brains
Accessory	XI	Head turning, shoulder shrugging	Motor	Matter
Hypoglossal	XII	Tongue movements	Motor	Most

Cranial nerves and passageways

Cribriform plate	I
Optic canal	II
Superior orbital fissure	III, IV, V_1, VI
Foramen rotundum	V_2
Foramen ovale	V_3
Internal auditory meatus	VII, VIII
Jugular foramen	IX, X, XI
Hypoglossal canal	XII

Brain stem anatomy

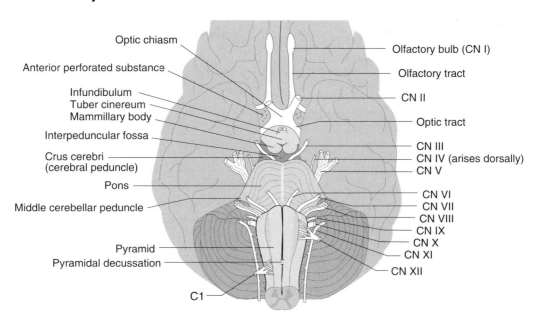

Optic chiasm
Anterior perforated substance
Infundibulum
Tuber cinereum
Mammillary body
Interpeduncular fossa
Crus cerebri (cerebral peduncle)
Pons
Middle cerebellar peduncle
Pyramid
Pyramidal decussation
C1

Olfactory bulb (CN I)
Olfactory tract
CN II
Optic tract
CN III
CN IV (arises dorsally)
CN V
CN VI
CN VII
CN VIII
CN IX
CN X
CN XI
CN XII

CNs that lie medially at brain stem: III, VI, XII. $3(\times 2) = 6(\times 2) = 12$.

Homunculus

Topographical representation of sensory and motor areas in the cerebral cortex. Use to localize lesion (e.g., in blood supply) leading to specific defects.

For example, lower extremity deficit in sensation or movement indicates involvement of the anterior cerebral artery (see following entry).

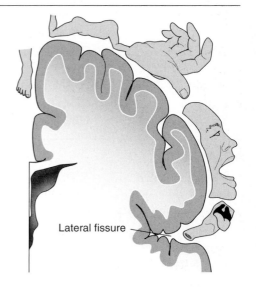

Lateral fissure

Circle of Willis

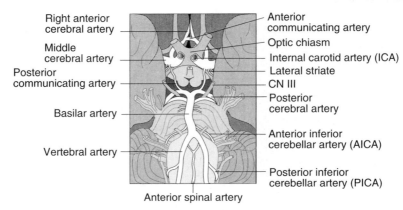

Right anterior cerebral artery
Middle cerebral artery
Posterior communicating artery
Basilar artery
Vertebral artery
Anterior spinal artery

Anterior communicating artery
Optic chiasm
Internal carotid artery (ICA)
Lateral striate
CN III
Posterior cerebral artery
Anterior inferior cerebellar artery (AICA)
Posterior inferior cerebellar artery (PICA)

Anterior cerebral artery—supplies medial surface of the brain, leg-foot area of motor and sensory cortices.

Middle cerebral artery—supplies lateral aspect of brain, Broca's and Wernicke's speech areas.

Anterior communicating artery—most common circle of Willis aneurysm; may cause visual-field defects.

Posterior communicating artery—common area of aneurysm; causes CN III palsy.

Lateral striate—"arteries of stroke"; supply internal capsule, caudate, putamen, globus pallidus.

In general, stroke of anterior circle → general sensory and motor dysfunction, aphasia; stroke of posterior circle → vertigo, ataxia, visual deficits, coma.

KLM sounds: kuh, la, mi

Kuh-kuh-kuh tests palate elevation (CN X—vagus).   Say it aloud.
La-la-la tests tongue (CN XII—hypoglossal).
Mi-mi-mi tests lips (CN VII—facial).

Vagal nuclei

Nucleus **S**olitarius	Visceral **S**ensory information (e.g., taste, gut distention, etc.).	VII, IX, **X.**
Nucleus a**M**biguus	**M**otor innervation of pharynx, larynx, and upper esophagus.	IX, **X,** XI.
Dorsal motor nucleus	Sends autonomic (parasympathetic) fibers to heart, lungs, and upper GI.	

Lesions and deviations

CN XII lesion (LMN)—tongue deviates **toward** side of lesion (lick your wounds).
CN V motor lesion—jaw deviates **toward** side of lesion.
Unilateral lesion of cerebellum—patient tends to fall **toward** side of lesion.
CN X lesion—uvula deviates **away** from side of lesion.
CN XI lesion—head turns to ipsilateral side of lesion.

Herniation syndromes

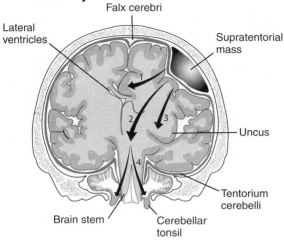

Lateral ventricles
Falx cerebri
Supratentorial mass
Uncus
Tentorium cerebelli
Brain stem
Cerebellar tonsil

1. Cingulate herniation under falx cerebri
2. Downward transtentorial (central) herniation
3. Uncal herniation
4. Cerebellar tonsillar herniation into the foramen magnum

Coma and death result when these herniations compress the brain stem

(Adapted, with permission, from Simon RP et al. *Clinical Neurology*, 4th ed. Stamford, CT: Appleton & Lange, 1999:314.)

Uncal herniation

Clinical signs	Cause
Ipsilateral dilated pupil/ptosis	Stretching of CN III
Contralateral homonymous hemianopsia	Compression of ipsilateral posterior cerebral artery
Ipsilateral paresis	Compression of contralateral crus cerebri (Kernohan's notch)
Duret hemorrhages— paramedian artery rupture	Caudal displacement of brain stem

Spinal cord and associated tracts

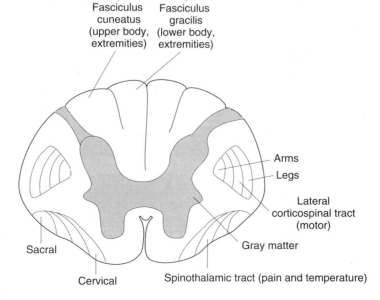

Dorsal columns (pressure, vibration, touch, proprioception)

Fasciculus cuneatus (upper body, extremities)
Fasciculus gracilis (lower body, extremities)

Arms
Legs
Lateral corticospinal tract (motor)
Gray matter
Spinothalamic tract (pain and temperature)
Sacral
Cervical

Spinal cord lesions

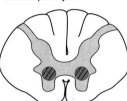

Poliomyelitis/Werdnig-Hoffmann disease: lower motor neuron lesions only, flaccid paralysis

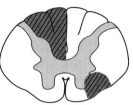

Multiple sclerosis: mostly white matter of cervical region; random and asymmetric lesions *Path3.23*

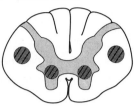

ALS: combined upper and lower motor neuron deficits with no sensory deficit *Path3.1*

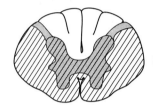

Complete occlusion of ventral artery; spares dorsal columns

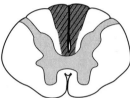

Tabes dorsalis: impaired proprioception and locomotor ataxia resulting from tertiary syphilis *Micro2.61*

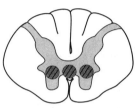

Syringomyelia: ventral white commissure and ventral horns *Path3.33*

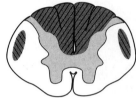

Vitamin B$_{12}$ neuropathy/Friedreich's ataxia: dorsal columns, lateral corticospinal tracts and spinocerebellar tracts *Path3.11*

UCV

Dorsal column organization	In dorsal columns, lower limbs are inside to avoid crossing the upper limbs on the outside. Fasciculus gracilis = legs. Fasciculus cuneatus = arms.	Dorsal column is organized like you are, with hands at sides—arms outside and legs inside.
Brown-Séquard syndrome 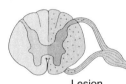 Lesion UCV *Anat.54*	Hemisection of spinal cord. Findings below the lesion: 1. Ipsilateral motor paralysis and spasticity (pyramidal tract)—not shown 2. Ipsilateral loss of tactile, vibration, proprioception sense (dorsal column) 3. Contralateral pain and temperature loss (spinothalamic tract) 4. Ipsilateral loss of all sensation at level of lesion If lesion occurs above T1, presents with Horner's syndrome.	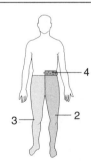
Lower motor neuron (LMN) signs	LMN injury signs—atrophy, flaccid paralysis, absent deep tendon reflexes. Fasciculations may be present.	**Lower** MN ≈ everything lowered (less muscle mass, ↓ muscle tone, ↓ reflexes, downgoing toes).
Upper motor neuron (UMN) signs	UMN injury signs—minor atrophy, spastic paralysis (clonus), hyperactive deep tendon reflexes, possible positive Babinski.	**Upper** MN ≈ everything **up** (tone, DTRs, toes).

Facial lesions

Central facial	Paralysis of the contralateral lower quadrant.	**AL**exander **Bell** with **STD**:
Bell's palsy	Peripheral ipsilateral facial paralysis with inability to close eye on involved side. *Anat.53*	**A**IDS, **L**yme, **S**arcoid, **T**umors, **D**iabetes.

Can occur idiopathically.

Seen as a complication in **A**IDS, **L**yme disease, **S**arcoidosis, **T**umors, **D**iabetes.

Complete destruction of the facial nucleus itself or its branchial efferent fibers (facial nerve proper) paralyzes all ipsilateral facial muscles.

UMN lesion	Lesion to internal capsule causes contralateral weakness of lower face only.
LMN lesion	Upper and lower lesion paralysis with weakness of upper and lower face.

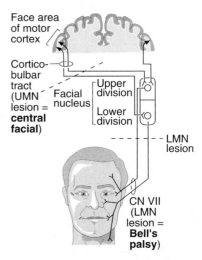

UCV

Spindle muscle control

Reflex arc	Muscle stretch → intrafusal stretch → stimulates Ia afferent→ stimulates α motor neuron → reflex extrafusal contraction.
Gamma loop	CNS stimulates γ motor neuron → contracts intrafusal fiber → increased sensitivity of reflex arc.

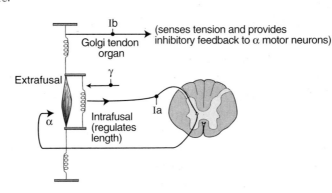

Brachial plexus

1. Waiter's tip
2. Claw hand
3. Wrist drop
4. Winged scapula
5. Deltoid paralysis
6. Saturday night palsy
7. Difficulty flexing elbow, variable sensory loss
8. Decreased thumb function
9. Intrinsic muscles of hand, Pope's blessing

Rad = radial nerve
Ax = axillary nerve
LT = long thoracic nerve
MC = musculocutaneous nerve
Med = median nerve
Uln = ulnar nerve

Upper limb nerve injury

Nerve	Injury/deficit in motion	Deficit in sensation
Radial	Shaft of humerus—loss of triceps brachii (triceps reflex), brachioradialis (brachioradialis reflex), and extensor carpi radialis longus (→ wrist drop); often 2° to humerus fracture	Posterior brachial cutaneous Posterior antebrachial cutaneous
Median	Supracondyle of humerus—no loss of power in any of the arm muscles; loss of forearm pronation, wrist flexion, finger flexion, and several thumb movements; eventually, thenar atrophy	Loss of sensation over the lateral palm and thumb and the radial $2\frac{1}{2}$ fingers
Ulnar	Medial epicondyle—impaired wrist flexion and adduction, and impaired adduction of thumb and the ulnar 2 fingers	Loss of sensation over the medial palm and ulnar $1\frac{1}{2}$ fingers
Axillary	Surgical neck of humerus or anterior shoulder dislocation—loss of deltoid action	
Musculocutaneous	Loss of function of coracobrachialis, biceps, and brachialis muscles (biceps reflex)	

Erb-Duchenne palsy	Traction or tear of the superior trunk of the brachial plexus (C5 and C6 roots); follows blow to shoulder or trauma during delivery. Findings: limb hangs by side (paralysis of abductors), medially rotated (paralysis of lateral rotators), forearm is pronated (loss of biceps).	"Waiter's tip" owing to appearance of arm.

Radial nerve	Known as the "great extensor nerve." Provides innervation of the **B**rachioradialis, **E**xtensors of the wrist and fingers, **S**upinator, and **T**riceps.	Radial nerve innervates the **BEST!** To **SUP**inate is to move as if carrying a bowl of **SOUP.**

Thoracic outlet syndrome	An embryologic defect; can compress subclavian artery and inferior trunk of brachial plexus (C8, T1), resulting in thoracic outlet syndrome: 1. Atrophy of the thenar and hypothenar eminences 2. Atrophy of the interosseous muscles 3. Sensory deficits on the medial side of the forearm and hand 4. Disappearance of the radial pulse upon moving the head toward the opposite side

Clinical reflexes	Biceps = C5 nerve root. Triceps = C7 nerve root. Patella = L4 nerve root. Achilles = S1 nerve root. Babinski—dorsiflexion of the big toe and fanning of other toes; sign of upper motor neuron lesion, but normal reflex in 1st year of life (upper motor neuron loss).

Biceps C5
Triceps C7
Patellar @ L4
Aen → S1

Behavioral Science

"It's psychosomatic. You need a lobotomy. I'll get a saw."
—Calvin, "Calvin & Hobbes"

A heterogeneous mix of epidemiology/biostatistics, psychiatry, psychology, sociology, psychopharmacology, and more falls under this heading. Many medical students do not study this discipline diligently because the material is felt to be "easy" or "common sense." In our opinion, this is a missed opportunity. Each question gained in behavioral science is equal to a question in any other section in determining the overall score.

Many students feel that some behavioral science questions are less concrete and require an awareness of the social aspects of medicine. For example: If a patient does or says something, what should you do or say in response? These so-called quote questions now constitute much of the behavioral science section. We have included several examples in the high-yield clinical vignettes. Medical ethics and medical law are also appearing with increasing frequency. In addition, the key aspects of the doctor-patient relationship (e.g., communication skills, open-ended questions, facilitation, silence) are high yield. Basic biostatistics and epidemiology are very learnable and high yield. Be able to apply biostatistical concepts such as specificity and predictive values in a problem-solving format. Also review the clinical presentation of personality disorders.

High-Yield Clinical Vignettes

High-Yield Topics

Epidemiology

Ethics

Life Cycle

Physiology

Psychiatry

Psychology

These abstracted case vignettes are designed to demonstrate the thought processes necessary to answer multistep clinical reasoning questions.

Vignette	Question	Answer
■ Woman with anxiety about a gynecologic exam is told to relax and to imagine going through the steps of the exam.	What process does this exemplify?	Systematic desensitization.
■ 65-year-old man is diagnosed with incurable metastatic pancreatic adenocarcinoma. His family asks you, the doctor, not to tell the patient.	What do you do?	Assess whether telling patient will negatively affect his health. If not, tell him.
■ Man admitted for chest pain is medicated for ventricular tachycardia. The next day he jumps out of bed and does 50 pushups to show the nurses he has not had a heart attack.	What defense mechanism is he using?	Denial.
■ You find yourself attracted to your 26-year-old patient.	What do you say?	Nothing! The tone of the interview must be very professional; it is not acceptable to have any sort of romantic relationship with patients. If you feel your actions may be misinterpreted, invite a chaperone into the room.
■ A large group of people is followed over 10 years. Every 2 years, it is determined who develops heart disease and who does not.	What type of study is this?	Cohort study.
■ Girl can groom herself, can hop on one foot, and has an imaginary friend.	How old is she?	4 years old.
■ Man has flashbacks about his girlfriend's death 2 months ago following a hit-and-run accident. He often cries and wishes for the death of the culprit.	What is the diagnosis?	Normal bereavement.
■ 36-year-old woman with strong family history of breast cancer refuses a mammogram because she heard it hurts.	What do you do?	Discuss the risks and benefits of not having a mammogram. Each patient must give their own informed consent to each procedure; if the patient refuses, you must abide by their wishes.

HIGH-YIELD FACTS

Behavioral Science

Vignette	Question	Answer
■ During a particular stage of sleep, man has variable blood pressure, penile tumescence, and variable EEG.	What stage of sleep is he in?	REM sleep.
■ 15-year-old girl of normal height and weight for her age has enlarged parotid glands but no other complaints. The mother confides that she found laxatives in the daughter's closet.	What is the diagnosis?	Bulimia.
■ 11-year-old girl exhibits Tanner stage 4 sexual development (almost full breasts and pubic hair).	What is the diagnosis?	Advanced stage, early development.
■ 4-year-old girl complains of a burning feeling in her genitalia; otherwise she behaves and sleeps normally. Smear of discharge shows N. *gonorrhoeae*.	How was she infected?	Sexual abuse.
■ 72-year-old man insists on stopping treatment for his heart condition because it makes him feel "funny."	What do you do?	Although you want to encourage the patient to take his medication, the patient has the final say in his own treatment regime. You should investigate the "funny" feeling and determine if there are drugs available that don't elicit this particular side effect.
■ Person demands only the best and most famous doctor in town.	What is the personality disorder?	Narcissism.
■ Nurse has episodes of hypoglycemia; blood analysis reveals no elevation in C protein.	What is the diagnosis?	Factitious disorder; self-scripted insulin.
■ 55-year-old businessman complains of lack of successful sexual contacts with women and lack of ability to reach full erection. Two years ago he had a heart attack.	What might be the cause of his problem?	Fear of sudden death during intercourse.

Epidemiology/Biostatistics

1. Differences in the incidence of disease among various ethnic groups.
2. Leading causes and types of cancers in men versus women.
3. Prevalence of common psychiatric disorders (e.g., alcoholism, major depression, schizophrenia).
4. Differences in mortality rates among ethnic and racial groups.
5. Definitions of morbidity, mortality, and case fatality rate.
6. Epidemiology of cigarette smoking, including prevalence and success rates for quitting.
7. Modes of human immunodeficiency virus (HIV) transmission among different populations (e.g., perinatal, heterosexual, homosexual, intravenous).
8. Simple pedigree analysis (understand symbols) for inheritance of genetic diseases (e.g., counseling, risk assessment).
9. Different types of studies (e.g., randomized clinical trial, cohort, case-control).
10. Definition and use of standard deviation, p value, r value, mean, mode, and median.
11. Effects of changing a test's criteria on number of false positives and number of false negatives.

Neurophysiology

1. Physiologic changes (e.g., neurotransmitter levels) in common neuropsychiatric disorders (e.g., Alzheimer's disease, Huntington's disease, schizophrenia, bipolar disorder).
2. Changes in cerebrospinal fluid composition with common psychiatric diseases (e.g., depression).
3. Physiologic, physical, and psychological changes associated with aging (e.g., memory, lung capacity, glomerular filtration rate, muscle mass, pharmacokinetics of drugs).
4. Differences between anterior and posterior lobes of the pituitary gland (e.g., embryology, innervation, hormones).

Psychiatry/Psychology

1. Indicators of prognosis in psychiatric disorders (e.g., schizophrenia, bipolar disorder).
2. Genetic components of common psychiatric disorders (e.g., schizophrenia, bipolar disorder).
3. Diseases associated with different personality types.
4. Clinical features and treatment of phobias.
5. Clinical features of child abuse (shaken-baby syndrome).
6. Clinical features of common learning disorders (e.g., dyslexia, mental retardation).
7. Therapeutic application of learning theories (e.g., classical and operant conditioning) to psychiatric illnesses (e.g., disulfiram therapy for alcoholics).
8. Problems associated with the physician-patient relationship (e.g., reasons for patient noncompliance).
9. Management of the suicidal patient.
10. Addiction: risk factors, family history, behavior, factors contributing to relapse.
11. How physicians and medical students should help peers with substance abuse problems.

Prevalence vs. incidence

Prevalence is total number of cases in a population at a given time.

Incidence is number of new cases in a population per unit time.

Incidence is new **incidents.**

Prevalence ≅ incidence × disease duration.

Prevalence > incidence for chronic diseases (e.g., diabetes).

Prevalence = incidence for acute disease (e.g., common cold).

Sensitivity

Number of true positives divided by number of all people with the disease.

False negative ratio is equal to 1 − sensitivity.

High sensitivity is desirable for a screening test.

PID = **P**ositive **I**n **D**isease (note that PID is a **sensitive** topic).

SNOUT = Se**N**sitivity rules **OUT.**

Specificity

Number of true negatives divided by number of all people without the disease.

False positive ratio is equal to 1 − specificity.

High specificity is desirable for a confirmatory test.

NIH = **N**egative **I**n **H**ealth.

SPIN = **SP**ecificity rules **IN.**

Predictive value

Positive predictive value

Number of true positives divided by number of people who tested positive for the disease.

The probability of having a condition, given a positive test.

Negative predictive value

Number of true negatives divided by number of people who tested negative for the disease.

The probability of not having the condition, given a negative test.

Unlike sensitivity and specificity, predictive values are dependent on the prevalence of the disease.

The higher the prevalence of a disease, the higher the positive predictive value of the test.

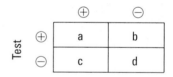

		Disease	
		⊕	⊖
Test	⊕	a	b
	⊖	c	d

$$\text{Sensitivity} = \frac{a}{a+c}$$

$$\text{Specificity} = \frac{d}{b+d}$$

$$\text{PPV} = \frac{a}{a+b}$$

$$\text{NPV} = \frac{d}{c+d}$$

Odds ratio and relative risk

Odds ratio

Approximates the relative risk if the prevalence of the disease is not too high. Used for case-control (retrospective) studies.

OR = ad/bc

Relative risk

Disease risk in exposed group/disease risk in unexposed group. Used for cohort studies.

		Disease	
		⊕	⊖
Exposure	⊕	a	b
	⊖	c	d

$$RR = \frac{\left[\dfrac{a}{a+b}\right]}{\left[\dfrac{c}{c+d}\right]} \qquad \text{Attributable risk} = \left[\frac{a}{a+b}\right] - \left[\frac{c}{c+d}\right]$$

If the 95% confidence interval for OR or RR includes 1, the study is inconclusive.

Standard deviation vs. error

n = sample size
σ = standard deviation
SEM = standard error of the mean
SEM = $\sigma/\sqrt{n}$
Therefore, SEM < σ and SEM decreases as n increases.

Normal (Gaussian) distribution:

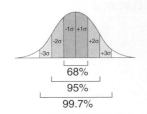
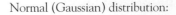

68%
95%
99.7%

Statistical distribution

Terms that describe statistical distributions:

Normal ≈ Gaussian ≈ bell-shaped (mean = median = mode).

Bimodal is simply 2 humps.

Positive skew is asymmetry with tail on the right (mean > median > mode).

Negative skew has tail on the left (mean < median < mode).

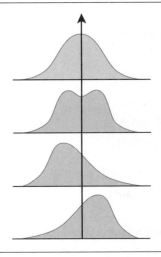

Precision vs. accuracy

Precision is:
1. The consistency and reproducibility of a test (reliability)
2. The absence of random variation in a test
Accuracy is the trueness of test measurements.

Random error—reduced precision in a test.
Systematic error—reduced accuracy in a test.

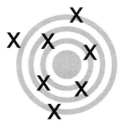
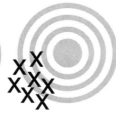
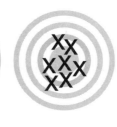
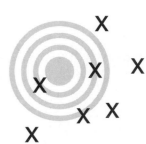

| Accuracy | Precision | Accuracy and precision | No accuracy, no precision |

Reliability and validity

Reliability—Reproducibility (dependability) of a test.
Validity—whether the test truly measures what it purports to measure. Appropriateness of a test.

Test is reliable if repeat measurements are the same.
Test is valid if it measures what it is supposed to measure.

Correlation coefficient (r)

r is always between −1 and 1. Absolute value indicates strength of correlation.
Coefficient of determination = r^2.

t-test vs. **ANOVA vs. χ^2**	**t**-test checks difference between 2 **mean**s. ANOVA analyzes variance of 3 or more variables. χ^2 checks difference between 2 or more percentages or proportions of categorical outcomes (not mean values).	Mr. **T** is **mean**. **ANOVA** = **AN**alysis Of **VA**riance of 3 or more variables. χ^2 = compare percentages (%) or proportions.
Meta-analysis	Pooling data from several studies (often via a literature search) to achieve greater statistical power.	Cannot overcome limitations of individual studies or bias in study selection.
Case-control study	Observational study. Sample chosen based on presence (cases) or absence (controls) of disease. Information collected about risk factors.	Often retrospective.
Cohort study	Observational study. Sample chosen based on presence or absence of risk factors. Subjects followed over time for development of disease.	The Framingham heart study was a large prospective cohort study.
Clinical trial	Experimental study. Compares therapeutic benefit of 2 or more treatments.	Highest-quality study when randomized and double-blind.
Bias	When one outcome is more likely to occur than another. 1. **Selection bias**—subjects choose group 2. **Recall bias**—knowledge of presence of disorder alters recall by subjects 3. **Sampling bias**—subjects are not representative; therefore the results are not generalizable	Way to reduce bias: 1. Blind studies (single vs. double) 2. Placebo responses 3. Crossover studies (each subject acts as own control) 4. Randomization

Statistical hypotheses

Null (H_0) — Hypothesis of no difference (e.g., there is no association between the disease and the risk factor in the population).

Alternative (H_1) — Hypothesis that there is some difference (e.g., there is some association between the disease and the risk factor in the population).

	Reality	
Study results	H_1	H_0
H_1	Power $(1 - \beta)$	α
H_0	β	

Type I error (α)	Stating that there **is** an effect or difference when there really is not (to mistakenly accept the experimental hypothesis and reject the null hypothesis). α is a preset level of significance, usually $p < .05$. p = probability of making a type I error.	If $p < .05$, then there is less than a 5% chance that the data will show something that is not really there. α = you "saw" a difference that did not exist—for example, convicting an innocent man.

Type II error (β)

Stating that there **is not** an effect or difference when there really is (to fail to reject the null hypothesis when in fact H_0 is false). β is the probability of making a type II error.

β = you did not "see" a difference that does exist— for example, setting a guilty man free.

$1 - \beta$ is "power" of study, or probability that study will see a difference if it is there.

Power

Probability of rejecting null hypothesis when it is in fact false. It depends on:
1. Total number of end points experienced by population
2. Difference in compliance between treatment groups (differences in the mean values between groups)

If you increase sample size, you increase power. There is power in numbers.
Power = $1 - \beta$.

Reportable diseases

Only some infectious diseases are reportable in all states, including AIDS, chickenpox, gonorrhea, hepatitis A and B, measles, mumps, rubella, salmonella, shigella, syphilis, and tuberculosis.
Other diseases (including HIV) vary by state.

B. A. SSSMMART
Chicken or you're **G**one:
Hep **B**
Hep **A**
Salmonella
Shigella
Syphilis
Measles
Mumps
AIDS
Rubella
Tuberculosis
Chickenpox
Gonorrhea

Leading causes of death in the United States by age

Infants	Congenital anomalies, short gestation/low birth weight, sudden infant death syndrome, maternal complications of pregnancy, respiratory distress syndrome.
Age 1–14	Injuries, cancer, congenital anomalies, homicide, heart disease.
Age 15–24	Injuries, homicide, suicide, cancer, heart disease.
Age 25–64	Cancer, heart disease, injuries, suicide, stroke.
Age 65+	Heart disease, cancer, stroke, COPD, pneumonia and influenza.

Disease prevention	1°—Prevent disease occurrence (e.g., vaccination).
	2°—Early detection of disease (e.g., Pap smear).
	3°—Reduce disability from disease (e.g., exogenous insulin for diabetes).

Additional Services for Specific Groups	
Risk factor	Preventive service(s) needed
Diabetes	Eye, foot exams; urine test
Drug abuse	HIV, TB tests; hepatitis immunization
Alcoholism	Influenza, pneumococcal immunizations; TB test
Overweight	Blood sugar test (test for diabetes mellitus)
Homeless, recent refugee or immigrant	TB test
High-risk sexual behavior	HIV, hep B, syphilis, gonorrhea, chlamydia tests

Risk factors for suicide completion	White, male, alone, prior attempts, presence and lethality of plan, medical illness, alcohol or drug use, on 3 or more prescription medications. Women try more often; men succeed more often.	**SAD PERSONS:** Sex (male), Age, Depression, Previous attempt, Ethanol, Rational thought, Sickness, Organized plan, No spouse, Social support lacking.
Most common surgeries	Dilation and curettage, hysterectomy, tonsillectomy, sterilization, hernia repair, oophorectomy, cesarean section, cholecystectomy.	Most done on women.
Medicare, Medicaid	Medicare and Medicaid are federal programs that originated from amendments to the Social Security Act. Medicare Part A = hospital; Part B = doctor bills. Medicaid is federal and state assistance for very poor people.	MedicarE is for Elderly. MedicaiD is for Destitute.

BEHAVIORAL SCIENCE—ETHICS

Autonomy	Obligation to respect patients as individuals and to honor their preferences in medical care.	
Informed consent	Legally requires: 1. Discussion of pertinent information 2. Obtaining the patient's agreement to the plan of care 3. Freedom from coercion	Patients must understand the risks, benefits, and alternatives, which include no intervention.
Exceptions to informed consent	1. Patient lacks decision-making capacity (not legally competent) 2. Implied consent in an emergency 3. Therapeutic privilege—withholding information when disclosure would severely harm the patient or undermine informed decision-making capacity 4. Waiver—patient waives the right of informed consent	

Decision-making capacity	1. Patient makes and communicates a choice 2. Patient is informed 3. Decision remains stable over time 4. Decision consistent with patient's values and goals 5. Decision not a result of delusions or hallucinations	The patient's family cannot require that a doctor withhold information from the patient.

Oral advance directive

Incapacitated patient's prior oral statements commonly used as guide. Problems arise from variance in interpretation of these statements. However, if patient was informed, directive is specific, patient makes a choice, and decision is repeated over time, the oral directive is more valid.

Written advance directive

Living wills—patient directs physician to withhold or withdraw life-sustaining treatment if the patient develops a terminal disease or enters a persistent vegetative state.

Durable power of attorney—patient designates a surrogate to make medical decisions in the event that the patient loses decision-making capacity. Patient may also specify decisions in clinical situations. More flexible than a living will.

Nonmaleficence

"Do no harm." However, if benefits of an intervention outweigh the risks, a patient may make an informed decision to proceed.

Beneficence

Physicians have a special ethical responsibility to act in the patient's best interest ("physician is a fiduciary"). Patient autonomy may conflict with beneficence. If the patient makes an informed decision, ultimately the patient has the right to decide.

Confidentiality

Confidentiality respects patient privacy and autonomy. Disclosing information to family and friends should be guided by what the patient would want. The patient may also waive the right to confidentiality (e.g., insurance companies).

Exceptions to confidentiality

1. Potential harm to others is serious
2. Likelihood of harm to self is great
3. No alternative means exist to warn or to protect those at risk
4. Physicians can take steps to prevent harm
   Examples include:
   1. Infectious diseases—physicians may have a duty to warn public officials and identifiable people at risk
   2. The Tarasoff decision—law requiring physician to directly inform and protect potential victim from harm; may involve breach of confidentiality
   3. Child and/or elder abuse
   4. Impaired automobile drivers
   5. Suicidal/homicidal patient

HIGH-YIELD FACTS

Behavioral Science

Malpractice	Civil suit under negligence requires:	Unlike a criminal suit, in which
	1. Physician breach of duty to patient	the burden of proof is "beyond
	2. Patient suffers harm	a reasonable doubt," the
	3. Breach of duty causes harm	burden of proof in a
		malpractice suit is "more
		likely than not."

BEHAVIORAL SCIENCE—LIFE CYCLE

Apgar score (at birth)	Score 0–2 at 1 and 5 minutes in each of 5 categories:	After Virginia **Apgar,** a famous anesthesiologist.
	1. Color (blue/pale, trunk pink, all pink)	**APGAR:**
	2. Heart rate (0, <100, 100+)	**A**ppearance (color)
	3. Reflex irritability (0, grimace, grimace + cough)	**P**ulse
	4. Muscle tone (limp, some, active)	**G**rimace
	5. Respiratory effort (0, irregular, regular)	**A**ctivity
	10 is perfect score.	**R**espiration

Low birth weight	Defined as less than 2500 g. Associated with greater incidence of physical and emotional problems. Caused by prematurity or intrauterine growth retardation. Complications include infections, respiratory distress syndrome, necrotizing enterocolitis, intraventricular hemorrhage, and persistent fetal circulation.	

Infant deprivation effects	Long-term deprivation of affection results in:	Studied by René Spitz. The **4 W's: W**eak, **W**ordless, **W**anting (socially), **W**ary. Deprivation for > 6 months can lead to irreversible changes.
	1. Decreased muscle tone	
	2. Poor language skills	
	3. Poor socialization skills	
	4. Lack of basic trust	
	5. Anaclitic depression	
	6. Weight loss	
	7. Physical illness	
	Severe deprivation can result in infant death.	

Anaclitic depression	Depression in an infant owing to continued separation from caregiver—can result in failure to thrive. Infant becomes withdrawn and unresponsive.	

Regression in children	Children regress to younger behavior under stress: physical illness, punishment, birth of a new sibling, tiredness. An example is bed-wetting in a previously toilet-trained child when hospitalized.	

Child abuse

	Physical abuse	**Sexual abuse**
Evidence	Healed fractures on x-ray, cigarette burns, subdural hematomas, multiple bruises, retinal hemorrhage or detachment	Genital/anal trauma, STDs, UTIs
Abuser	Usually female and the 1° caregiver	Known to victim, usually male
Epidemiology	~3000 deaths/year in the United States	Peak incidence 9–12 years of age

Developmental milestones

	Approximate age	Milestone
Infant	3 mo	Holds head up, social smile, Moro reflex disappears
	4–5 mo	Rolls front to back, sits when propped
	7–9 mo	Stranger anxiety, sits alone, orients to voice
	12–14 mo	Upgoing Babinski disappears
	15 mo	Walking, few words, separation anxiety
Toddler	12–24 mo	Object permanence
	18–24 mo	Rapprochement
	24–48 mo	Parallel play
	24–36 mo	Core gender identity
Preschool	30–36 mo	Toilet training
	3 yrs	Group play, rides tricycle, copies line or circle drawing
	4 yrs	Cooperative play, simple drawings (stick figure), hops on 1 foot
School age	6–11 yrs	Development of conscience (superego), same-sex friends, identification with same-sex parent
Adolescence (puberty)	11 yrs (girls) 13 yrs (boys)	Abstract reasoning (formal operations), formation of personality

Reflexes present at birth

1. Moro reflex—extension of limbs when startled
2. Rooting reflex—nipple seeking
3. Palmar reflex—grasps objects in palm
4. Babinski reflex—large toe dorsiflexes with plantar stimulation

Normally disappear within 1st year.

Changes in the elderly

1. Sexual changes—sexual interest does not decrease
   Men: slower erection/ejaculation, longer refractory period
   Women: vaginal shortening, thinning, and dryness
2. Sleep patterns— $\downarrow$ REM sleep, $\downarrow$ slow-wave sleep, $\uparrow$ sleep latency, $\uparrow$ awakenings during the night
3. Common medical conditions—arthritis, hypertension, heart disease
4. Psychiatric problems (e.g., depression) become more prevalent
5. Suicide rate increases

Kübler-Ross dying stages

Denial, Anger, Bargaining, Grieving, Acceptance.
Stages do not necessarily occur in this order, and
  > 1 stage can be present at once.

Death Arrives Bringing Grave Adjustments.

Grief

Normal bereavement characterized by shock, denial, guilt, and somatic symptoms.
  Typically lasts 6 months to 1 year.   *BehSci.57*
Pathologic grief includes excessively intense or prolonged grief or grief that is delayed,
  inhibited, or denied.   *BehSci.58*

UCV

Neurotransmitter changes with disease	Anxiety—↑ NE, ↓ GABA, ↓ serotonin. Depression—↓ NE and serotonin (5-HT). Alzheimer's dementia—↓ ACh. Huntington's disease—↓ GABA, ↓ ACh. Schizophrenia—↑ dopamine. Parkinson's disease—↓ dopamine.
Frontal lobe functions	Concentration, orientation, language, abstraction, judgment, motor regulation, mood. Lack of social judgment is most notable in frontal lobe lesion.

Sleep stages

Stage (% of total sleep time in young adults)	Description	Waveform
	Awake (eyes open), alert, active mental concentration	Beta (highest frequency, lowest amplitude)
	Awake (eyes closed)	Alpha
1 (5%)	Light sleep	Theta
2 (45%)	Deeper sleep	Sleep spindles and K-complexes
3–4 (25%)	Deepest, non-REM sleep; sleepwalking; night terrors, bed-wetting (slow-wave sleep)	Delta (lowest frequency, highest amplitude)
REM (25%)	Dreaming, loss of motor tone, possibly a memory processing function, erections, ↑ brain O_2 use	Beta At night, **BATS** D**rink** B**lood**.

1. Serotonergic predominance of raphe nucleus key to initiating sleep
2. Norepinephrine reduces REM sleep
3. Extraocular movements during REM due to activity of PPRF (paramedian pontine reticular formation/conjugate gaze center)
4. REM sleep having the same EEG pattern as while awake and alert has spawned the terms "paradoxical sleep" and "desynchronized sleep"
5. Benzodiazepines shorten stage 4 sleep; thus useful for night terrors and sleepwalking
   BehSci.39, 87
6. Imipramine is used to treat enuresis since it decreases stage 4 sleep   *BehSci.36*

UCV

REM sleep	↑ and variable pulse, rapid eye movements (REM), ↑ and variable blood pressure, penile/clitoral tumescence. 25% of total sleep. Occurs every 90 minutes; duration ↑ through the night. REM sleep ↓ with age. Acetylcholine is the principal neurotransmitter involved in REM sleep.	REM sleep is like sex: ↑ pulse, penile/ clitoral tumescence, ↓ with age.

Sleep apnea	Central sleep apnea—no respiratory effort.	Treatment: weight loss, CPAP, surgery.
	Obstructive sleep apnea—respiratory effort against airway obstruction.	
	Person stops breathing for at least 10 seconds repeatedly during sleep.	
	Associated with obesity, loud snoring, systemic/pulmonary hypertension, arrhythmias, and possibly sudden death.	
	Individuals may become chronically tired.	

Narcolepsy

UCV *BehSci.7*

Person falls asleep suddenly. May include hypnagogic (just before sleep) or hypnopompic (just before awakening) hallucinations. The person's nocturnal and narcoleptic sleep episodes start off with REM sleep. **Cataplexy** (sudden collapse while awake) in some patients. Strong genetic component. Treat with stimulants (e.g., amphetamines).

Sleep patterns of depressed patients

Patients with depression typically have the following changes in their sleep stages:
1. ↓ slow-wave sleep
2. ↓ REM latency
3. Early-morning awakening (important screening question)

Stress effects

Stress induces production of free fatty acids, 17-OH corticosteroids, lipids, cholesterol, catecholamines; affects water absorption, muscular tonicity, gastrocolic reflex, and mucosal circulation.

Sexual dysfunction

UCV *BehSci.91*

Differential diagnosis includes:
1. Drugs (e.g., antihypertensives, neuroleptics, SSRIs, ethanol)
2. Diseases (e.g., depression, diabetes)
3. Psychological (e.g., performance anxiety)

HIGH-YIELD FACTS

Behavioral Science

Orientation

Is the patient aware of him- or herself as a person?
Does the patient know his or her own name?
Anosognosia—unaware that one is ill.
Autotopagnosia—unable to locate one's own body parts.
Depersonalization—body seems unreal or dissociated.

Order of loss: 1st—time;
2nd—place; last—person.

Amnesia types

*Antero*grade amnesia is being unable to remember
things that occurred after a CNS insult (no new
memory).
Korsakoff's amnesia is a classic anterograde amnesia
that is caused by thiamine deficiency (bilateral
destruction of the mammillary bodies), is seen in
alcoholics, and is associated with confabulations.
*Retro*grade amnesia is inability to remember things
that occurred before a CNS insult. Complication of
ECT.

Antero = after.

Retro = before.

Substance dependence

Maladaptive pattern of substance use defined as 3 or more of the following signs in 1 year:
1. Tolerance
2. Withdrawal
3. Substance taken in larger amounts than intended
4. Persistent desire or attempts to cut down
5. Lots of energy spent trying to obtain substance
6. Important social, occupational, or recreational activities given up or reduced because of substance use
7. Use continued in spite of knowing the problems that it causes

Substance abuse

Maladaptive pattern leading to clinically significant impairment or distress. Symptoms have not met criteria for substance dependence. 1 or more of the following in 1 year:
1. Recurrent use resulting in failure to fulfill major obligations at work, school, or home
2. Recurrent use in physically hazardous situations
3. Recurrent substance-related legal problems
4. Continued use in spite of persistent problems caused by use

HIGH-YIELD FACTS

Behavioral Science

Signs and symptoms of substance abuse

Drug	Intoxication	Withdrawal
Alcohol	Disinhibition, emotional lability, slurred speech, ataxia, coma, blackouts. *BehSci.96*	Tremor, tachycardia, hypertension, malaise, nausea, seizures, delirium tremens (DTs), tremulousness, agitation, hallucinations.
Opioids	CNS depression, nausea and vomiting, constipation, pupillary constriction (pinpoint pupils), seizures (overdose is life-threatening).	Anxiety, insomnia, anorexia, sweating, dilated pupils, piloerection ("cold turkey"), fever, rhinorrhea, nausea, stomach cramps, diarrhea ("flu-like" symptoms), yawning.
Amphetamines	Psychomotor agitation, impaired judgment, pupillary dilation, hypertension, tachycardia, euphoria, prolonged wakefulness and attention, cardiac arrhythmias, delusions, hallucinations, fever.	Post-use "crash," including depression, lethargy, headache, stomach cramps, hunger, hypersomnolence.
Cocaine	Euphoria, psychomotor agitation, impaired judgment, tachycardia, pupillary dilation, hypertension, hallucinations (including tactile), paranoid ideations, angina and sudden cardiac death.	Post-use "crash" including severe depression and suicidality, hypersomnolence, fatigue, malaise, severe psychological craving.
PCP	Belligerence, impulsiveness, fever, psychomotor agitation, vertical and horizontal nystagmus, tachycardia, ataxia, homicidality, psychosis, delirium. *BehSci.97*	Recurrence of intoxication symptoms due to reabsorption in GI tract; sudden onset of severe, random, homicidal violence.
LSD	Marked anxiety or depression, delusions, visual hallucinations, flashbacks, pupil dilation.	
Marijuana	Euphoria, anxiety, paranoid delusions, perception of slowed time, impaired judgment, social withdrawal, increased appetite, dry mouth, hallucinations.	
Barbiturates	Low safety margin, respiratory depression.	Anxiety, seizures, delirium, life-threatening cardiovascular collapse.
Benzodiazepines	Amnesia, ataxia, somnolence, minor respiratory depression. Addictive effects with alcohol. Greater safety margin.	Rebound anxiety, seizures, tremor, insomnia.
Caffeine	Restlessness, insomnia, increased diuresis, muscle twitching, cardiac arrhythmias.	Headache, lethargy, depression, weight gain.
Nicotine	Restlessness, insomnia, anxiety, arrhythmias.	Irritability, headache, anxiety, weight gain, craving, tachycardia.

UCV

Delirium tremens   Life-threatening alcohol withdrawal syndrome that peaks 2–5 days after last drink.
In order of appearance—autonomic system hyperactivity (tachycardia, tremors, anxiety), psychotic symptoms (hallucinations, delusions), confusion.
Treat with benzodiazepines.

Heroin addiction	Approximately 500,000 U.S. addicts. Heroin is Schedule I (not prescribable). Also look for track marks (needle sticks in veins). Related diagnoses are hepatitis, abscesses, overdose, hemorrhoids, AIDS, and right-sided endocarditis.	Naloxone (Narcan) and naltrexone competitively inhibit opioids. Methadone (long-acting oral opiate) for heroin detoxification or long-term maintenance.
Delirium UCV *BehSci.3-4*	↓ attention span and level of arousal, disorganized thinking, hallucinations, illusions, misperceptions, disturbance in sleep-wake cycle, cognitive dysfunction. Key to diagnosis: waxing and waning level of consciousness; develops rapidly. Often due to substance use/abuse or medical illness.	DeliRIUM = changes in sensoRIUM. Most common psychiatric illness on medical and surgical floors. Often reversible. Check for drugs with anticholinergic effects.
Dementia UCV *BehSci.5, 6*	Development of multiple cognitive deficits—memory, aphasia, apraxia, agnosia, loss of abstract thought, behavioral/personality changes, impaired judgment. Key to diagnosis: rule out delirium—patient is alert, no change in level of consciousness. More often gradual onset. In elderly patients, depression may present like dementia.	DeMEMtia characterized by MEMory loss. Commonly irreversible.

Major depressive episode
 	
UCV *BehSci.53-55, 56*
	Characterized by 5 of the following for 2 weeks, including (1) depressed mood or (2) anhedonia:
	  1. Sleep disturbances
	  2. Loss of Interest
	  3. Guilt
	  4. Loss of Energy
	  5. Loss of Concentration
	  6. Change in Appetite
	  7. Psychomotor retardation
	  8. Suicidal ideations
	  9. Depressed mood
	Major depressive disorder, recurrent—requires 2 or more episodes with a symptom-free interval of 2 months. Lifetime prevalence—5–12% male, 10–25% female.
	Dysthymia is a milder form of depression lasting at least 2 years.
		SIG E CAPS.

Electroconvulsive therapy	Treatment option for major depressive disorder refractory to other treatment. ECT is painless and produces a seizure. Complications can result from anesthesia. The major adverse effects of ECT are disorientation and anterograde and retrograde amnesia.	

HIGH-YIELD FACTS

Behavioral Science

Manic episode

Distinct period of abnormally and persistently elevated, expansive, or irritable mood lasting at least 1 week.
During mood disturbance, 3 or more of the following are present:

1. **D**istractibility

   DIG FAST.
2. **I**nsomnia— ↓ need for sleep
3. **G**randiosity—inflated self-esteem
4. **F**light of ideas
5. Increase in goal-directed **A**ctivity/ psychomotor agitation
6. Pressured **S**peech
7. **T**houghtlessness—seeks pleasure without regard to consequences

UCV *BehSci.50*

Hypomanic episode

Like manic episode except mood disturbance not severe enough to cause marked impairment in social and/or occupational functioning or to necessitate hospitalization; there are no psychotic features.

Bipolar disorder

6 separate criteria sets exist for bipolar disorders with combinations of manic (bipolar I), hypomanic (bipolar II), and depressed episodes. 1 manic or hypomanic episode defines bipolar disorder. Lithium is drug of choice.
Cyclothymic disorder is a milder form lasting at least 2 years.

UCV *BehSci.50-52*

Malingering

Patient consciously fakes or claims to have a disorder in order to attain a specific gain (e.g., financial).

UCV *BehSci.47*

Factitious disorder

Consciously creates symptoms in order to assume "sick role" and to get medical attention. **Munchausen's syndrome** is manifested by a chronic history of multiple hospital admissions and willingness to receive invasive procedures. **Munchausen's syndrome by proxy** is seen when illness in a child is caused by the parent. Motivation is unconscious.

UCV *BehSci.48*

Somatoform disorders

Both illness production and motivation are unconscious drives. Several types:

1. Conversion—symptoms suggest motor or sensory neurologic or physical disorder, but tests and physical exam are negative   *BehSci.89*
2. Somatoform pain disorder—pain that is not explained completely by illness   *BehSci.94*
3. Hypochondriasis—misinterpretation of normal physical findings, leading to preoccupation with and fear of having a serious illness in spite of medical reassurance   *BehSci.90*
4. Somatization disorder—variety of complaints in multiple organ systems   *BehSci.93*
5. Body dysmorphic disorder—patient convinced that part of own anatomy is malformed   *BehSci.88*
6. Pseudocyesis—false belief of being pregnant associated with objective signs of pregnancy   *BehSci.92*

UCV

Gain: 1°, 2°, 3°

1° gain—what the symptom does for the patient's internal psychic economy.

2° gain—what the symptom gets the patient (sympathy, attention).

3° gain—what the caretaker gets (like an MD on an interesting case).

Panic disorder

Discrete periods of intense fear and discomfort peaking
    in 10 minutes with 4 of the following:

1. **P**alpitations
2. **A**bdominal distress
3. **N**ausea
4. **I**ncreased perspiration
5. **C**hest pain, chills, and choking

PANIC.

Panic disorder must be diagnosed in context of
    occurrence (e.g., panic disorder with agoraphobia).

High prevalence during Step 1 exam.

UCV *BehSci.29*

Specific phobia

Fear that is excessive or unreasonable, cued by presence or anticipation of a specific
    object or entity. Exposure provokes anxiety response. Person recognizes fear is
    excessive (insight). Fear interferes with normal routine. Treatment options
    include systematic desensitization. Examples include:

1. Gamophobia (*gam* = gamete)—fear of marriage
2. Algophobia (*alg* = pain)—fear of pain
3. Acrophobia (*acro* = height)—fear of heights
4. Agoraphobia (*agora* = open market)—fear of open places

UCV *BehSci.31*

Post-traumatic stress disorder

Person experienced or witnessed event that involved actual or threatened death or serious
    injury. Response involves intense fear, helplessness, or horror. Traumatic event is
    persistently reexperienced; person persistently avoids stimuli associated with the trauma
    and experiences persistent symptoms of increased arousal. Disturbance lasts > 1 month
    and causes distress or social/occupational impairment.

UCV *BehSci.30, 37*

Personality

Personality trait—an enduring pattern of perceiving, relating to, and thinking about the
    environment and oneself that is exhibited in a wide range of important social and
    personal contexts.

Personality disorder—when these patterns become inflexible and maladaptive, causing
    impairment in social or occupational functioning or subjective distress; person is usually
    not aware of problem.

Cluster A personality disorders

Odd or eccentric; cannot develop meaningful social
    relationships. No psychosis; genetic association
    with schizophrenia.

"Weird."

Types:

1. Paranoid—distrust and suspiciousness; projection is
    main defense mechanism
2. Schizoid—voluntary social withdrawal, limited
    emotional expression
3. Schizotypal—interpersonal awkwardness, odd
    thought patterns and appearance

UCV *BehSci.73, 75, 76*

Cluster B personality disorders	Dramatic, emotional, or erratic; genetic association with mood disorders. Types: 1. Antisocial—disregard for and violation of rights of others, criminality; males > females; conduct disorder if < 18 years 2. Borderline—unstable mood and behavior, impulsiveness, sense of emptiness; females > males 3. Histrionic—excessive emotionality, somatization, attention seeking, sexually provocative 4. Narcissistic—grandiosity, sense of entitlement; may demand "top" physician/best health care	"Wild."
UCV BehSci.66, 68, 70, 71		
Cluster C personality disorders	Anxious or fearful; genetic association with anxiety disorders. Types: 1. Avoidant—sensitive to rejection, socially inhibited, timid, feelings of inadequacy 2. Obsessive-compulsive—preoccupation with order, perfectionism, and control 3. Dependent—submissive and clinging, excessive need to be taken care of, low self-confidence	"Worried."
UCV BehSci.67, 69, 72, 74		
Hallucination vs. illusion vs. delusion	Hallucinations are perceptions in the absence of external stimuli. Illusions are misinterpretations of actual external stimuli. Delusions are false beliefs not shared with other members of culture/subculture that are firmly maintained in spite of obvious proof to the contrary.	
UCV BehSci.78		
Delusion vs. loose association	A delusion is a disorder in the content of thought (the actual idea). A loose association is a disorder in the form of thought (the way ideas are tied together).	
Hallucination types	Visual and auditory hallucinations are common in schizophrenia. Olfactory hallucination often occurs as an aura of a psychomotor epilepsy. Gustatory hallucination is rare. Tactile hallucination (e.g., formication) is common in delirium tremens. Also seen in cocaine abusers ("cocaine bugs"). Hypnagogic hallucination occurs while going to sleep. Hypnopompic hallucination occurs while waking from sleep.	

Schizophrenia	Periods of psychosis and disturbed behavior lasting > 6 months.
	Positive symptoms—hallucinations, delusions, strange behavior, loose associations.
	Negative symptoms—flat affect, social withdrawal, thought blocking, lack of motivation.

The **4 A's** described by Bleuler:
1. **A**mbivalence (uncertainty)
2. **A**utism (self-preoccupation and lack of communication)
3. **A**ffect (blunted)
4. **A**ssociations (loose)

5th A should be **A**uditory hallucinations.

Genetic factors outweigh environmental factors in the etiology of schizophrenia.

Lifetime prevalence—1.5% (males/females, blacks/whites). Presents earlier in men.

Five subtypes:
1. Disorganized
2. Catatonic
3. Paranoid
4. Undifferentiated
5. Residual

Schizoaffective disorder—a combination of schizophrenia and a mood disorder.

UCV *BehSci.80-85*

BEHAVIORAL SCIENCE—PSYCHOLOGY

Structural theory of the mind	Freud's three structures of the mind.
Id	Primal urges, sex, and aggression. (I want it.)
Superego	Moral values, conscience. (You know you can't have it.)
Ego	Bridge and mediator between the unconscious mind and the external world. (Deals with the conflict.)
Topographic theory of the mind	Conscious—what you are aware of.
	Preconscious—what you are able to make conscious with effort (like your phone number).
	Unconscious—what you are not aware of; the central goal of Freudian psychoanalysis is to make the patient aware of what is hidden in his/her unconscious.
Oedipus complex	Repressed sexual feelings of a child for the opposite-sex parent, accompanied by rivalry with same-sex parent. First described by Freud.

Ego defenses

All ego defenses are automatic and unconscious reactions to psychological stress.

Mature

Altruism	Guilty feelings alleviated by unsolicited generosity toward others.	Mafia boss makes large donation to charity.
Humor	Appreciating the amusing nature of an anxiety-provoking or adverse situation.	Nervous medical student jokes about the boards.
Sublimation	Process whereby one replaces an unacceptable wish with a course of action that is similar to the wish but does not conflict with one's value system.	Aggressive impulses used to succeed in business ventures.
Suppression	Voluntary (unlike other defenses) withholding of an idea or feeling from conscious awareness.	Choosing not to think about the USMLE until the week of the exam.

Mature women wear a **SASH:** Sublimation, Altruism, Suppression, Humor.

Immature

Acting out	Unacceptable feelings and thoughts are expressed through actions.	Tantrums.
Dissociation	Temporary, drastic change in personality, memory, consciousness, or motor behavior to avoid emotional stress.	Extreme forms can result in multiple personalities (dissociative identity disorder).
Denial	Avoidance of awareness of some painful reality.	A common reaction in newly diagnosed AIDS and cancer patients.
Displacement	Process whereby avoided ideas and feelings are transferred to some neutral person or object.	Mother yells at child because she is angry at her husband.
Fixation	Partially remaining at a more childish level of development.	Men fixating on sports games.
Identification	Modeling behavior after another person.	Abused child becomes an abuser.
Isolation	Separation of feelings from ideas and events.	Describing murder in graphic detail with no emotional response.
Projection	An unacceptable internal impulse is attributed to an external source.	A man who wants another woman thinks his wife is cheating on him.
Rationalization	Proclaiming logical reasons for actions actually performed for other reasons, usually to avoid self-blame.	Saying the job was not important anyway, after getting fired.
Reaction formation	Process whereby a warded-off idea or feeling is replaced by an (unconsciously derived) emphasis on its opposite.	A patient with libidinous thoughts enters a monastery.
Regression	Turning back the maturational clock and going back to earlier modes of dealing with the world.	Seen in children under stress (e.g., bed-wetting) and in patients on dialysis (e.g., crying).
Repression	Involuntary withholding of an idea or feeling from conscious awareness. The basic mechanism underlying all others.	
Splitting	Belief that people are either good or bad.	A patient says that all the nurses are cold and insensitive but that the doctors are warm and friendly.

Transference and countertransference

Transference	Patient projects feelings stemming from personal life onto physician.
Countertransference	Doctor projects feelings stemming from personal life onto patient.

Classical conditioning

Learning in which a natural response (salivation) is elicited by a conditioned (learned) stimulus (bell) that previously was presented in conjunction with an unconditioned stimulus (food).

Programmed by association, not necessarily reward. As in Pavlov's classical experiments with dogs (ringing the bell provoked salivation).

Operant conditioning

Learning in which a particular action is elicited because it produces a reward.

Positive reinforcement—desired reward produces action (mouse presses button to get food).

Negative reinforcement—removal of aversive stimulus increases behavior (mouse presses button to avoid shock). Do not confuse with punishment.

Reinforcement schedules

Pattern of reinforcement determines how quickly a behavior is learned and extinguished.

Continuous	Behavior shows the most rapid extinction when not rewarded.	This explains why people continue to play slot machines at casinos (variable ratio) and yet get upset when vending machines (continuous) don't work.
Variable ratio	Behavior shows the slowest extinction when not rewarded.	

Intelligence testing

Stanford-Binet and Wechsler are the most famous tests.

Mean is defined at 100, with standard deviation of 15.

IQ < 70 (or 2 standard deviations below the mean) is one of the criteria for diagnosis of mental retardation.

IQ scores are correlated with genetic factors but are more highly correlated with school achievement.

Intelligence tests are objective (not projective) tests.

Biochemistry

"Biochemistry is the study of carbon compounds that crawl."
—Mike Adams

This high-yield material includes molecular biology, genetics, cell biology, and principles of metabolism (especially vitamins, cofactors, minerals, and single-enzyme-deficiency diseases). When studying metabolic pathways, emphasize important regulatory steps and enzyme deficiencies that result in disease. For example, understanding the defect in Lesch-Nyhan syndrome and its clinical consequences is higher yield than memorizing every intermediate in the purine salvage pathway. Do not spend time on hard-core organic chemistry, mechanisms, and physical chemistry. Detailed chemical structures are infrequently tested. Familiarity with the latest biochemical techniques that have medical relevance—such as enzyme-linked immunosorbent assay (ELISA), immunoelectrophoresis, Southern blotting, and PCR—is useful. Beware if you placed out of your medical school's biochemistry class, for the emphasis of the test differs from the emphasis of many undergraduate courses. Review the related biochemistry when studying pharmacology or genetic diseases as a way to reinforce and integrate the material.

High-Yield Clinical Vignettes

High-Yield Topics

DNA/RNA

Lab Tests/Techniques

Genetics

Cellular

Metabolism

Nutrition

Vignette	Question	Answer
■ Full-term neonate of uneventful delivery becomes mentally retarded and hyperactive and has a musty odor.	What is the diagnosis?	PKU.
■ A stressed executive comes home from work, consumes 7 or 8 martinis in rapid succession before dinner, and becomes hypoglycemic.	What is the mechanism?	NADH increase prevents gluconeogenesis by shunting pyruvate and oxaloacetate to lactate and malate.

DNA/RNA/Protein

1. Molecular biology: tools and techniques (e.g., cloning, cDNA libraries, PCR, restriction fragment length polymorphism, restriction enzymes, sequencing).
2. Transcriptional regulation: the operon model (lac, trp operons) of transcription, eukaryotic transcription (e.g., TATA box, enhancers, effects of steroid hormones, transcription factors).
3. Protein synthesis: steps, regulation, energy (Which step requires ATP? GTP?), differences between prokaryotes and eukaryotes (N-formyl methionine), post-translational modification (targeting to organelles, secretion).
4. Acid-base titration curve of amino acids, proteins.

Genetics

1. Inherited hyperlipidemias: types, clinical manifestations, specific changes in serum lipids.
2. Glycogen and lysosomal storage diseases (e.g., type III glycogen storage disease), I-cell disease.
3. Porphyrias: defects, clinical presentation, effect of barbiturates.
4. Inherited defects in amino acid metabolism.

Metabolism

1. Glycogen synthesis: regulation, inherited defects.
2. Oxygen consumption, carbon dioxide production, and ATP production for fats, proteins, and carbohydrates.
3. Amino acid degradation pathways (urea cycle, tricarboxylic acid cycle).
4. Effect of enzyme phosphorylation on metabolic pathways.
5. Rate-limiting enzymes in different metabolic pathways (e.g., pyruvate decarboxylase).
6. Sites of different metabolic pathways (What organ? Where in the cell?).
7. Fed state versus fasting state: forms of energy used, direction of metabolic pathways.
8. Tyrosine kinases and their effects on metabolic pathways (insulin receptor, growth factor receptors).

9. Anti-insulin (gluconeogenic) hormones (e.g., glucagon, GH, cortisol).
10. Synthesis and metabolism of neurotransmitters (e.g., acetylcholine, epinephrine, norepinephrine, dopamine).
11. Purine/pyrimidine degradation.
12. Carnitine shuttle: function, inherited defects.
13. Cellular/organ effects of insulin secretion.

Chromatin structure

Condensed by (−) charged DNA looped twice around (+) charged H2A, H2B, H3, and H4 histones (nucleosome bead). H1 ties nucleosomes together in a string (30-nm fiber). In mitosis, DNA condenses to form mitotic chromosomes.

Think of beads on a string.

Heterochromatin — Condensed, transcriptionally inactive.
Euchromatin — Less condensed, transcriptionally active.

Eu = true, "truly transcribed."

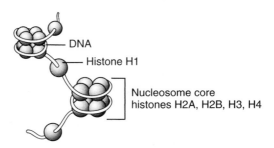

Nucleotides

Purines (**A, G**) have 2 rings. Pyrimidines (**C, T, U**) have 1 ring. Guanine has a ketone. Thymine has a methyl.
Uracil found in RNA; thymine in DNA.
G-C bond (3 H-bonds) stronger than A-T bond (2 H-bonds).

PURe **A**s Gold: **PUR**ines.
CUT the **PY** (pie): **PY**rimidines.
THYmine has a me**THY**l.

Transition vs. transversion

Transition—substituting purine for purine or pyrimidine for pyrimidine.
Transversion—substituting purine for pyrimidine or vice versa.

Transversion—
Transconversion (1 type to another).

Genetic code features

Unambiguous—each codon specifies only 1 amino acid.
Degenerate—more than 1 codon may code for same amino acid.
Commaless, nonoverlapping (except some viruses).
Universal (exceptions include mitochondria, archaeobacteria, *Mycoplasma*, and some yeasts).

Mutations in DNA	Silent—same aa, often base change in 3rd position of codon. Missense—changed aa (conservative—new aa is similar in chemical structure). Nonsense—change resulting in early stop codon. Frame shift—change resulting in misreading of all nucleotides downstream, usually resulting in a truncated protein.	Severity of damage: nonsense > missense > silent.
Prokaryotic DNA replication and DNA polymerases	Origin of replication—continuous DNA synthesis on leading strand and discontinuous (Okazaki fragments) on lagging strand. **Primase** makes an RNA **primer** on which DNA polymerase III can initiate replication. **DNA polymerase III** reaches primer of preceding fragment; $5' \rightarrow 3'$ exonuclease activity of DNA polymerase I degrades RNA primer; **DNA ligase** seals; $3' \rightarrow 5'$ exonuclease activity of DNA polymerase III "proofreads" each added nucleotide. **DNA topoisomerases** create a nick in the helix to relieve supercoils.	Eukaryotic genome has multiple origins of replication. Bacteria, viruses, and plasmids have only 1 origin of replication. DNA polymerase III has $5' \rightarrow 3'$ synthesis and $3' \rightarrow 5'$ exonuclease proofreading ability. DNA polymerase I excises RNA primer.

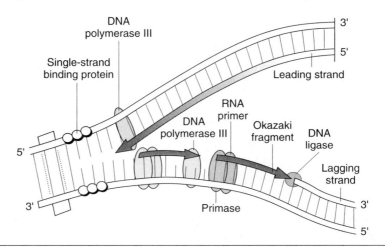

Eukaryotic DNA polymerases	α replicates lagging strand; synthesizes RNA primer. β repairs DNA. γ replicates mitochondrial DNA. δ replicates leading-strand DNA. ε repairs DNA.	
DNA repair: single strand	Single-strand, excision repair–specific glycosylase recognizes and removes damaged base. Endonuclease makes a break several bases to the 5′ side. Exonuclease removes short stretch of nucleotides. DNA polymerase fills gap. DNA ligase seals.	If both strands are damaged, repair may proceed via recombination with undamaged homologous chromosome.

DNA repair defects
UCV Bio.51, 74

Xeroderma pigmentosum (skin sensitivity to UV light), ataxia-telangiectasia (x-rays), Bloom's syndrome (radiation), and Fanconi's anemia (cross-linking agents).

Xeroderma pigmentosum
UCV Bio.74

Defective excision repair such as uvr ABC exonuclease. Results in inability to repair thymidine dimers, which form in DNA when exposed to UV light. Associated with dry skin and with melanoma and other cancers.

Autosomal recessive.

DNA/RNA/protein synthesis direction

DNA and RNA are both synthesized $5' \rightarrow 3'$. Remember that the 5' of the incoming nucleotide bears the triphosphate (energy source for bond). The 3' hydroxyl of the nascent chain is the target. Protein synthesis also proceeds in the 5' to 3' direction.

Imagine the incoming nucleotide bringing a gift (triphosphate) to the 3' host. "**BYOP** (phosphate) from **5** to **3**." Amino acids are linked N to C.

Types of RNA

mRNA is the **largest** type of RNA.
rRNA is the most **abundant** type of RNA.
tRNA is the **smallest** type of RNA.

Massive, **R**ampant, **T**iny.

RNA polymerases

Eukaryotes

RNA polymerase I makes **r**RNA.
RNA polymerase II makes **m**RNA.
RNA polymerase III makes **t**RNA.
No proofreading function, but can initiate chains.
RNA polymerase II opens DNA at promoter site (A-T-rich upstream sequence—TATA and CAAT).
α-amanitin inhibits RNA polymerase II.

I, II, and III are numbered as their products are used in protein synthesis. OR **1, 2, 3** = **RMT** (rhyme).

Prokaryotes

RNA polymerase makes all 3 kinds of RNA.

Start and stop codons

AUG (or rarely GUG) is the mRNA initiation codon. AUG codes for methionine, which may be removed before translation is completed. In prokaryotes the initial AUG codes for a formyl-methionine (f-met).
Stop codons: UGA, UAA, UAG.

AUG in**AUG**urates protein synthesis.

UGA = **U** **G**o **A**way.
UAA = **U** **A**re **A**way.
UAG = **U** **A**re **G**one.

Regulation of gene expression

Promoter

Site where RNA polymerase and multiple other transcription factors bind to DNA upstream from gene locus.

Promoter mutation commonly results in dramatic decrease in amount of gene transcribed.

Enhancer

Stretch of DNA that alters gene expression by binding transcription factors. May be located close to, far from, or even within (in an intron) the gene whose expression it regulates.

Introns vs. exons	Exons contain the actual genetic information coding for protein. Introns are intervening noncoding segments of DNA.	INtrons stay IN the nucleus, whereas EXons EXit and are EXpressed.

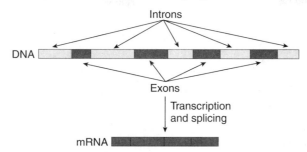

Splicing of mRNA	Introns are precisely spliced out of 1° mRNA transcripts. A lariat-shaped intermediate is formed. Small nuclear ribonucleoprotein particles (snRNP) facilitate splicing by binding to 1° mRNA transcripts and forming spliceosomes.

RNA processing (eukaryotes)	Occurs in nucleus. After transcription: 1. Capping on 5′ end (7-methyl-G) 2. Polyadenylation on 3′ end (≈ 200 A's) 3. Splicing out of introns Initial transcript is called heterogeneous nuclear RNA (hnRNA). Capped and tailed transcript is called mRNA.	Only processed RNA is transported out of the nucleus.

tRNA structure	75–90 nucleotides, cloverleaf form, anticodon end is opposite 3′ aminoacyl end. All tRNAs, both eukaryotic and prokaryotic, have CCA at 3′ end along with a high percentage of chemically modified bases. The amino acid is covalently bound to the 3′ end of the tRNA.

tRNA charging	Aminoacyl-tRNA synthetase (1 per aa, uses ATP) scrutinizes aa before and after it binds to tRNA. If incorrect, bond is hydrolyzed by synthetase. The aa-tRNA bond has energy for formation of peptide bond. A mischarged tRNA reads usual codon but inserts wrong amino acid.	Aminoacyl-tRNA synthetase and binding of charged tRNA to the codon are responsible for accuracy of amino acid selection.

tRNA wobble	Accurate base pairing is required only in the first 2 nucleotide positions of an mRNA codon, so codons differing in the 3rd "wobble" position may code for the same tRNA/amino acid.

Protein synthesis: ATP vs. GTP	P site—peptidyl; A site—aminoacyl. ATP is used in tRNA charging, whereas GTP is used in binding of tRNA to ribosome and for translocation.	ATP—tRNA Activation. GTP—tRNA Gripping and Going places.

Polymerase chain reaction (PCR)	Molecular biology laboratory procedure that is used to synthesize many copies of a desired fragment of DNA.
	Steps:
	1. DNA is denatured by heating to generate 2 separate strands
	2. During cooling, excess premade primers anneal to a specific sequence on each strand to be amplified
	3. Heat-stable DNA polymerase replicates the DNA sequence following each primer
	These steps are repeated multiple times for DNA sequence amplification.

Molecular biology techniques

Southern blot	A **DNA** sample is electrophoresed on a gel and then transferred to a filter. The filter is then soaked in a denaturant and subsequently exposed to a labeled DNA probe that recognizes and anneals to its complementary strand. The resulting double-stranded labeled piece of DNA is visualized when the filter is exposed to film.	DNA-DNA hybridization. **S**outhern = **S**ame.
Northern blot	Similar technique, except that Northern blotting involves radioactive DNA probe binding to sample **RNA.**	DNA-RNA hybridization.
Western blot	Sample protein is separated via gel electrophoresis and transferred to a filter. Labeled antibody is used to bind to relevant **protein.**	Antibody-protein hybridization.
Southwestern blot	Protein sample is run on a gel, transferred to a filter, and exposed to labeled DNA. Used to detect DNA-protein interactions as with transcription factors (e.g., p53, *jun*).	DNA-protein interaction.

| **Enzyme-linked immunosorbent assay (ELISA)** | A rapid immunologic technique in which an antibody or an antigen is coupled to an enzyme as a means of detecting an antigenic match—it is a test of **antigen-antibody** reactivity. The test challenges patients' blood samples either with an antigen to see if their immune system recognizes it or with an antibody to see whether a particular antigen is present in their system. If the target substance is present in the sample, the test solution will have an intense color reaction indicating a positive test result. | ELISA is used in many laboratories to determine whether a particular antibody (e.g., anti-HIV) is present in a patient's blood sample. Both the sensitivity and the specificity of ELISA approach 100%, but both false-positive and false-negative results do occur. |

Modes of inheritance

Autosomal dominant

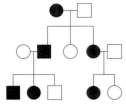

Often due to defects in structural genes. Many generations, both male and female, affected.

Often pleiotropic and, in many cases, present clinically after puberty. Family history crucial to diagnosis.

Autosomal recessive

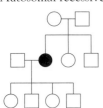

25% of offspring from 2 carrier parents are affected. Often due to enzyme deficiencies. Usually seen in only 1 generation.

Commonly more severe than dominant disorders; patients often present in childhood.

X-linked recessive

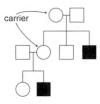

Sons of heterozygous mothers have a 50% chance of being affected. No male-to-male transmission.

Commonly more severe in males. Heterozygous females may be affected.

Mitochondrial inheritance

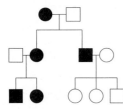

Transmitted only through mother. All offspring of affected females may show signs of disease.

Leber's hereditary optic neuropathy; mitochondrial myopathies.

Genetic terms

Variable expression	Nature and severity of the phenotype varies from 1 individual to another.
Incomplete penetrance	Not all individuals with a mutant genotype show the mutant phenotype.
Pleiotropy	1 gene has > 1 effect on an individual's phenotype.
Imprinting	Differences in phenotype depend on whether the mutation is of maternal or paternal origin (e.g., Angelman's syndrome [maternal], Prader-Willi syndrome [paternal]).
Anticipation	Severity of disease worsens or age of onset of disease is earlier in succeeding generations (e.g., Huntington's disease).
Loss of heterozygosity	If a patient inherits or develops a mutation in a tumor suppressor gene, the complementary allele must be deleted/mutated before cancer develops. This is not true of oncogenes.
Dominant negative mutation	Exerts a **dominant** effect because the body cannot produce enough of the normal gene product with only 1 allele functioning normally (e.g., COL1A1 gene mutation associated with osteogenesis imperfecta).
Linkage disequilibrium	Tendency for certain alleles at 2 linked loci to occur together more often than expected by chance. Measured in a population, not in a family, and often varies in different populations.

Hardy-Weinberg population genetics

If a population is in Hardy-Weinberg equilibrium, then:

$$p^2 + 2pq + q^2 = 1$$
$$p + q = 1$$

p and q are separate alleles; 2pq = heterozygote prevalence.

Hardy-Weinberg law assumes:

1. There is no mutation occurring at the locus
2. There is no selection for any of the genotypes at the locus
3. Mating is completely random
4. There is no migration into or out of the population being considered

Genetic errors

Disorder	Phenotype	Genetic mechanism	Prevalence
Down syndrome	Mental and growth retardation, dysmorphic features, internal organ anomalies	Chromosomal imbalance caused by trisomy 21	≈ 1:800; ↑ risk with advanced maternal age
Fragile X–associated mental retardation	Mental retardation, characteristic facial features, large testes	X-linked; progressive expansion of unstable DNA causes failure to express gene-encoding RNA-binding protein	≈ 1:1500 males; can be manifest in females; multistep mechanism
Sickle cell anemia	Recurrent painful crises, ↑ susceptibility to infections	Autosomal recessive; caused by a single missense mutation in β globin	≈ 1:400 African-Americans
Cystic fibrosis	Recurrent pulmonary infections, exocrine pancreatic insufficiency, infertility	Autosomal recessive; caused by multiple loss-of-function mutations in a chloride channel	≈ 1:2000 whites; very rare in Asians
Neurofibromatosis	Multiple café-au-lait spots, neurofibromas, ↑ tumor susceptibility	Autosomal dominant; caused by multiple loss-of-function mutations in a signaling molecule	≈ 1:3000; about 50% are new mutations
Duchenne's muscular dystrophy	Muscular weakness and degeneration	X-linked recessive; caused by multiple loss-of-function mutations in a muscle protein	≈ 1:3000; about 33% are new mutations
Osteogenesis imperfecta	↑ susceptibility to fractures, connective tissue fragility	Phenotypically and genetically heterogeneous	≈ 1:10,000
Phenylketonuria	Mental and growth retardation	Autosomal recessive; caused by multiple loss-of-function mutations in phenylalanine hydroxylase	≈ 1:10,000

(Adapted, with permission, from McPhee S et al. *Pathophysiology of Disease: An Introduction to Clinical Medicine,* 3rd ed. New York: McGraw-Hill, 2000:7.)

HIGH-YIELD FACTS

Biochemistry

Lysosomal storage diseases

Each is caused by a deficiency in one of the many lysosomal enzymes.

Fabry's disease	Caused by deficiency of α-galactosidase A, resulting in accumulation of ceramide trihexoside. Finding: renal failure. *Bio.48*	X-linked recessive.
Krabbe's disease	Absence of galactosylceramide β-galactosidase leads to the accumulation of galactocerebroside in the brain. Optic atrophy, spasticity, early death. *Bio.61*	Autosomal recessive.
Gaucher's disease	Caused by deficiency of β-glucocerebrosidase, leading to glucocerebroside accumulation in brain, liver, spleen, and bone marrow (Gaucher's cells with characteristic "crinkled paper" enlarged cytoplasm). Type I, the more common form, is compatible with a normal life span. *Bio.54*	Autosomal recessive.
Niemann-Pick disease	Deficiency of sphingomyelinase causes buildup of **sphingo**myelin and cholesterol in reticuloendothelial and parenchymal cells and tissues. Patients die by age 3. *Bio.65*	Autosomal recessive. No **man PICK**s (Niemann-**PICK**) his nose with his **sphing**er.
Tay-Sachs disease	Absence of hexosaminidase A results in GM_2 ganglioside accumulation. Death occurs by age 3. Cherry-red spot visible on macula. Carrier rate is 1 in 30 in Jews of European descent (1 in 300 for others). *Bio.72*	Autosomal recessive. **Tay-saX** lacks he**X**osaminidase.
Metachromatic leukodystrophy	Deficiency of arylsulfatase A results in the accumulation of sulfatide in the brain, kidney, liver, and peripheral nerves. *Bio.64*	Autosomal recessive.
Hurler's syndrome	Deficiency of α-L-iduronidase results in corneal clouding and mental retardation. *Bio.58*	Autosomal recessive.
Hunter's syndrome	Deficiency of iduronate sulfatase. Mild form of Hurler's with no corneal clouding and mild mental retardation. *Bio.57*	X-linked recessive. Hunters aim for the **X.**

UCV

Enzyme kinetics

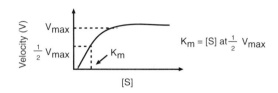

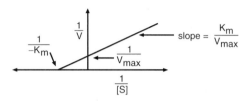

$$K_m = [S] \text{ at } \tfrac{1}{2} V_{max}$$

$$\text{slope} = \frac{K_m}{V_{max}}$$

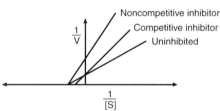

The lower the K_m, the higher the affinity.

Competitive inhibitors: Resemble substrates; bind reversibly to active sites of enzymes. High substrate concentration overcomes effect of inhibitor. V_{max} remains unchanged; K_m ↑ compared to uninhibited.

Noncompetitive inhibitors: Do not resemble substrate; bind to enzyme but not necessarily at active site. Inhibition cannot be overcome by high substrate concentration. V_{max} ↓; K_m remains unchanged compared to uninhibited.

HINT: Competitive inhibitors cross each other competitively, while noncompetitive inhibitors don't.

Enzyme regulation methods

Enzyme concentration alteration (synthesis and/or destruction), covalent modification (e.g., phosphorylation), proteolytic modification (zymogen), allosteric regulation (e.g., feedback inhibition), and transcriptional regulation (e.g., steroid hormones).

Cell cycle phases

M (mitosis: prophase–metaphase–anaphase–telophase)

G_1 (growth)

S (synthesis of DNA)

G_2 (growth)

G_0 (quiescent G_1 phase)

G_1 and G_0 are of variable duration. Mitosis is usually shortest phase. Most cells are in G_0.

Rapidly dividing cells have a shorter G_1.

G stands for Gap or Growth; S for Synthesis.

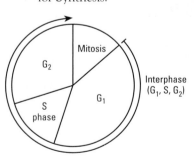

Plasma membrane composition

Plasma membranes contain cholesterol ($\approx 50\%$, promotes membrane stability), phospholipids ($\approx 50\%$), sphingolipids, glycolipids, and proteins. Only noncytoplasmic side of membrane contains glycosylated lipids or proteins (i.e., the plasma membrane is an asymmetric, fluid bilayer).

Phosphatidylcholine function

Phosphatidylcholine (lecithin) is a major component of RBC membranes, of myelin, of bile, and of surfactant (DPPC—dipalmitoyl phosphatidylcholine). Also used in esterification of cholesterol.

Sodium pump

Na^+-K^+ATPase is located in the plasma membrane with ATP site on cytoplasmic side. For each ATP consumed, 3 Na^+ go out and 2 K^+ come in. During cycle, pump is phosphorylated. Ouabain inhibits by binding to K^+ site. Cardiac glycosides (digoxin, digitoxin) also inhibit the Na^+-K^+ATPase, causing ↑ cardiac contractility.

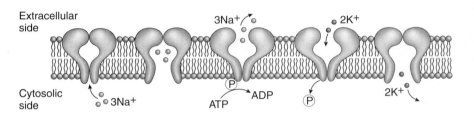

G-protein-linked 2nd messengers

Receptor	G-protein class	Major functions
α_1	q	↑ vascular smooth muscle contraction
α_2	i	↓ sympathetic outflow, ↓ insulin release
β_1	s	↑ heart rate, ↑ contractility, ↑ renin release, ↑ lipolysis, ↑ aqueous humor formation
β_2	s	Vasodilation, bronchodilation, ↑ glucagon release
M_1	q	CNS
M_2	i	↓ heart rate
M_3	q	↑ exocrine gland secretions
D_1	s	Relaxes renal vascular smooth muscle
D_2	i	Modulates transmitter release, especially in brain
H_1	q	↑ nasal and bronchial mucus production, contraction of bronchioles, pruritus, and pain
H_2	s	↑ gastric acid secretion
V_1	q	↑ vascular smooth muscle contraction
V_2	s	↑ H_2O permeability and reabsorption in the collecting tubules of the kidney

$\alpha_1, M_1, M_3,$ H_1, V_1 Receptor $\xrightarrow{G_q}$ Phospholipase C $\longrightarrow$ Lipids ↓ PIP_2 $\longrightarrow$ IP_3 $\longrightarrow$ ↑ $[Ca^{2+}]_{in}$; DAG $\longrightarrow$ Protein kinase C

$\beta_1, \beta_2, D_1,$ H_2, V_2 Receptor $\xrightarrow{G_s}$ Adenylcyclase $\longrightarrow$ ATP ↓ cAMP $\longrightarrow$ Protein kinase A

α_2, M_2, D_2 Receptor $\xrightarrow{G_i}$ Adenylcyclase $\longrightarrow$ cAMP ↓ $\longrightarrow$ Protein kinase A ↓

Arachidonic acid products	Phospholipase A_2 liberates arachidonic acid from cell membrane.	
	Lipoxygenase pathway yields Leukotrienes.	**L** for **L**ipoxygenase and **L**eukotriene.
	LT B_4 is a neutrophil chemotactic agent.	
	LT C_4, D_4, and E_4 (SRS-A) function in bronchoconstriction, vasoconstriction, contraction of smooth muscle, and increased vascular permeability.	
	Cyclooxygenase pathway yields thromboxanes, prostaglandins, and prostacyclin.	
	Tx A_2 stimulates platelet aggregation and vasoconstriction.	
	PGI$_2$ inhibits platelet aggregation and promotes vasodilation.	**P**latelet-**G**athering **I**nhibitor.

Microtubule	Cylindrical structure 24 nm in diameter and of variable length. A helical array of polymerized dimers of α- and β-tubulin (13 per circumference). Each dimer has 2 GTP bound. Incorporated into flagella, cilia, mitotic spindles. Grows slowly, collapses quickly. Microtubules are also involved in slow axoplasmic transport in neurons.	Drugs that act on microtubules: Mebendazole/thiabendazole (antihelminthic) Taxol (anti–breast cancer) Griseofulvin (antifungal) Vincristine/vinblastine (anti-cancer) Colchicine (anti-gout)

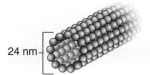
24 nm

Collagen synthesis and structure	Hydroxylation of specific prolyl and lysyl residues in the endoplasmic reticulum requires vitamin C.
	Procollagen molecules are exocytosed into extracellular space. Procollagen peptidases cleave terminal regions of procollagen, transforming procollagen into insoluble tropocollagen, which aggregates to form collagen fibrils.
	Fibrillar structure is reinforced by the formation of covalent lysine-hydroxylysine cross-links between tropocollagen molecules.
	Collagen fibril—many staggered collagen molecules (linked by lysyl oxidase). Collagen molecule—3 collagen α chains (usually Gly-X-Y, X and Y—proline, hydroxyproline, or hydroxylysine).

Ehlers-Danlos syndrome	Faulty collagen synthesis causing:
	1. Hyperextensible skin
	2. Tendency to bleed
	3. Hypermobile joints
	10 types. Inheritance varies from autosomal dominant (type IV) to autosomal recessive (type VI) to X-linked recessive (type IX).

Osteogenesis imperfecta

Clinically characterized by **multiple fractures** occurring with minimal trauma (brittle bone disease), which may occur during the birth process, as well as by **blue sclerae** due to the translucency of the connective tissue over the choroid. Caused by a variety of gene defects resulting in abnormal collagen synthesis.

The most common form is autosomal dominant with abnormal collagen type I synthesis.

May be confused with child abuse.

UCV *Bio.89*

Sphingolipid components

Components of nerve tissue. See lysosomal storage diseases.

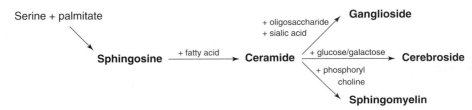

Serine + palmitate

Sphingosine — + fatty acid → Ceramide

+ oligosaccharide / + sialic acid → **Ganglioside**

+ glucose/galactose → **Cerebroside**

+ phosphoryl choline

→ **Sphingomyelin**

ATP

Base (adenine), ribose, 3 phosphoryls. 2 phosphoanhydride bonds, 7 kcal/mol each.
Aerobic metabolism of glucose produces 38 ATP via malate shuttle, 36 ATP via G3P shuttle.
Anaerobic glycolysis produces only 2 ATP per glucose molecule.
ATP hydrolysis can be coupled to energetically unfavorable reactions.

Activated carriers

Phosphoryl (ATP)
Electrons (NADH, NADPH, $FADH_2$)
Acyl (coenzyme A, lipoamide)
CO_2 (biotin)
1-carbon units (tetrahydrofolates)
CH_3 groups (SAM)
Aldehydes (TPP)
Glucose (UDP-glucose)
Choline (CDP-choline)

HIGH-YIELD FACTS

Biochemistry

| **S-adenosyl-methionine** | ATP + methionine → **SAM.** SAM transfers methyl units to a wide variety of acceptors (e.g., in synthesis of phosphocreatine, a high-energy phosphate active in muscle ATP production). Regeneration of methionine (and thus SAM) is dependent on vitamin B_{12}. | **SAM** the methyl donor man. |

| **Signal molecule precursors** | ATP → cAMP via adenylate cyclase.
 GTP → cGMP via guanylate cyclase.
 Glutamate → GABA via glutamate decarboxylase (requires vitamin B_6).
 Choline → ACh via choline acetyltransferase (ChAT).
 Arachidonate → prostaglandins, thromboxanes, leukotrienes via cyclooxygenase/ lipoxygenase.
 Fructose-6-P → fructose-1,6-bis-P via phosphofructokinase (PFK), the rate-limiting enzyme of glycolysis.
 1,3-BPG → 2,3-BPG via bisphosphoglycerate mutase. | |

| **NAD⁺/NADPH** | **NAD⁺** is generally used in **catabolic** processes to carry reducing equivalents away as NADH. **NADPH** is used in **anabolic** processes as a supply of reducing equivalents. | NADPH is a product of the HMP shunt and the malate dehydrogenase reaction.
 NADPH is used in:
 1. Anabolic processes
 2. Respiratory burst
 3. P450 |

Oxygen-dependent respiratory burst

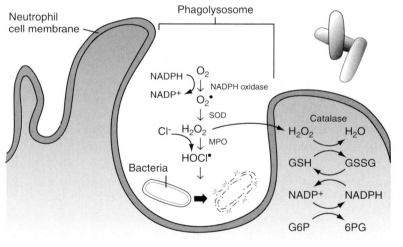

SOD = superoxide dismutase
MPO = myeloperoxidase
G6P = glucose-6-phosphate dehydrogenase

GSH/GSSG = glutathione (reduced/oxidized)
HOCl• = bleach

| **Hexokinase vs. glucokinase** | Hexokinase is found throughout body.
 Glucokinase (lower affinity [$\uparrow K_m$] but higher capacity [$\uparrow V_{max}$]) is predominantly found in the liver. | Only hexokinase is feedback inhibited by G6P. |

HIGH-YIELD FACTS

Biochemistry

Glycolysis regulation, irreversible enzymes

D-glucose $\xrightarrow{\text{Hexokinase/glucokinase*}}$ Glucose-6-phosphate

Glucose-6-P $\ominus$

Fructose-6-P $\xrightarrow[\substack{\text{Phosphofructokinase}\\\text{(rate-limiting step)}}]{}$ Fructose-1,6-BP

ATP $\ominus$, AMP $\oplus$, citrate $\ominus$, fructose-2,6-BP $\oplus$

Phosphoenolpyruvate $\xrightarrow{\text{Pyruvate kinase}}$ Pyruvate

ATP $\ominus$, alanine $\ominus$, fructose-1,6-BP $\oplus$

Pyruvate $\xrightarrow[\substack{\text{Pyruvate}\\\text{dehydrogenase}}]{}$ Acetyl-CoA

ATP $\ominus$, NADH $\ominus$, acetyl-CoA $\ominus$.

* Glucokinase in liver; hexokinase in all other tissues.

Glycolytic enzyme deficiency

Hexokinase, glucose phosphate isomerase, aldolase, triosephosphate isomerase, phosphate glycerate kinase, enolase, and pyruvate kinase deficiencies are associated with hemolytic anemia.

RBCs metabolize glucose anaerobically (no mitochondria) and thus depend solely on glycolysis.

Pyruvate dehydrogenase complex

The complex contains 3 enzymes that require 5 cofactors: pyrophosphate (from thiamine), lipoic acid, CoA (from pantothenate), FAD (riboflavin), NAD (niacin).

Reaction: pyruvate + NAD$^+$ + CoA $\rightarrow$ acetyl-CoA + CO_2 + NADH.

The complex is similar to the α-ketoglutarate dehydrogenase complex (same cofactors, similar substrate and action).

Cofactors are the first 4 B vitamins plus lipoic acid:
  B$_1$ (thiamine; TPP)
  B$_2$ (FAD)
  B$_3$ (NAD)
  B$_5$ (pantothenate $\rightarrow$ CoA)
  Lipoic acid

Pyruvate dehydrogenase deficiency

Causes backup of substrate (pyruvate and alanine), resulting in lactic acidosis. Can be seen in alcoholics due to B$_1$ deficiency.

Findings: neurologic defects.

Treatment: $\uparrow$ intake of ketogenic nutrients (e.g., high fat content).

Lysine and Leucine—the only purely ketogenic amino acids.

Pyruvate metabolism

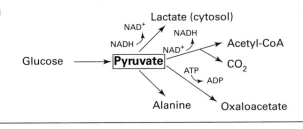

6 ATP equivalents are needed to generate glucose from pyruvate.

Cori cycle

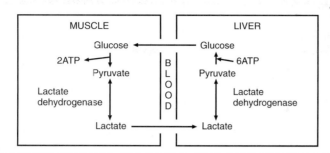

Transfers excess reducing equivalents from RBCs and muscle to liver, allowing muscle to function anaerobically (net 2 ATP).

TCA cycle

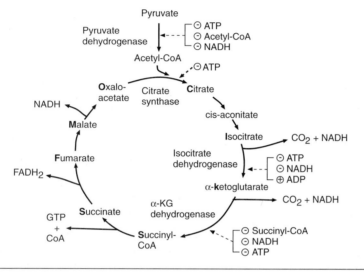

Produces 3 NADH, 1 FADH$_2$, 2 CO$_2$, 1 GTP per acetyl CoA = 12 ATP/acetyl-CoA (2× everything per glucose)

α-ketoglutarate dehydrogenase complex requires same cofactors as the pyruvate dehydrogenase complex.

Cindy **I**s **K**inky **S**o **S**he **F**ornicates **M**ore **O**ften.

Electron transport chain and oxidative phosphorylation

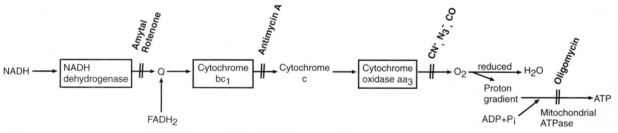

Electron transport chain

1 NADH → 3 ATP; 1 FADH$_2$ → 2 ATP

Oxidative phosphorylation poisons

1. Electron transport inhibitors (rotenone, antimycin A, CN$^-$, CO) directly inhibit electron transport, causing a ↓ of proton gradient and block of ATP synthesis.
2. ATPase inhibitor (oligomycin) directly inhibits mitochondrial ATPase, causing an ↑ of proton gradient, but no ATP is produced because electron transport stops.
3. Uncoupling agents (2,4-DNP) increase permeability of membrane, causing a ↓ of proton gradient and ↑ oxygen consumption. ATP synthesis stops. Electron transport continues.

HIGH-YIELD FACTS

Biochemistry

Gluconeogenesis, irreversible enzymes

Pyruvate carboxylase	In mitochondria. Pyruvate → oxaloacetate.	Requires biotin, ATP. Activated by acetyl-CoA.
PEP carboxykinase	In cytosol. Oxaloacetate → phosphoenolpyruvate.	Requires GTP.
Fructose-1,6-bisphosphatase	In cytosol. Fructose-1,6-bisphosphate → fructose-6-P.	**P**athway **P**roduces **F**resh **G**lucose.
Glucose-6-phosphatase	In cytosol. Glucose-6-P → glucose.	

Above enzymes found only in liver, kidney, intestinal epithelium. Muscle cannot participate in gluconeogenesis.

Hypoglycemia is caused by a deficiency of these key gluconeogenic enzymes listed above (e.g., von Gierke's disease, which is caused by a lack of glucose-6-phosphatase in the liver).

UCV *Bio.68, 73*

Pentose phosphate pathway (HMP shunt)

Produces ribose-5-P from G6P for nucleotide synthesis.

Produces NADPH from NADP⁺ for fatty acid and steroid biosynthesis and for maintaining reduced glutathione inside RBCs.

All reactions of this pathway occur in the cytoplasm.

Sites: lactating mammary glands, liver, adrenal cortex—all sites of fatty acid or steroid synthesis.

Glucose-6-phosphate dehydrogenase deficiency

G6PD is a rate-limiting enzyme in HMP shunt (which yields NADPH). NADPH is necessary to keep glutathione reduced, which in turn detoxifies free radicals and peroxides. ↓ NADPH in RBCs leads to **hemolytic anemia** due to poor RBC defense against oxidizing agents (fava beans, sulfonamides, primaquine) and antituberculosis drugs. X-linked recessive disorder.

G6PD deficiency is more prevalent among blacks.

Heinz bodies—altered Hemoglobin precipitates within RBCs.

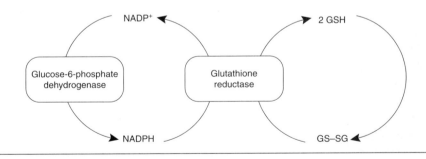

UCV *Bio.78*

Disorders of fructose metabolism

Fructose intolerance	Hereditary deficiency of aldolase B (recessive). Fructose-1-phosphate accumulates, causing a ↓ in available phosphate, which results in inhibition of glycogenolysis and gluconeogenesis.
	Symptoms: hypoglycemia, jaundice, cirrhosis.
	Treatment: must ↓ intake of both fructose and sucrose (glucose + fructose).
Essential fructosuria	Involves a defect in fructokinase and is a benign, asymptomatic condition.
	Symptoms: fructose appears in blood and urine.

FRUCTOSE METABOLISM (LIVER)

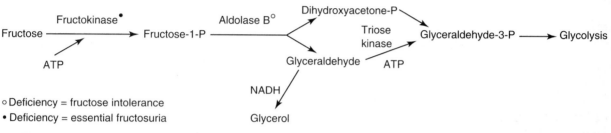

○ Deficiency = fructose intolerance
● Deficiency = essential fructosuria

UCV Bio.55

Disorders of galactose metabolism

Galactosemia	Absence of galactose-1-phosphate uridyltransferase. Autosomal recessive. Damage is caused by accumulation of toxic substances (including galactitol) rather than absence of an essential compound.
	Symptoms: cataracts, hepatosplenomegaly, mental retardation.
	Treatment: exclude galactose and lactose (galactose + glucose) from diet.
Galactokinase deficiency	Causes galactosemia and galactosuria, galactitol accumulation if galactose is present in diet.

GALACTOSE METABOLISM

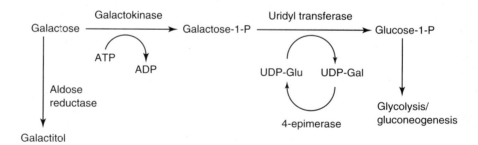

Lactase deficiency	Age-dependent and/or hereditary lactose intolerance (blacks, Asians).
	Symptoms: bloating, cramps, osmotic diarrhea.
	Treatment: avoid milk or add lactase pills to diet.

Essential amino acids	Ketogenic: Leu, Lys.	All essential amino acids:
	Glucogenic/ketogenic: Ile, Phe, Trp.	**PriVaTe TIM HALL.**
	Glucogenic: Met, Thr, Val, Arg, His.	Arg and His are required during periods of growth.

Acidic and basic amino acids

At body pH (7.4), acidic amino acids Asp and Glu are negatively charged; basic amino acids Arg and Lys are positively charged. Basic amino acid His at pH 7.4 has no net charge.

Arginine is the most basic amino acid. Arg and Lys are found in high amounts in histones, which bind to negatively charged DNA.

Asp = aspartic ACID, Glu = glutamic ACID.
Arg and Lys have an extra NH_3 group.

Transport of ammonium by alanine and glutamine

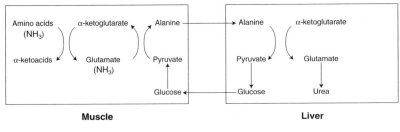

Muscle **Liver**

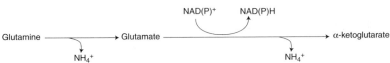

Urea cycle

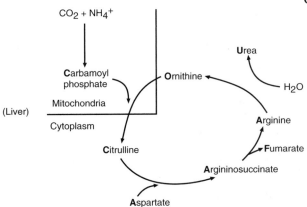

Ordinarily, Careless Crappers Are Also Frivolous About Urination.

Amino acid derivatives

Phenylalanine ⟶ Tyrosine ⟶ Thyroxine

Tyrosine ⟶ Dopa ⟶ Dopamine ⟶ NE ⟶ Epi

Dopamine ⟶ Melanin

Tryptophan ⟶ Niacin ⟶ NAD⁺/NADP⁺

Tryptophan ⟶ Serotonin

Tryptophan ⟶ Melatonin

Histidine ⟶ Histamine

Glycine ⟶ Porphyrin ⟶ Heme

Arginine ⟶ Creatine

Arginine ⟶ Urea

Arginine ⟶ Nitric oxide

Phenylketonuria UCV Bio.67	Normally, phenylalanine is converted into tyrosine (nonessential aa). In PKU, there is ↓ phenylalanine hydroxylase or ↓ tetrahydrobiopterin cofactor. Tyrosine becomes essential and phenylalanine builds up, leading to excess phenylketones. Findings: mental retardation, fair skin, eczema, musty body odor. Treatment: ↓ phenylalanine (contained in Nutrasweet) and ↑ tyrosine in diet.	Screened for at birth. Phenylketones—phenylacetate, phenyllactate, and phenylpyruvate in urine.
Alkaptonuria UCV Bio.44	Congenital deficiency of homogentisic acid oxidase in the degradative pathway of tyrosine. Resulting alkapton bodies cause **dark urine.** Also, the connective tissue is dark. Benign disease. May have arthralgias.	
Albinism UCV Bio.43	Congenital deficiency of tyrosinase. Results in an inability to synthesize melanin from tyrosine. Can result from a lack of migration of neural crest cells.	Lack of melanin results in an ↑ risk of skin cancer.
Homocystinuria UCV Bio.56	Defect in cystathionine synthase and/or methionine synthase. 2 forms: 1. Deficiency (treatment: ↓ Met and ↑ Cys in diet) 2. ↓ affinity of synthase for pyridoxal phosphate (treatment: ↑↑ vitamin B_6 in diet)	Results in excess homocystine in the urine. Cysteine becomes essential. Can cause mental retardation, osteoporosis, and lens dislocation.
Cystinuria UCV Bio.46	Common (1/7000) inherited defect of tubular amino acid transporter for **C**ystine, **O**rnithine, **L**ysine, and **A**rginine in kidneys. Excess cystine in urine can lead to the precipitation of cystine kidney stones.	**COLA.** Treat with acetazolamide to alkalinize the urine.

Maple syrup urine disease

Blocked degradation of **branched** amino acids (Ile, Val, Leu) due to ↓ α-ketoacid dehydrogenase.
Causes severe CNS defects, mental retardation, and death.

Urine smells like maple syrup.
I Love **V**ermont maple syrup.

UCV *Bio.63*

Purine salvage deficiencies

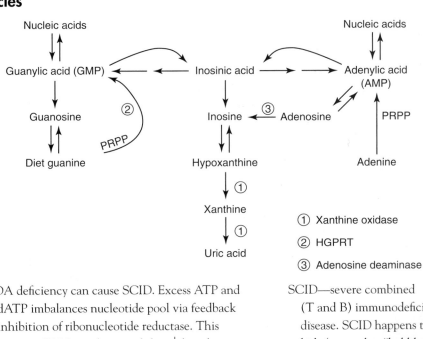

① Xanthine oxidase
② HGPRT
③ Adenosine deaminase

Adenosine deaminase deficiency	ADA deficiency can cause SCID. Excess ATP and dATP imbalances nucleotide pool via feedback inhibition of ribonucleotide reductase. This prevents DNA synthesis and thus ↓ lymphocyte count. 1st disease to be treated by experimental human gene therapy.	SCID—severe combined (T and B) immunodeficiency disease. SCID happens to kids (remember "bubble boy").
Lesch-Nyhan syndrome	Purine salvage problem owing to absence of HGPRTase, which converts hypoxanthine to inosine monophosphate (IMP) and guanine to guanosine monophosphate (GMP). X-linked recessive. Results in excess uric acid production. Findings: retardation, self-mutilation, aggression, hyperuricemia, gout, and choreoathetosis.	**LNS**—**L**acks **N**ucleotide **S**alvage (purine).

UCV *Bio.62*

Fatty acid metabolism sites

Fatty acid synthesis = cytosol.
Fatty acid degradation = mitochondria.
Fatty acid entry into mitochondrion is via carnitine shuttle (inhibited by cytoplasmic malonyl-CoA).
Fatty acid entry into cytosol is via citrate shuttle.

Fatty acid degradation occurs where its products will be consumed—in the mitochondrion.

Liver: fed state vs. fasting state

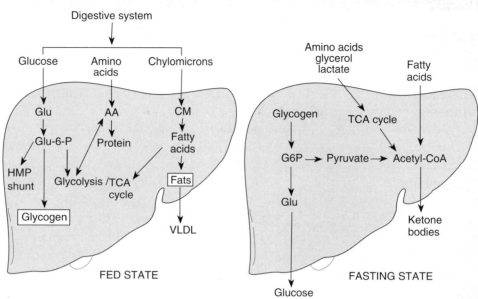

Glycogen storage diseases

12 types, all resulting in abnormal glycogen metabolism and an accumulation of glycogen within cells.

Type I	Von Gierke's disease—glucose-6-phosphatase deficiency. Findings: severe fasting hypoglycemia, ↑↑ glycogen in liver. *Bio.73*	The liver becomes a muscle. (Think about it.)
Type II	Pompe's disease—lysosomal α-1,4-glucosidase deficiency. Findings: cardiomegaly and systemic findings, leading to early death. *Bio.69*	Pompe's trashes the Pump (heart, liver, and muscle).
Type III	Cori's—deficiency of debranching enzyme α-1,6-glucosidase.	
Type V	McArdle's disease—skeletal muscle glycogen phosphorylase deficiency. Findings: ↑ glycogen in muscle but cannot break it down, leading to painful cramps, myoglobinuria with strenuous exercise.	McArdle's: Muscle. Very Poor Carbohydrate Metabolism.

UCV

Ketone bodies

In liver: fatty acid and amino acids → acetoacetate + β-hydroxybutyrate (to be used in muscle and brain). Ketone bodies found in prolonged starvation and diabetic ketoacidosis. Excreted in urine. Made from HMG-CoA. Ketone bodies are metabolized by the brain to 2 molecules of acetyl-CoA.

Breath smells like acetone (fruity odor). Urine test for ketones does not detect β-hydroxybutyrate (favored by high redox state).

UCV *Bio.8*

Insulin

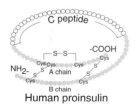

Made in β cells of pancreas. No effect on glucose uptake by brain, RBCs, and hepatocytes. Required for adipose and skeletal muscle uptake of glucose. GLUT2 receptors are found in β cells and GLUT4 in muscle and fat. Inhibits glucagon release by α cells of pancreas. Serum C-peptide is not present with exogenous insulin intake.

Brain, liver, and RBCs take up glucose independent of insulin. Insulin moves glucose Into cells.

Insulin vs. glucagon

Glucagon phosphorylates stuff → turns glycogen synthase OFF and phosphorylase ON.
Insulin dephosphorylates stuff → turns glycogen synthase ON and phosphorylase OFF.

Cholesterol synthesis

Rate-limiting step is catalyzed by HMG-CoA reductase, which converts HMG-CoA to mevalonate.
⅔ of plasma cholesterol is esterified by lecithin-cholesterol acyltransferase (LCAT).

Lovastatin inhibits HMG-CoA reductase.

Lipoproteins

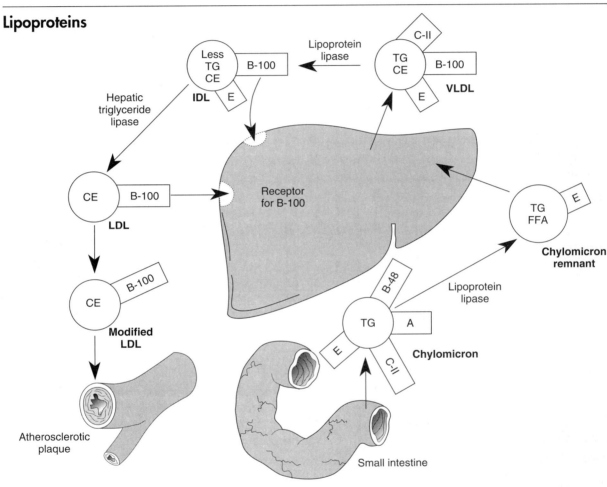

TG = triglyceride, CE = cholesterol, FFA = free fatty acid

Lipoprotein lipase—fatty acid uptake into cells from chylomicrons and VLDLs.
Hormone-sensitive lipase—degradation of stored triacylglycerols.

Major apolipoproteins

A-I: **A**ctivates LCAT.
B-100: **B**inds to LDL receptor.
C-II: **C**ofactor for lipoprotein lipase.
E: Mediates **E**xtra (remnant) uptake.

Lipoprotein functions

	Function and route	Apolipoproteins
Chylomicron	Delivers dietary triglycerides to peripheral tissues and dietary cholesterol to liver. Secreted by intestinal epithelial cells. Excess causes pancreatitis, lipemia retinalis, and eruptive xanthomas.	B-48 mediates secretion. A's are used for formation of new HDL. C-II activates lipoprotein lipase. E mediates remnant uptake by liver.
VLDL	Delivers hepatic triglycerides to peripheral tissues. Secreted by liver. Excess causes pancreatitis.	B-100 mediates secretion. C-II activates lipoprotein lipase. E mediates remnant uptake by liver.
LDL	Delivers hepatic cholesterol to peripheral tissues. Formed by lipoprotein lipase modification of VLDL in the peripheral tissue. Taken up by target cells via receptor-mediated endocytosis. Excess causes atherosclerosis, xanthomas, and arcus corneae.	B-100 mediates binding to cell surface receptor for endocytosis.
HDL	Mediates centripetal transport of cholesterol (reverse cholesterol transport, from periphery to liver). Acts as a repository for apoC and apoE (which are needed for chylomicron and VLDL metabolism). Secreted from both liver and intestine.	A's help form HDL structure. A-I in particular activates LCAT (which catalyzes esterification of cholesterol). CETP mediates transfer of cholesteryl esters to other lipoprotein particles.
	LDL and HDL carry most cholesterol. LDL transports cholesterol from liver to tissue; HDL transports it from periphery to liver.	HDL is Healthy. LDL is Lousy.

Familial hyper-cholesterolemia (IIa)

Autosomal-dominant genetic defect in LDL receptor resulting in xanthomas and earlier onset of atherosclerosis. Homozygotes can have MIs by age 30.

Metabolism sites

Mitochondria	Fatty acid oxidation (β-oxidation), acetyl-CoA production, Krebs cycle.
Cytoplasm	Glycolysis, fatty acid synthesis, HMP shunt, protein synthesis (RER), steroid synthesis (SER).
Both	Gluconeogenesis, urea cycle, heme synthesis.

Regulation of metabolic pathways

Pathway	Major Regulatory Enzyme(s)	Activator	Inhibitor	Effector Hormone	Remarks
Citric acid cycle	Citrate synthase		ATP, long-chain acyl-CoA		Regulated mainly by the need for ATP and therefore by the supply of NAD^+
Glycolysis and pyruvate oxidation	Phosphofructokinase	AMP, fructose-2,6-bisphosphate in liver, fructose-1,6-bisphosphate in muscle	Citrate (fatty acids, ketone bodies), ATP, cAMP	Glucagon ↓	Induced by insulin
	Pyruvate dehydrogenase	CoA, NAD, ADP, pyruvate	Acetyl-CoA, NADH, ATP (fatty acids, ketone bodies)	Insulin ↑ (in adipose tissue)	Also important in regulating the citric acid cycle
Gluconeogenesis	Pyruvate carboxylase Phosphoenolpyruvate carboxykinase	Acetyl-CoA	ADP		Induced by glucocorticoids, glucagon, cAMP
	Fructose-1,6-bisphosphatase	cAMP	AMP, fructose-2,6-bisphosphate	Glucagon	Suppressed by insulin
Glycogenesis	Glycogen synthase		Phosphorylase (in liver) cAMP, Ca^{2+} (muscle)	Insulin ↑ Glucagon ↓ (liver) Epinephrine ↓	Induced by insulin
Glycogenolysis	Phosphorylase	cAMP, Ca^{2+} (muscle)		Insulin ↓ Glucagon ↑ (liver) Epinephrine ↑	
Pentose phosphate pathway	Glucose-6-phosphate dehydrogenase	$NADP^+$	NADPH		Induced by insulin
Lipogenesis	Acetyl-CoA carboxylase	Citrate	Long-chain acyl-CoA, cAMP	Insulin ↑ Glucagon ↓ (liver)	Induced by insulin
Cholesterol synthesis	HMG-CoA reductase		Cholesterol, cAMP	Insulin ↑ Glucagon ↓ (liver)	Inhibited by certain drugs, e.g., lovastatin

Metabolism in major organs

Organ	Major Function	Major Pathways	Main Substrates	Major Products	Specialist Enzymes
Liver	Service for the other organs and tissues	Most represented, including gluconeogenesis; β-oxidation; ketogenesis; lipoprotein formation; urea, uric acid, and bile acid formation; cholesterol synthesis	Free fatty acids, glucose (well fed), lactate, glycerol, fructose, amino acids (Ethanol)	Glucose, VLDL (triacylglycerol), HDL, ketone bodies, urea, uric acid, bile acids, plasma proteins (Acetate)	Glucokinase, glucose-6-phosphatase, glycerol kinase, phosphoenolpyruvate carboxykinase, fructokinase, arginase, HMG-CoA synthase and lyase, 7α-hydroxylase
Brain	Coordination of the nervous system	Glycolysis, amino acid metabolism	Glucose (main substrate), amino acids, ketone bodies (in starvation) Polyunsaturated fatty acids in neonate	Lactate	
Heart	Pumping of blood	Aerobic pathways, e.g., β-oxidation and citric acid cycle	Free fatty acids, lactate, ketone bodies, VLDL and chylomicron triacylglycerol, some glucose		Lipoprotein lipase Respiratory chain well developed
Adipose tissue	Storage and breakdown of triacylglycerol	Esterification of fatty acids and lipolysis	Glucose, lipoprotein triacylglycerol	Free fatty acids, glycerol	Lipoprotein lipase, hormone-sensitive lipase
Muscle Fast twitch Slow twitch	Rapid movement Sustained movement	Glycolysis Aerobic pathways, e.g., β-oxidation and citric acid cycle	Glucose Ketone bodies, triacylglycerol in VLDL and chylomicrons, free fatty acids	Lactate	Lipoprotein lipase Respiratory chain well developed

HIGH-YIELD FACTS

Biochemistry

Aminolevulinate (ALA) synthase	Rate-limiting step for heme synthesis. The end-product (heme) feedback inhibits this enzyme. Found in the mitochondria, where it converts succinyl-CoA and glycine to ALA.	
Heme synthesis UCV *Bio.42*	Occurs in the liver and bone marrow. Committed step is glycine + succinyl-CoA → δ-aminolevulinate. Catalyzed by ALA synthase. Accumulation of intermediates causes porphyrias. Lead inhibits ALA dehydratase and ferrochelatase, preventing incorporation of iron and causing anemia and porphyria.	Underproduction of heme causes microcytic hypochromic anemia.
Heme catabolism	Heme is scavenged from RBCs and Fe^{2+} is reused. Heme → biliverdin → bilirubin (sparingly water soluble, toxic to CNS, transported by albumin). Bilirubin is removed from blood by liver, conjugated with glucuronate, and excreted in bile. In the intestine it is processed into its excreted form. Some urobilinogen, an intestinal intermediate, is reabsorbed into blood and excreted as urobilin into urine.	
Hemoglobin	Hemoglobin is composed of 4 polypeptide subunits (2 α and 2 β) and exists in 2 forms: 1. T (taut) form has low affinity for oxygen. 2. R (relaxed) form has high affinity for oxygen (300×). Hemoglobin exhibits positive cooperativity and negative allostery (accounts for the sigmoid-shaped O_2 dissociation curve for hemoglobin), unlike myoglobin.	Carbon monoxide has a 200× greater affinity for hemoglobin than for oxygen.
Hb structure regulation	↑ Cl^-, H^+, CO_2, DPG, and temperature favor T form over **R** form (shifts dissociation curve to right, leading to ↑ O_2 unloading). T form has low affinity for O_2.	When you're **R**elaxed, you do your job better (carry O_2).
Methemoglobinemia UCV *Bio.81*	Iron in hemoglobin is in a reduced state (ferrous, Fe^{2+}). Methemoglobin is an oxidized form of hemoglobin (ferric, Fe^{3+}) that does not bind oxygen as readily.	
CO_2 transport in blood	CO_2 binds to amino acids in globin chain (at N terminus) but not to heme. CO_2 binding favors T (taut) form of hemoglobin (and thus promotes O_2 unloading).	CO_2 must be transported from tissue to lungs, the reverse of O_2.

Vitamins

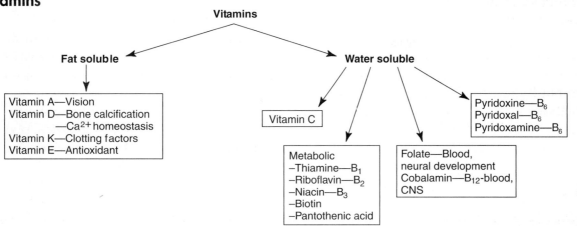

Vitamins: fat soluble	A, D, E, K. Absorption dependent on gut (ileum) and pancreas. Toxicity more common than for water-soluble vitamins, because these accumulate in fat.	Malabsorption syndromes (steatorrhea), such as cystic fibrosis and sprue, or mineral oil intake can cause fat-soluble vitamin deficiencies.
Vitamins: water soluble	B_1 (thiamine: TPP) B_2 (riboflavin: FAD, FMN) B_3 (niacin: NAD^+) B_5 (pantothenate: CoA) B_6 (pyridoxine: PP) B_{12} (cobalamin) C (ascorbic acid) Biotin Folate	All wash out easily from body except B_{12} (stored in liver). B-complex deficiencies often result in dermatitis, glossitis, and diarrhea.

Vitamin A (retinol)

Deficiency	Night blindness and dry skin. .	Retinol is vitamin A, so think Retin-A (used topically for wrinkles and acne).
Function	Constituent of visual pigments (retinal).	
Excess	Arthralgias, fatigue, headaches, skin changes, sore throat, alopecia.	

UCV *Bio.32*

Vitamin B_1 (thiamine)

Deficiency	Beriberi and Wernicke-Korsakoff syndrome. Seen in alcoholism and malnutrition.	Beriberi characterized by polyneuritis, cardiac pathology, and edema. Spell beriberi as **Ber1Ber1.**
Function	In thiamine pyrophosphate, a cofactor for oxidative decarboxylation of α-keto acids (pyruvate, α-ketoglutarate) and a cofactor for transketolase in the HMP shunt.	Wet beriberi may lead to high-output cardiac failure (dilated cardiomyopathy).

UCV *Bio.33*

HIGH-YIELD FACTS

Biochemistry

Vitamin B$_2$ (riboflavin)

Deficiency	Angular stomatitis, **C**heilosis, **C**orneal vascularization.	The 2 **C**'s.
Function	Cofactor in oxidation and reduction (e.g., FADH$_2$).	**FAD** and **FMN** are derived from ribo**F**lavin (B$_2$ = **2** ATP).

Vitamin B$_3$ (niacin)

Deficiency	Pellagra can be caused by Hartnup disease, malignant carcinoid syndrome, and INH.	Pellagra's symptoms are the **3 D's:** **D**iarrhea, **D**ermatitis, **D**ementia (also beefy glossitis).
Function	Constituent of NAD$^+$, NADP$^+$ (used in redox reactions). Derived from tryptophan.	**N**AD derived from **N**iacin (B$_3$ = **3** ATP).

UCV *Bio.34*

Vitamin B$_5$ (pantothenate)

Deficiency	Dermatitis, enteritis, alopecia, adrenal insufficiency.	
Function	Constituent of CoA, part of fatty acid synthase. Cofactor for acyl transfers.	Pantothen-**A** is in Co-**A**.

Vitamin B$_6$ (pyridoxine)

Deficiency	Convulsions, hyperirritability (deficiency inducible by INH and oral contraceptives).
Function	Converted to pyridoxal phosphate, a cofactor used in transamination (e.g., ALT and AST), decarboxylation, and trans-sulfuration.

Biotin

Deficiency	Dermatitis, enteritis. Caused by antibiotic use, ingestion of raw eggs.	"**AVID**in in egg whites **AVID**ly binds biotin."
Function	Cofactor for carboxylations: 1. Pyruvate → oxaloacetate 2. Acetyl-CoA → malonyl-CoA 3. Proprionyl-CoA → methylmalonyl-CoA	

Folic acid

Deficiency Most common vitamin deficiency in the United States.
Macrocytic, megaloblastic anemia (often no neurologic symptoms, as opposed to vitamin B_{12} deficiency), sprue.

Function Coenzyme for 1-carbon transfer; involved in methylation reactions.
Important for the synthesis of nitrogenous bases in DNA and RNA.

FOLate from **FOL**iage.
Eat green leaves (because folic acid is not stored very long). Supplemental folic acid in early pregnancy reduces neural tube defects.
PABA is the folic acid precursor in bacteria. Sulfa drugs and dapsone are PABA analogs.

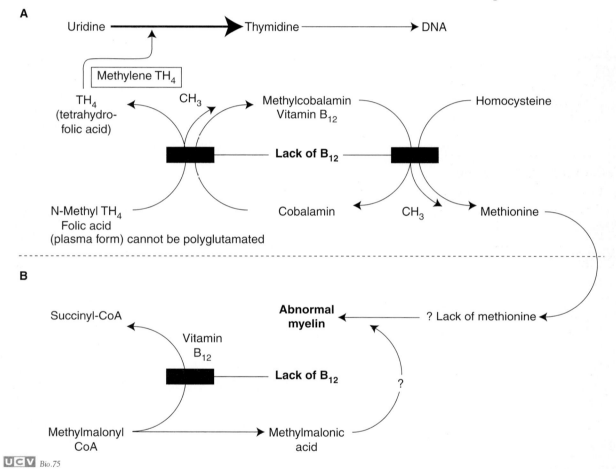

A.

Uridine ⟶ Thymidine ⟶ DNA

Methylene TH_4

TH_4 (tetrahydrofolic acid) CH_3 Methylcobalamin Vitamin B_{12} Homocysteine

Lack of B_{12}

N-Methyl TH_4 Folic acid (plasma form) cannot be polyglutamated Cobalamin CH_3 Methionine

B.

Succinyl-CoA Abnormal myelin ? Lack of methionine

Vitamin B_{12}

Lack of B_{12} ?

Methylmalonyl CoA ⟶ Methylmalonic acid

UCV *Bio.75*

(**A.** Adapted, with permission, from McPhee S et al. *Pathophysiology of Disease: An Introduction to Clinical Medicine*, 3rd ed. New York: McGraw-Hill, 2000:113.
B. Adapted, with permission, from McPhee S et al. *Pathophysiology of Disease: An Introduction to Clinical Medicine*, 3rd ed. New York: McGraw-Hill, 2000:113, as modified from Chandrasoma P et al. *Concise Pathology*, 3rd ed. Stamford, CT: Appleton & Lange, 1998.)

HIGH-YIELD FACTS

Biochemistry

Vitamin B$_{12}$ (cobalamin)

Deficiency	Macrocytic, megaloblastic anemia; neurologic symptoms (optic neuropathy, subacute combined degeneration, paresthesia); glossitis.	Found only in animal products. Vitamin B$_{12}$ deficiency is usually caused by malabsorption (sprue, enteritis, *Diphyllobothrium latum*), lack of intrinsic factor (pernicious anemia), or absence of terminal ileum (Crohn's disease). Use Schilling test to detect deficiency.
Function	Cofactor for homocysteine methylation and methylmalonyl-CoA handling. Stored primarily in the liver. Synthesized only by microorganisms.	

Vitamin C (ascorbic acid)

Deficiency	Scurvy.	Vitamin **C** Cross-links **C**ollagen. British sailors carried limes to prevent scurvy (origin of the word "limey").
Function	Necessary for hydroxylation of proline and lysine in collagen synthesis. Facilitates iron absorption by keeping iron in Fe^{+2} reduced state (more absorbable) Necessary as a cofactor for dopamine → norepinephrine. Scurvy findings: swollen gums, bruising, anemia, poor wound healing.	

UCV Bio.35

Vitamin D

	D$_2$ = ergocalciferol, consumed in milk. D$_3$ = cholecalciferol, formed in sun-exposed skin. 25-OH D$_3$ = storage form. 1,25 (OH)$_2$ D$_3$ = active form.	Remember that drinking milk (fortified with vitamin D) is good for bones. Causes of hypercalcemia:
Deficiency	Rickets in children (bending bones), osteomalacia in adults (soft bones), and hypocalcemic tetany.	1. Vitamin D intoxication 2. Malignancy
Function	Increases intestinal absorption of calcium and phosphate.	3. Hyperparathyroidism 4. Milk-alkali syndrome
Excess	Hypercalcemia, loss of appetite, stupor. Seen in sarcoidosis, a disease where the epithelioid macrophages convert vitamin D into its active form.	5. Sarcoidosis 6. Paget's disease of bone

UCV Bio.29

Vitamin E

Deficiency	Increased fragility of erythrocytes.	Vitamin **E** is for **E**rythrocytes.
Function	Antioxidant (protects erythrocytes from hemolysis).	

Vitamin K

Deficiency	Neonatal hemorrhage with ↑ PT and ↑ aPTT but normal bleeding time.	**K** for **K**oagulation. Note that the vitamin K–dependent clotting factors are II, VII, IX, X, and protein C and S. Warfarin is a vitamin K antagonist.
Function	Catalyzes γ-carboxylation of glutamic acid residues on various proteins concerned with blood clotting. Synthesized by intestinal flora. Therefore, vitamin K deficiency can occur after the prolonged use of broad-spectrum antibiotics.	

UCV Bio.36

Ethanol metabolism

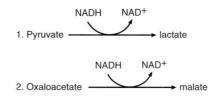

Ethanol $\xrightarrow{\text{Alcohol dehydrogenase}}$ Acetaldehyde $\xrightarrow{\text{Acetaldehyde dehydrogenase}}$ Acetate

NAD$^+$ → NADH   NAD$^+$ → NADH

NAD^+ is the limiting reagent.

Alcohol dehydrogenase operates via zero-order kinetics.

Disulfiram (Antabuse) inhi acetaldehyde dehydrogenase (acetaldehyde accumulates, contributing to hangover symptoms).

Ethanol hypoglycemia

Ethanol metabolism increases NADH/NAD$^+$ ratio in liver, causing diversion of pyruvate to lactate and OAA to malate, thereby inhibiting gluconeogenesis and leading to hypoglycemia. This altered NADH/NAD+ ratio is responsible for the hepatic fatty change (hepatocellular steatosis) seen in chronic alcoholics (shunting away from glycolysis and toward fatty acid synthesis).

NADH → NAD$^+$

1. Pyruvate ⟶ lactate

NADH → NAD$^+$

2. Oxaloacetate ⟶ malate

Kwashiorkor vs. marasmus

Kwashiorkor—protein malnutrition resulting in skin lesions, edema, liver malfunction (fatty change). Clinical picture is small child with swollen belly.

Marasmus—protein-calorie malnutrition resulting in tissue wasting.

Kwashiorkor results from a protein-deficient **MEAL:**
- **M**alabsorption
- **E**dema
- **A**nemia
- **L**iver (fatty)

Microbiology

"What lies behind us and what lies ahead of us are tiny matters
compared to what lives within us."
—Oliver Wendell Holmes

This high-yield material covers the basic concepts of microbiology and immunology. The emphasis in previous examinations has been approximately 40% bacteriology (20% basic, 20% quasi-clinical), 25% immunology, 25% virology (10% basic, 15% quasi-clinical), 5% parasitology, and 5% mycology. Learning the distinguishing characteristics, target organs, and method of spread of—as well as relevant laboratory tests for—major pathogens can improve your score substantially.

Many students preparing for this part of the boards make the mistake of studying bacteriology thoroughly without devoting sufficient time to the other topics. For this reason, learning immunology and virology thoroughly is high yield. Learn the components and mechanistic details of the immune response, including T cells, B cells, and the structure and function of immunoglobulins. Also learn the major immunodeficiency diseases (e.g., AIDS, agammaglobulinemia, DiGeorge syndrome). Knowledge of viral structures and genomes remains important as well.

High-Yield Clinical Vignettes
High-Yield Images
High-Yield Topics
Clinical Bacteriology
Bacteriology
Mycology
Parasitology
Virology
Systems
Immunology

These abstracted case vignettes are designed to demonstrate the thought processes necessary to answer multistep clinical reasoning questions.

Vignette	Question	Answer
■ An alcoholic vomits gastric contents and develops foul-smelling sputum.	What organisms are most likely?	Anaerobes.
■ Middle-age male presents with acute-onset monoarticular joint pain and bilateral Bell's palsy.	What is the likely disease and how did he get it?	Lyme disease; bite from *Ixodes* tick.
■ Patient with *Mycoplasma pneumoniae* exhibits cryo-agglutinins during recovery phase.	What types of immunoglobulins are reacting?	IgM.
■ Urinalysis of patient shows WBC casts.	What is the diagnosis?	Pyelonephritis.
■ Young child presents with tetany and candidiasis. Hypocalcemia and immunosuppression are found.	What cell is deficient?	T cell (DiGeorge).
■ Patient presents with rose gardener's scenario (thorn prick with ulcers along lymphatic drainage).	What is the infectious bug?	*Sporothrix schenckii*.
■ 25-year-old medical student has a burning feeling in his gut after meals. Biopsy of gastric mucosa shows gram-negative rods.	What is the likely organism?	H. pylori.
■ 32-year-old male has "cauliflower" skin lesions. Tissue biopsy shows broad-based budding yeasts.	What is the likely organism?	*Blastomyces*.
■ Breast-feeding woman suddenly develops redness and swelling of her right breast. On examination, it is found to be a fluctuant mass.	What is the diagnosis?	Mastitis caused by *S. aureus*.
■ Young child has recurrent lung infections and granulomatous lesions.	What is the defect in neutrophils?	NADPH oxidase (chronic granulomatous disease).
■ 20-year-old college student presents with lymphadenopathy, fever, and hepatosplenomegaly. His serum agglutinates sheep red blood cells.	What cell is infected?	B cell (EBV; infectious mononucleosis).

Vignette	Question	Answer
■ 1 hour after eating custard at a picnic, a whole family began to vomit. After 10 hours, they were better.	What is the organism?	*S. aureus* (produces preformed enterotoxin).
■ Infant becomes flaccid after eating honey.	What organism is implicated, and what is the mechanism of action?	*Clostridium botulinum*; inhibited release of acetylcholine.
■ Man presents with squamous cell carcinoma of penis.	He had exposure to what virus?	HPV.
■ Patient develops endocarditis 3 weeks after receiving prosthetic heart valve.	What organism is suspected?	*S. aureus* or *S. epidermidis*.

The high-yield images referenced below may not all appear in this chapter or in the high-yield glossy photo insert; however, they are still worthy of consideration.

1. Patient who visited Mexico presents with bloody diarrhea → what infectious form is found in the stool? → erythrocyte-ingesting trophozoite → *Entamoeba histolytica*.
2. Glossy photograph of cardiac valve with cauliflower growth → diagnosis? → bacterial endocarditis.
3. Adolescent with cough and rusty sputum → what does Gram stain of sputum show? → gram-positive diplococci (*Streptococcus pneumoniae*/pneumococci).
4. HIV-positive patient with CSF showing 75/mm³ lymphocytes suddenly dies. Picture of yeast in meninges → diagnosis? → cryptococcal meningitis.

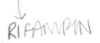
RIFAMPIN

HIGH-YIELD FACTS

Microbiology

Microbiology

1. Principles and interpretation of bacteriologic lab tests (culture, drug sensitivity, specific growth requirements).
2. Dermatologic manifestations of bacterial and viral infections (e.g., syphilis, Rocky Mountain spotted fever, meningococcemia, herpes zoster, coxsackievirus infection).
3. Common sexually transmitted diseases (e.g., syphilis, AIDS, HSV, gonorrhea, chlamydia).
4. Viral gastroenteritis in the pediatric and adult populations.
5. Common causes of community-acquired and nosocomial pneumonia.
6. Protozoa that frequently cause disease in the U.S. (e.g., *Entamoeba histolytica*, *Giardia*).
7. Parasites (protozoa, helminths) that cause disease more commonly outside the United States (e.g., malaria, Chagas' disease, elephantiasis).
8. Herpes simplex encephalitis (temporal lobe lesion, mental status changes, treat with acyclovir).
9. Tests available for diagnosis of viral infections (e.g., plaque assay, PCR).
10. Microscopic appearance of organisms.

Immunology

1. Principles and interpretation of immunologic tests (e.g., ELISA, complement-fixation tests, direct and indirect Coombs' tests).
2. Immune complex diseases (e.g., poststreptococcal glomerulonephritis, systemic lupus erythematosus, serum sickness).
3. Genetics of immunoglobulin variety and specificity (class switching, VDJ recombination, affinity maturation).
4. Mechanisms of antigenic variation and immune system evasion employed by bacteria, fungi, protozoa, and viruses.
5. How different types of immune deficiencies lead to different susceptibilities to infection (e.g., T-cell defects and viral/fungal infection; splenectomy and encapsulated organisms).
6. MHC/HLA haplotypes: transplant compatibility, disease associations, familial inheritance.
7. Allergies: common antigens, antigen-IgE–mast cell complex, presumed mechanism of immunotherapy (blocking antibodies).
8. Granulomas: role of macrophages, foreign body versus immune granulomas, caseating (TB) versus noncaseating (sarcoid) granulomas, common causes (e.g., TB, sarcoid, fungi).
9. Components of vaccines and how they produce immunity.
10. Characteristics and functions of macrophages and NK (natural killer) cells.

Bacterial structures

Structure	Function	Chemical composition
Peptidoglycan	Gives rigid support, protects against osmotic pressure.	Sugar backbone with cross-linked peptide side chains.
Cell wall/cell membrane (gram positives)	Major surface antigen.	Teichoic acid induces TNF and IL-1.
Outer membrane (gram negatives)	Site of endotoxin (lipopolysaccharide); major surface antigen.	Lipid A induces TNF and IL-1; polysaccharide is the antigen.
Plasma membrane	Site of oxidative and transport enzymes.	Lipoprotein bilayer.
Ribosome	Protein synthesis.	RNA and protein in 50S and 30S subunits.
Periplasm	Space between the cytoplasmic membrane and outer membrane in gram-negative bacteria.	Contains many hydrolytic enzymes, including β-lactamases.
Capsule	Protects against phagocytosis.	Polysaccharide (except *Bacillus anthracis*, which contains D-glutamate).
Pilus/fimbria	Mediates adherence of bacteria to cell surface; sex pilus forms attachment between 2 bacteria during conjugation.	Glycoprotein.
Flagellum	Motility.	Protein.
Spore	Provides resistance to dehydration, heat, and chemicals.	Keratin-like coat; dipicolinic acid.
Plasmid	Contains a variety of genes for antibiotic resistance, enzymes, and toxins.	DNA.
Glycocalix	Mediates adherence to surfaces, especially foreign surfaces (e.g., indwelling catheters).	Polysaccharide.

Cell walls

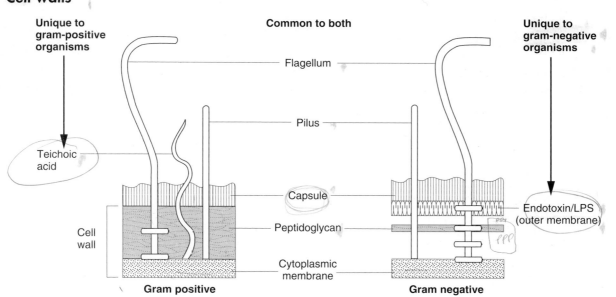

(Adapted, with permission, from Levinson W, Jawetz E. *Medical Microbiology and Immunology: Examination and Board Review,* 6th ed. New York: McGraw-Hill, 2000:7.)

HIGH-YIELD FACTS

Microbiology

Bacterial growth curve

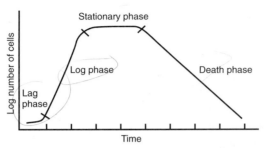

(Adapted, with permission, from Levinson W, Jawetz E. *Medical Microbiology and Immunology: Examination and Board Review*, 6th ed. New York: McGraw-Hill, 2000:14.)

Main features of exotoxins and endotoxins

Property	Exotoxin	Endotoxin
Source	Certain species of some gram-positive and gram-negative bacteria	Cell wall of most gram-negative bacteria
Secreted from cell	Yes	No
Chemistry	Polypeptide	Lipopolysaccharide
Location of genes	Plasmid or bacteriophage	Bacterial chromosome
Toxicity	High (fatal dose on the order of 1 μg)	Low (fatal dose on the order of hundreds of micrograms)
Clinical effects	Various effects (see text)	Fever, shock
Mode of action	Various modes (see text)	Includes TNF and IL-1
Antigenicity	Induces high-titer antibodies called antitoxins	Poorly antigenic
Vaccines	Toxoids used as vaccines	No toxoids formed and no vaccine available
Heat stability	Destroyed rapidly at 60°C (except staphylococcal enterotoxin)	Stable at 100°C for 1 hour
Typical diseases	Tetanus, botulism, diphtheria	Meningococcemia, sepsis by gram-negative rods

(Adapted, with permission, from Levinson W, Jawetz E. *Medical Microbiology and Immunology: Examination and Board Review*, 6th ed. New York: McGraw-Hill, 2000:34.)

Bugs with exotoxins

Gram-positive bugs

	Mode of action
Corynebacterium diphtheriae	Inactivates EF-2 by ADP ribosylation (similar to exotoxin A of *Pseudomonas*); causes pharyngitis and "pseudomembrane" in throat.
Clostridium tetani	Blocks the release of the inhibitory neurotransmitter glycine; causes "lockjaw."
Clostridium botulinum	Blocks the release of acetylcholine; causes anticholinergic symptoms, CNS paralysis; spores found in canned food, honey (causes floppy baby).
Clostridium perfringens	α toxin is a lecithinase; causes gas gangrene; get double zone of hemolysis on blood agar.
Bacillus anthracis	1 toxin in the toxin complex is an adenylate cyclase.
Staphylococcus aureus	Toxin is a superantigen that binds to class II MHC protein and T-cell receptor, inducing IL-1 and IL-2 synthesis in toxic shock syndrome; also causes food poisoning.
Streptococcus pyogenes	Erythrogenic toxin (causes rash of scarlet fever) and streptolysin O (antigen for ASO antibody is found in rheumatic fever). Erythrogenic toxin is a superantigen; streptolysin O is a hemolysin.

Gram-negative bugs

Escherichia coli	Heat-labile toxin stimulates adenylate cyclase by ADP ribosylation of G protein; causes watery diarrhea.
	Heat-stable toxin stimulates guanylate cyclase.
Vibrio cholerae	Stimulates adenylate cyclase by ADP ribosylation of G protein; increases pumping of Cl⁻ and H_2O into gut; causes voluminous rice-water diarrhea.
Bordetella pertussis	Stimulates adenylate cyclase by ADP ribosylation; causes whooping cough; inhibits chemokine receptor, causing lymphocytosis.

Endotoxin

A lipopolysaccharide found in cell wall of gram-negative bacteria.

N-dotoxin is an integral part of gram-Negative cell wall. Endotoxin is heat stable.

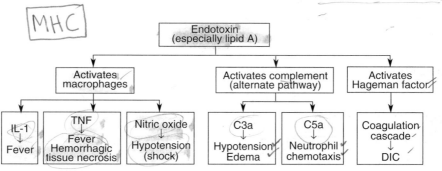

(Adapted, with permission, from Levinson W, Jawetz E. *Medical Microbiology and Immunology: Examination and Board Review*, 6th ed. New York: McGraw-Hill, 2000:39.)

Gram stain limitations

These bugs do not Gram stain well:

Treponema (too thin to be visualized).

Rickettsia (intracellular parasite).
Mycobacteria (high-lipid-content cell wall requires acid-fast stain).
Mycoplasma (no cell wall).
Legionella pneumophila (primarily intracellular).
Chlamydia (intracellular parasite).

[handwritten: LRC intracellular]

These **R**ascals **M**ay **M**icroscopically **L**ack **C**olor.
Treponemes—darkfield microscopy and fluorescent antibody staining.

Mycobacteria—acid fast.

Legionella—silver stain.
[handwritten: → legions → cornage → silver]

Fermentation patterns of *Neisseria*

The pathogenic *Neisseria* species are differentiated on the basis of sugar fermentation.

Menin**G**ococci ferment **M**altose and **G**lucose.
Gonococci ferment **G**lucose.

Pigment-producing bacteria

Staphylococcus aureus produces a yellow pigment.
Pseudomonas aeruginosa produces a blue-green pigment.
Serratia marcescens produces a red pigment.

Aureus (Latin) = gold.

Serratia marcescens = maraschino cherries are red.

IgA proteases

IgA proteases allow these organisms to colonize mucosal surfaces: *Streptococcus pneumoniae, Neisseria meningitidis, Neisseria gonorrhoeae, Haemophilus influenzae.*

Gram-positive lab algorithm

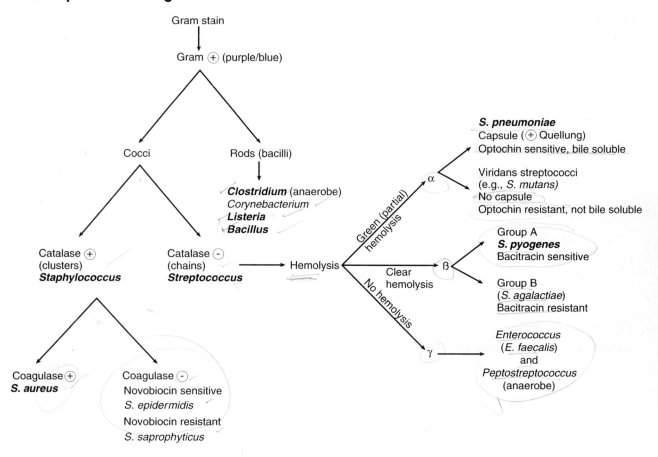

Important pathogens are in **bold type.**

Note: *Enterococcus* is either α- or γ-hemolytic.

Gram-negative lab algorithm

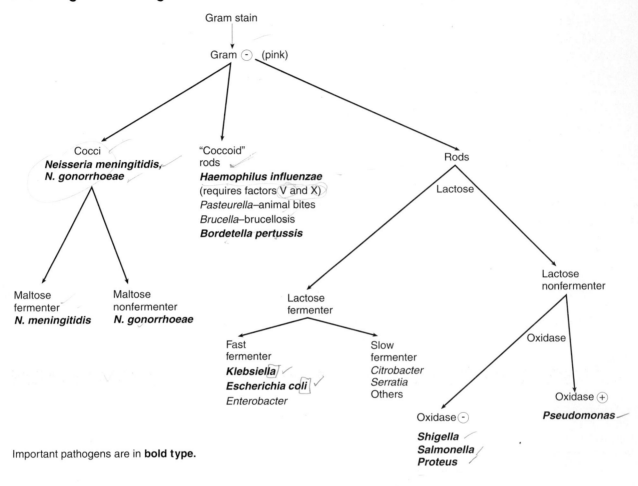

Important pathogens are in **bold type**.

Special culture requirements

Bug	Media used for isolation
H. influenzae	Chocolate agar with factors V (NAD) and X (hematin)
N. gonorrhoeae	Thayer-Martin (VCN) media
B. pertussis	Bordet-Gengou (potato) agar
C. diphtheriae	Tellurite plate, Loffler's medium, blood agar
M. tuberculosis	Löwenstein-Jensen agar
Lactose-fermenting enterics (e.g., Escherichia, Klebsiella, and Enterobacter)	Pink colonies on MacConkey's agar
Legionella pneumophila	Charcoal yeast extract agar buffered with increased iron and cysteine
Fungi	Sabouraud's agar

Stains

Congo red	Amyloid; apple-green birefringence in polarized light.
Giemsa's	*Borrelia, Plasmodium,* trypanosomes, *Chlamydia.*
PAS (periodic acid Schiff)	Stains glycogen, mucopolysaccharides; used to diagnose Whipple's disease.
Ziehl-Neelsen	Acid-fast bacteria.
India ink	*Cryptococcus neoformans.*

Conjugation, transduction, and transformation

Transfer procedure	Process	Types of cells involved	Nature of DNA transferred
Conjugation	DNA transferred from 1 bacterium to another	Prokaryotic	Chromosomal or plasmid
Transduction	DNA transferred by a virus from 1 cell to another	Prokaryotic	Any gene in generalized transduction; only certain genes in specialized transduction
Transformation	Purified DNA taken up by a cell	Prokaryotic or eukaryotic (e.g., human)	Any DNA

(Adapted, with permission, from Levinson W, Jawetz E. *Medical Microbiology and Immunology: Examination and Board Review,* 6th ed. New York: McGraw-Hill, 2000:18.)

MICROBIOLOGY—BACTERIOLOGY

Obligate aerobes	Use an O_2-dependent system to generate ATP. Examples include **N**ocardia, **P**seudomonas *aeruginosa,* **M**ycobacterium *tuberculosis,* and **B**acillus. Mycobacterium tuberculosis has a predilection for the apices of the lung, which have the highest PO_2.	P. **AER**uginosa is an **AER**obe seen in burn wounds, nosocomial pneumonia, and pneumonias in cystic fibrosis patients. **N**agging **P**ests **M**ust **B**reathe.
Obligate anaerobes	Examples include *Clostridium, Bacteroides,* and *Actinomyces.* They lack catalase and/or superoxide dismutase and thus are susceptible to oxidative damage. They are generally foul smelling (short-chain fatty acids), are difficult to culture, and produce gas in tissue (CO_2 and H_2).	Anaerobes are normal flora in GI tract, pathogenic elsewhere. AminO_2glycosides are ineffective against anaerobes because these antibiotics require O_2 to enter into bacterial cell.

Intracellular bugs

Obligate intracellular	*Rickettsia, Chlamydia.* Can't make own ATP.	Stay inside (cells) when it is **R**eally **C**old.
Facultative intracellular	*Mycobacterium, Brucella, Francisella, Listeria, Yersinia, Legionella, Salmonella.*	

HIGH-YIELD FACTS

Microbiology

Encapsulated bacteria

Examples are *Streptococcus pneumoniae* (pneumococcus), *Haemophilus influenzae* (especially b serotype), *Neisseria meningitidis* (meningococcus), and *Klebsiella pneumoniae*.

Polysaccharide capsule is an antiphagocytic virulence factor.

Positive **Quellung** reaction: If encapsulated bug is present, capsule **swells** when specific anticapsular antisera are added.

IgG_2 necessary for immune response. Capsule serves as antigen in vaccines (Pneumovax, *H. influenzae* b, meningococcal vaccines).

Quellung = capsular **"swelling."**

Pneumococcus associated with "rusty" sputum, sepsis in sickle cell anemia, and splenectomy.

Spores: bacterial

Only certain gram-positive rods form spores when nutrients are limited. Spores are highly resistant to destruction by heat and chemicals. Have dipicolinic acid in their core. Have no metabolic activity. Must autoclave to kill spores (as is done to surgical equipment).

Gram-positive soil bugs ≈ spore formers (*Bacillus anthracis*, *Clostridium perfringens*, *C. tetani*).

α-hemolytic bacteria

Include the following organisms:
1. *Streptococcus pneumoniae* (catalase negative and optochin sensitive)
2. Viridans streptococci (catalase negative and optochin resistant)

β-hemolytic bacteria

Include the following organisms:
1. *Staphylococcus aureus* (catalase and coagulase positive)
2. *Streptococcus pyogenes* (catalase negative and bacitracin sensitive)
3. *Streptococcus agalactiae* (catalase negative and bacitracin resistant)
4. *Listeria monocytogenes* (tumbling motility, meningitis in newborns, unpasteurized milk)

Catalase/coagulase (gram-positive cocci)

Catalase degrades H_2O_2, an antimicrobial product of PMNs. H_2O_2 is a substrate for myeloperoxidase.

Staphylococci make catalase, whereas streptococci do not.

S. aureus makes coagulase, whereas *S. epidermidis* and *S. saprophyticus* do not.

Staph make catalase because they have more "staff." Bad staph (*aureus*, because *epidermidis* is skin flora) make coagulase and toxins.

Staphylococcus aureus 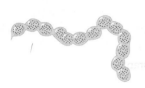 UCV *Micro2.106*	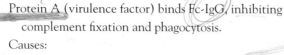 Protein A (virulence factor) binds Fc-IgG, inhibiting complement fixation and phagocytosis. Causes: 1. Inflammatory disease—skin infections, organ abscesses, pneumonia 2. Toxin-mediated disease—toxic shock syndrome (TSST-1 toxin), scalded skin syndrome (exfoliative toxin), rapid-onset food poisoning (enterotoxins)	TSST is a superantigen that binds to class II MHC and T-cell receptor, resulting in polyclonal T-cell activation. *S. aureus* food poisoning is due to ingestion of preformed toxin. *Micro2.18* Causes acute bacterial endocarditis.
Streptococcus pyogenes (group A β-hemolytic streptococci) sequelae UCV *Micro1.26, Micro2.83*	Causes: 1. Pyogenic—pharyngitis, cellulitis, impetigo 2. Toxigenic—scarlet fever, TSS 3. Immunologic—rheumatic fever, acute glomerulonephritis Bacitracin sensitive. Antibody to **M protein** enhances host defenses against *S. pyogenes*.	Pharyngitis gives you rheumatic "phever." Rheumatic fever = **PECCS**: Polyarthritis, Erythema marginatum, Chorea, Carditis, Subcutaneous nodules.
Enterococci	Enterococci (*Enterococcus faecalis* and *E. faecium*) are penicillin G resistant and cause UTI and subacute endocarditis. Lancefield group D includes the enterococci and the nonenterococcal group D streptococci. Lancefield grouping is based on differences in the C carbohydrate on the bacterial cell wall. Variable hemolysis.	*Entero* = intestine, *faecalis* = feces, *strepto* = twisted (chains), *coccus* = berry. Enterococci, hardier than nonenterococcal group D, can thus grow in 6.5% NaCl (lab test).
Viridans group streptococci	Viridans streptococci are α-hemolytic. They are normal flora of the oropharynx and cause dental caries (*Streptococcus mutans*) and subacute bacterial endocarditis (*S. sanguis*). Resistant to optochin, differentiating them from *S. pneumoniae*, which is α-hemolytic but is optochin sensitive.	*Sanguis* (Latin) = blood. There is lots of blood in the heart (endocarditis). Viridans group strep live in the mouth because they are not afraid **of-the-chin** (**op-to-chin** resistant).
Clostridia (with exotoxins) UCV	Gram-positive, spore-forming, obligate anaerobic bacilli. *Clostridium tetani* produces an exotoxin causing tetanus. *Micro2.62* *C. botulinum* produces a preformed, heat-labile toxin that inhibits ACh release, causing botulism. *Micro1.66* *C. perfringens* produces α toxin, a hemolytic lecithinase that causes myonecrosis or gas gangrene. *Micro1.88* *C. difficile* produces a cytotoxin, an exotoxin that kills enterocytes, causing pseudomembranous colitis. Often 2° to antibiotic use, especially clindamycin or ampicillin. *Pharm.31*	**TET**anus is **TET**anic paralysis (blocks glycine release [inhibitory neurotransmitter] from Renshaw cells in spinal cord. **BOT**ulinum is from bad **BOT**tles of food (causes a flaccid paralysis). **PERF**ringens **PERF**orates a gangrenous leg. **DI**fficile causes **DI**arrhea. Treat with metronidazole.

Diphtheria (and exotoxin)

Caused by *Corynebacterium diphtheriae* via exotoxin encoded by β-prophage. Potent exotoxin inhibits protein synthesis via ADP ribosylation of EF-2. Symptoms include pseudomembranous pharyngitis (grayish-white membrane) with lymphadenopathy. Lab diagnosis based on gram-positive rods with metachromatic granules.

UCV *Micro1.82*

Coryne = club shaped.
Grows on tellurite agar.
ABCDEFG:
　ADP ribosylation
　Beta-prophage
　Corynebacterium
　Diphtheriae
　Elongation Factor 2
　Granules

Anthrax

Caused by *Bacillus anthracis*, a gram-positive, spore-forming rod that produces anthrax toxin.
Contact → malignant pustule (painless ulcer); can progress to bacteremia and death.
Inhalation of spores can cause life-threatening pneumonia (woolsorters' disease).

UCV *Micro1.58*

Black skin lesions—vesicular papules covered by black eschar.

Actinomyces vs. *Nocardia*

Both are gram-positive rods forming long branching filaments resembling fungi.
Actinomyces israelii, a gram-positive anaerobe, causes oral/facial abscesses with "sulfur granules" that may drain through sinus tracts in skin. Normal oral flora.
Nocardia asteroides, a gram-positive and also a weakly acid-fast aerobe in soil, causes pulmonary infection in immunocompromised patients.

UCV *Micro2.29, Micro1.50*

A. israelii forms yellow "sulfur granules" in sinus tracts.
SNAP:
　Sulfa for
　Nocardia;
　Actinomyces use
　Penicillin

Penicillin and gram-negative bugs

Gram-negative bugs are resistant to benzyl penicillin G but may be susceptible to penicillin derivatives such as ampicillin. The gram-negative outer membrane layer inhibits entry of penicillin G and vancomycin.

Bugs causing food poisoning

Vibrio parahaemolyticus and *V. vulnificus* in contaminated seafood.
Bacillus cereus in reheated rice.
Staphylococcus aureus in meats, mayonnaise, custard.
Clostridium perfringens in reheated meat dishes.
Clostridium botulinum in improperly canned foods (bulging cans).
E. coli 0157:H7 in undercooked meat.
Salmonella in poultry, meat, and eggs.

S. aureus food poisoning starts quickly and ends quickly. "Food poisoning from reheated rice? **Be serious!**" (**B. cereus**).

Diarrhea

Species	Typical findings
Escherichia coli	Ferments lactose
Vibrio cholerae	Comma-shaped organisms
Salmonella	Does not ferment lactose, motile
Shigella	Does not ferment lactose, nonmotile, very low ID_{50}
Campylobacter jejuni	Comma- or S-shaped organisms; growth at 42°C
Vibrio parahaemolyticus	Transmitted by seafood
Yersinia enterocolitica	Usually transmitted from pet feces (e.g., puppies)

Bugs causing watery diarrhea	Include *Vibrio cholerae* (associated with rice-water stools), enterotoxigenic *E. coli*, viruses (e.g., rotaviruses), and protozoans (e.g., *Cryptosporidium* and *Giardia*).
Bugs causing bloody diarrhea	Include *Salmonella*, *Shigella*, *Campylobacter jejuni*, enterohemorrhagic/enteroinvasive (0157:H7) *E. coli*, *Yersinia enterocolitica*, and *Entamoeba histolytica* (a protozoan).
Enterobacteriaceae	Diverse family including *E. coli*, *Salmonella*, *Klebsiella*, *Enterobacter*, *Serratia*, *Proteus*. All species have somatic (O) antigen (which is the polysaccharide of endotoxin). The capsular (K) antigen is related to the virulence of the bug. The flagellar (H) antigen is found in motile species. All ferment glucose and are oxidase negative.	Think **COFFEe:** **C**apsular **O** antigen **F**lagellar antigen **F**erment glucose **E**nterobacteriaceae
Haemophilus influenzae **UCV** Micro1.87, 1.24, 1.93	Ha**EMOP**hilus causes **E**piglottitis, **M**eningitis, **O**titis media, and **P**neumonia. Small gram-negative (coccobacillary) rod. Aerosol transmission. Most invasive disease caused by capsular type b. Produces IgA protease. Culture on chocolate agar requires factors **V** (NAD) and **X** (hematin) for growth. Treat meningitis with ceftriaxone. Rifampin prophylaxis in close contacts. Does not cause the flu (influenza virus does).	When a child has "flu," mom goes to five (**V**) and dime (**X**) store to buy some chocolate. Vaccine contains type b capsular polysaccharide conjugated to diphtheria toxoid or other protein. Given between 2 and 18 months of age.
Legionella pneumophila **UCV** Micro2.13	Legionnaires' disease. Gram-negative rod. Gram stains poorly—use silver stain. Grow on charcoal yeast extract culture with iron and cysteine. Aerosol transmission from environmental water source habitat. No person-to-person transmission. Treat with erythromycin.	Think of a French legionnaire (soldier) with his silver helmet, sitting around a campfire (charcoal) with his iron dagger—he is no sissy (cysteine).

Pseudomonas aeruginosa	*PSEUdomonas* causes wound and burn infections, Pneumonia (especially in cystic fibrosis), Sepsis (black lesions on skin), External otitis (swimmer's ear), UTI, and hot tub folliculitis. Aerobic gram-negative rod. Non–lactose fermenting, oxidase positive. Produces pyocyanin (blue-green) pigment. Water source. Produces endotoxin (fever, shock) and exotoxin A (inactivates EF-2). Treat with aminoglycoside plus extended-spectrum penicillin (e.g., piperacillin, ticarcillin).	AERuginosa—AERobic. Think water connection and blue-green pigment. Think *Pseudomonas* in burn victims.
Helicobacter pylori Micro1.35	Causes gastritis and up to 90% of duodenal ulcers. Risk factor for peptic ulcer and gastric carcinoma. Gram-negative rod. Urease positive (e.g., urease breath test). Creates alkaline environment. Treat with triple therapy: (1) bismuth (Pepto-Bismol), metronidazole, and either tetracycline or amoxicillin; or (2) (more costly) metronidazole, omeprazole, and clarithromycin.	Pylori—think pylorus of stomach. *Proteus* and *H. pylori* are both urease positive (cleave urea to ammonia).
Lactose-fermenting enteric bacteria	These bacteria grow pink colonies on MacConkey's agar. Examples include *Klebsiella*, *E. coli*, *Enterobacter*, and *Citrobacter*.	Lactose is **KEE.**
Salmonella* vs. *Shigella	Both are non–lactose fermenters; both invade intestinal mucosa and can cause bloody diarrhea. Only *Salmonella* is motile and can invade further and disseminate hematogenously. Symptoms of salmonellosis may be prolonged with antibiotic treatments, and there is typically a monocyte response. *Shigella* is more virulent (10^1 organisms) than *Salmonella* (10^5 organisms).	Salmon swim (motile and disseminate). *Salmonella* has an animal reservoir; *Shigella* does not and is transmitted via "food, fingers, feces, and flies."
Cholera and pertussis toxins UCV	*Vibrio cholerae* toxin permanently activates G_s, causing rice-water diarrhea. Micro1.74 Pertussis toxin permanently disables G_i, causing whooping cough. Micro2.76 Both toxins act via ADP ribosylation that permanently activates adenyl cyclase (resulting in increased cAMP).	Cholera turns the "on" on. Pertussis turns the "off" off. Pertussis toxin also promotes lymphocytosis by inhibiting chemokine receptors.

Zoonotic bacteria

Species	Disease	Transmission and source	
Borrelia burgdorferi	Lyme disease	Tick bite; *Ixodes* ticks that live on deer and mice	**B**ugs **F**rom **Y**our **P**et
Brucella spp.	Brucellosis/ Undulant fever	Dairy products, contact with animals	**U**ndulate and **U**npasteurized dairy products give you
Francisella tularensis	Tularemia	Tick bite; rabbits, deer	**U**ndulant fever.
Yersinia pestis	Plague	Flea bite; rodents, especially prairie dogs	
Pasteurella multocida	Cellulitis	Animal bite; cats, dogs	

Gardnerella vaginalis

A coccobacillus that causes vaginosis—greenish vaginal discharge with fishy smell; nonpainful. Treat with metronidazole. Clue cells, or vaginal epithelial cells covered with bacteria, are visible under the microscope.

Neisseria

Gram-negative cocci.

Gonococci	**Meningococci**
No polysaccharide capsule	Polysaccharide capsule
No maltose fermentation	Maltose fermentation
No vaccine	Vaccine
Causes: gonorrhea, septic arthritis, neonatal conjunctivitis, PID	Causes: meningococcemia and meningitis, Waterhouse-Friderichsen syndrome

1° and 2° tuberculosis

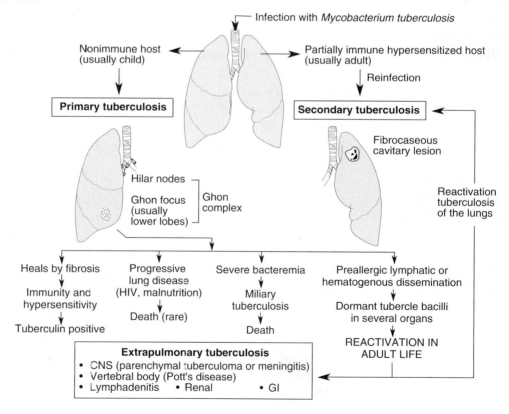

(Adapted, with permission, from Chandrasoma P, Taylor CR. *Concise Pathology*, 3rd ed. Stamford, CT: Appleton & Lange, 1998:523.)

HIGH-YIELD FACTS

Microbiology

Mycobacteria

Mycobacterium tuberculosis (TB, often resistant to multiple drugs).

M. kansasii (pulmonary TB-like symptoms).

M. scrofulaceum (cervical lymphadenitis in kids).

M. avium–intracellulare (often resistant to multiple drugs; causes disseminated disease in AIDS).

All mycobacteria are acid-fast organisms.

TB symptoms include fever, night sweats, weight loss, and hemoptysis.

Leprosy (Hansen's disease)

Caused by Mycobacterium leprae, an acid-fast bacillus that likes cool temperatures (infects skin and superficial nerves) and cannot be grown in vitro. Reservoir in United States: armadillos.

Treatment: long-term oral dapsone; toxicity is hemolysis and methemoglobinemia.

Alternate treatments include rifampin and combination of clofazimine and dapsone.

UCV *Micro2.16, Micro2.15*

Hansen's disease has two forms: lepromatous and tuberculoid; lepromatous is worse (failed cell-mediated immunity), tuberculoid is self-limited.

LEpromatous = LEthal.

Rickettsiae

Rickettsiae are obligate intracellular parasites and need CoA and NAD. All except Coxiella are transmitted by an arthropod vector and cause headache, fever, and rash; Coxiella is an atypical rickettsia because it is transmitted by aerosol.

Tetracycline is the treatment of choice for most rickettsial infections.

Classic triad—headache, fever, rash (vasculitis).

Rickettsial diseases and vectors

Rocky Mountain spotted fever (tick)—Rickettsia rickettsii.

Endemic typhus (fleas)—R. typhi.

Epidemic typhus (human body louse)—R. prowazekii.

Q fever (inhaled aerosols)—Coxiella burnetii.

Treatment for all: tetracycline.

TyPHus has centriPHugal (outward) spread of rash; sPotted fever is centriPetal (inward). Q fever is Queer because it has no rash, has no vector, and has negative Weil-Felix, and its causative organism can survive outside for a long time and does not have Rickettsia as its genus name.

Rocky Mountain spotted fever

Caused by Rickettsia rickettsii.

Symptoms: rash on palms and soles (migrating to wrists, ankles, then trunk), headache, fever.

Endemic to East Coast (in spite of name).

UCV *Micro2.44*

Palm and sole rash is seen in Rocky Mountain spotted fever, syphilis, and coxsackievirus A infection (hand, foot, and mouth disease).

Weil-Felix reaction

Weil-Felix reaction assays for antirickettsial antibodies, which cross-react with Proteus antigen. Weil-Felix is usually positive for typhus and Rocky Mountain spotted fever but negative for Q fever.

Mycoplasma pneumoniae 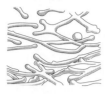 	Classic cause of atypical "walking" pneumonia (insidious onset, headache, nonproductive cough, diffuse interstitial infiltrate). X-ray looks worse than patient. High titer of cold agglutinins (IgM). Grown on Eaton's agar. Treatment: tetracycline or erythromycin (bugs are penicillin resistant because they have no cell wall).	No cell wall. Only bacterial membrane containing cholesterol. Mycoplasma pneumonia is more common in patients younger than age 30. Frequent outbreaks in military recruits and prisons.
Chlamydiae	Chlamydiae are obligate intracellular parasites that cause mucosal infections. 2 forms: 1. **E**lementary body (small, dense), which **E**nters cell via endocytosis 2. Initial or **R**eticulate body, which **R**eplicates in cell by fission Chlamydiae cause arthritis, conjunctivitis, pneumonia, and nongonococcal urethritis. The peptidoglycan wall is unusual in that it lacks muramic acid. Treatment: erythromycin or tetracycline.	_Chlamys_ = cloak (intracellular). _Chlamydia psittaci_—notable for an avian reservoir. _C. trachomatis_ causes arthritis and _C. pneumoniae_—infect only humans. _C. pneumoniae_—causes atypical pneumonia; transmitted by aerosol. Lab diagnosis: cytoplasmic inclusions seen on Giemsa or fluorescent antibody–stained smear.
Chlamydia trachomatis serotypes 	Types A, B, and C—chronic infection, causes blindness in Africa, ectopic pregnancy. Types D–K—urethritis/PID, neonatal pneumonia, or neonatal conjunctivitis. Types L1, L2, and L3—lymphogranuloma venereum (acute lymphadenitis—positive Frei test).	**ABC** = **A**frica/**B**lindness/**C**hronic infection. **L**1–3 = **L**ymphogranuloma venereum. D–K = everything else. Neonatal disease acquired by passage through infected birth canal. Treat with erythromycin eye drops.
Spirochetes 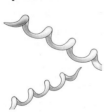	The spirochetes are spiral-shaped bacteria with axial filaments and include _Borrelia_ (big size), _Leptospira_, and _Treponema_. Only _Borrelia_ can be visualized using aniline dyes (Wright's or Giemsa stain) in light microscopy. _Treponema_ is visualized by dark-field microscopy.	**BLT**. **B** is **B**ig.

HIGH-YIELD FACTS

Microbiology

Lyme disease

Classic symptom is erythema chronicum migrans, an expanding "bull's eye" red rash with central clearing. Also affects joints, CNS, and heart.

Caused by *Borrelia burgdorferi,* which is transmitted by the tick *Ixodes.*

Mice are important reservoirs. Deer required for tick life cycle.

Treat with tetracycline.

Named after Lyme, Connecticut; disease is common in northeastern United States.

Transmission is most common in summer months.

UCV *Micro2.19*

3 stages of Lyme disease:
Stage 1—erythema chronicum migrans, flu-like symptoms.
Stage 2—neurologic and cardiac manifestations.
Stage 3—autoimmune migratory polyarthritis.

Treponemal disease

Treponemes are spirochetes.

Treponema pallidum causes syphilis.

T. pertenue causes yaws (a tropical infection that is not an STD, although VDRL test is positive).

Syphilis

1° syphilis

2° syphilis

3° syphilis

Caused by spirochete *Treponema pallidum.*

Presents with painless chancre (localized disease).

Disseminated disease with constitutional symptoms, maculopapular rash, condylomata lata.

Gummas, aortitis, neurosyphilis (tabes dorsalis), Argyll Robertson pupil.

UCV *Micro2.58-60, 61*

Treat with penicillin G.

Secondary syphilis = **S**ystemic.

VDRL vs. FTA-ABS

FTA-ABS is specific for treponemes, turns positive earliest in disease, and remains positive longest during disease. VDRL is less specific.

FTA-ABS = **F**ind **T**he **A**ntibody-**ABS**olutely:
1. Most specific
2. Earliest positive
3. Remains positive the longest

VDRL false positives

VDRL detects nonspecific Ab that reacts with beef cardiolipin. Used for diagnosis of syphilis, but many biologic false positives, including viral infection (mononucleosis, hepatitis), some drugs, rheumatic fever, rheumatoid arthritis, SLE, and leprosy.

VDRL:
Viruses (mono, hepatitis)
Drugs
Rheumatic fever and rheumatic arthritis
Lupus and leprosy

198

Spores: fungal	Most fungal spores are asexual. Both coccidioidomycosis and histoplasmosis are transmitted by inhalation of asexual spores.	Conidia—asexual fungal spores (e.g., blastoconidia, arthroconidia).
Candida albicans	Systemic or superficial fungal infection (budding yeast with pseudohyphae, germ tube formation at 37°C). Thrush in throat with immunocompromised patients (neonates, steroids, diabetes, AIDS), endocarditis in IV drug users, vaginitis (post-antibiotic), diaper rash. Treatment: nystatin for superficial infection; amphotericin B for serious systemic infection.	*Alba* = white.

UCV *Micro1.69*

Systemic mycoses

Disease	Endemic location	Notes
Coccidioidomycosis	Southwestern United States, California. *Micro1.78*	San Joaquin Valley or desert (desert bumps) "valley fever."
Histoplasmosis	Mississippi and Ohio river valleys. *Micro2.7*	Bird or bat droppings; intracellular (frequently seen inside macrophages).
Paracoccidioidomy-cosis	Rural Latin America.	"Captain's wheel" appearance.
Blastomycosis	States east of Mississippi River and Central America. *Micro1.65*	**B**ig, **B**road-**B**ased **B**udding.

Broad-based budding

	All of the above are caused by **dimorphic** fungi, which are mold in soil (at lower temperature) and yeast in tissue (at higher/body temperature: 37°C) except coccidioidomycosis, which is a spherule in tissue. Treat with fluconazole or ketoconazole for local infection; amphotericin B for systemic infection. Systemic mycoses can mimic TB (granuloma formation).	**Cold = Mold.** **Heat = Yeast.** Culture on Sabouraud's agar.

UCV

Cutaneous mycoses

Tinea versicolor	Caused by *Malassezia furfur*. Causes hypopigmented skin lesions. Occurs in hot, humid weather. Treat with topical miconazole, selenium sulfide (Selsun).
Tinea nigra	Caused by *Cladosporium werneckii*. Infection of keratinized layer of skin. Appears as brownish spot. Treat with topical salicylic acid.
Tinea pedis, tinea cruris, tinea corporis, tinea capitis	Pruritic lesions with central clearing resembling a ring, caused by dermatophytes (microsporum, trichophyton, and spidermophyton). See mold hyphae in KOH prep, not dimorphic. Pets are a reservoir for microsporum and can be treated with topical azoles.

Opportunistic fungal infections

Candida albicans	Thrush in immunocompromised (neonates, steroids, diabetes, AIDS), vulvovaginitis (high pH, diabetes, use of antibiotics), disseminated candidiasis (to any organ), chronic mucocutaneous candidiasis. *Micro1.69*
Aspergillus fumigatus	Allergic bronchopulmonary aspergillosis, lung cavity aspergilloma ("fungus ball"), invasive aspergillosis. **Mold** with septate hyphae that branch at a V-shaped (45°) angle. Not dimorphic. *Micro1.59, Micro1.60*
Cryptococcus neoformans	Cryptococcal meningitis, cryptococcosis. Heavily encapsulated **yeast.** Not dimorphic. Found in soil, pigeon droppings. Culture on Sabouraud's agar. Stains with India ink. Latex agglutination test detects polysaccharide capsular antigen.
Mucor and *Rhizopus* species	Mucormycosis. **Mold** with irregular nonseptate hyphae branching at wide angles (≥ 90°). Disease mostly in ketoacidotic diabetic and leukemic patients. Fungi also proliferate in the walls of blood vessels and cause infarction of distal tissue. *Micro2.25*

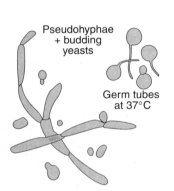

Pseudohyphae + budding yeasts

Germ tubes at 37°C

Candida

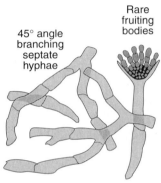

45° angle branching septate hyphae

Aspergillus

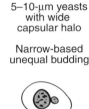

Rare fruiting bodies

5–10-μm yeasts with wide capsular halo

Narrow-based unequal budding

Cryptoccus

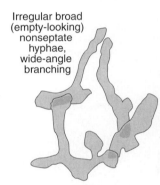

Irregular broad (empty-looking) nonseptate hyphae, wide-angle branching

Mucor

UCV

Pneumocystis carinii

Causes pneumonia (PCP). Yeast (originally classified as protozoan). Inhaled. Most infections asymptomatic. Immunosuppression (e.g., AIDS) predisposes to disease. Silver stain of lung tissue. Treat with TMP-SMX, pentamidine. Start prophylaxis when CD4 drops < 200 cells/mL in HIV patients.

UCV *Micro2.36*

Sporothrix schenckii

Yeast forms, unequal budding

Sporotrichosis. Dimorphic fungus that lives on vegetation. When traumatically introduced into the skin, typically by a thorn ("rose gardener's" disease), causes local pustule or ulcer with nodules along draining lymphatics (ascending lymphangitis). Little systemic illness. Cigar-shaped budding yeast visible in pus. Treat with itraconazole or potassium iodide.

UCV *Micro2.55*

Medically important protozoa

Organism	Disease	Transmission	Diagnosis	Treatment
Entamoeba histolytica Micro1.55	Amebiasis: bloody diarrhea, (dysentery), liver abscess, RUQ pain	Cysts in water	Serology and/or trophozoites or cysts in stool	Metronidazole and iodoquinol
Giardia lamblia Micro1.89	Giardiasis: bloating, flatulence, foul-smelling diarrhea	Cysts in water	Trophozoites or cysts in stool	Metronidazole
Cryptosporidium Micro1.81	Severe diarrhea in AIDS Mild disease (watery diarrhea) in non-HIV	Cysts in water	Cysts on acid-fast stain	None
Toxoplasma Micro2.65	Brain abscess in HIV, birth defects	Cysts in meat or cat feces	Serology, biopsy	Sulfadiazine + pyrimethamine
Pneumocystis carinii Micro2.36	Diffuse interstitial pneumonia in HIV	Inhalation	Lung biopsy or lavage; methenamine silver stain	TMP-SMX or dapsone or pentamidine
Plasmodium P. vivax P. ovale P. malariae P. falciparum Micro2.22	Malaria: cyclic fever, headache, anemia, splenomegaly Malaria—severe (cerebral)	Mosquito (Anopheles)	Blood smear	Chloroquine (primaquine for P. vivax, P. ovale), sulfadoxine + pyrimethamine, mefloquine, quinine
Trichomonas vaginalis	Vaginitis: foul-smelling, greenish discharge; itching and burning	Sexual	Trophozoites on wet mount	Metronidazole
Trypanosoma cruzi	Chagas' disease (heart disease) Micro1.71	Reduviid bug	Blood smear	Nifurtimox
Trypanosoma T. gambiense T. rhodesiense	African sleeping sickness Micro1.53	Tsetse fly	Blood smear	Suramin for blood-borne disease or melarsoprol for CNS penetration
Leishmania donovani	Visceral leishmaniasis (kala-azar)	Sandfly	Macrophages containing amastigotes	Sodium stibogluconate
Babesia	Babesiosis	Ixodes tick	Blood smear, no RBC pigment, appears as "maltese cross"	Quinine, clindamycin
Naegleria	Rapidly fatal meningoencephalitis	Swimming in freshwater lakes	Amebas in spinal fluid	None

UCV

HIGH-YIELD FACTS

Microbiology

Medically important helminths

Organism	Transmission/disease	Treatment
Cestodes (tapeworms)		
Taenia solium Micro2.88	Undercooked pork tapeworm; causes mass lesions in the brain, cysticercosis.	Praziquantel/niclosamide; albendazole for cysticercosis
Echinococcus granulosus Micro1.83	Eggs in dog feces when ingested can cause cysts in liver; causes anaphylaxis if echinococcal antigens are released from cysts.	Albendazole
Trematodes (flukes)		
Schistosoma Micro2.51, 2.52	Snails are host; cercariae penetrate skin of humans; causes granulomas, fibrosis, and inflammation of the spleen and liver.	Praziquantel
Clonorchis sinensis	Undercooked fish; causes inflammation of the biliary tract.	Praziquantel
Paragonimus westermani	Undercooked crab meat; causes inflammation and 2° bacterial infection of the lung.	Praziquantel
Nematodes (roundworms)		
Ancylostoma duodenale (hookworm) Micro1.32	Larvae penetrate skin of feet; intestinal infection can cause anemia.	Mebendazole/pyrantel pamoate
Ascaris lumbricoides	Eggs are visible in feces; intestinal infection.	Mebendazole/pyrantel pamoate
Enterobius vermicularis (pinworm) Micro1.36	Food contaminated with eggs; intestinal infection; causes anal pruritus.	Mebendazole/pyrantel pamoate
Strongyloides stercoralis Micro2.56	Larvae in soil penetrate the skin; intestinal infection.	Ivermectin/thiabendazole
Trichinella spiralis Micro2.66	Undercooked meat, usually pork; inflammation of muscle, periorbital edema.	Thiabendazole
Dracunculus medinensis	In drinking water; skin inflammation and ulceration.	Niridazole
Loa loa	Transmitted by deer fly; causes swelling in skin (can see worm crawling in conjunctiva).	Diethylcarbamazine
Onchocerca volvulus Micro2.31	Transmitted by female blackflies; causes river blindness.	Ivermectin
Toxocara canis	Food contaminated with eggs; causes granulomas (if in retina → blindness).	Diethylcarbamazine
Wuchereria bancrofti Micro2.20	Female mosquito; causes blockage of lymphatic vessels (elephantiasis).	Diethylcarbamazine

UCV

DNA viral genomes	All DNA viruses except the Parvoviridae are dsDNA. All are linear except papovaviruses and hepadnaviruses (circular).	All are dsDNA (like our cells), except **"part-of-a-virus"** (**parvovirus**) is ssDNA.
RNA viral genomes	All RNA viruses except Reoviridae are ssRNA.	All are ssRNA (like our mRNA), except "repeato-virus" (**reovirus**) is dsRNA.

DNA viruses

Viral Family	Envelope	DNA Structure	Medical Importance

Hepadnavirus
 	
Micro1.30
	Yes	DS – partial circular	Hepatitis B virus
			  Acute or chronic hepatitis
			  Vaccine available—use has increased tremendously
			  Not a retrovirus but has reverse transcriptase

Herpesviruses	Yes	DS – linear	HSV-1—oral (and some genital) lesions, keratoconjunctivitis HSV-2—genital (and some oral) lesions Varicella-zoster virus—chickenpox, zoster, shingles Epstein-Barr virus—mononucleosis, Burkitt's lymphoma Cytomegalovirus—infection in immunosuppressed patients, especially transplant recipients HHV-6—roseola (exanthem subitum) HHV-7—monkey bites (fatal in humans) HHV-8 (KSHV)—Kaposi's sarcoma–associated herpesvirus
Adenovirus *Micro1.25*	No	DS – linear	Febrile pharyngitis—sore throat Pneumonia Conjunctivitis—"pink eye"

Parvovirus
 	
Micro1.46
	No	SS – linear (–)
		(smallest DNA virus)
			B19 virus—aplastic crises in sickle cell disease
			  —"slapped cheeks" rash—erythema infectiosum
			  (fifth disease)
			AAV—adeno-associated virus

Papovavirus	No	DS – circular	HPV—warts, CIN, cervical cancer JC—progressive multifocal leukoencephalopathy (PML) in HIV BK—in kidney transplant patients
Poxvirus	Yes	DS – linear (largest DNA virus)	Smallpox though eradicated could be used in germ warfare Vaccinia—cowpox ("milkmaid's blisters") *Molluscum contagiosum*

UCV

DNA virus characteristics

Some general rules—all DNA viruses:

1. Are **HHAPPP**y viruses

   Hepadna, Herpes, Adeno, Pox, Parvo, Papova.

2. Are double stranded

   EXCEPT **Parvo** (single stranded).

3. Are linear

   EXCEPT **Papovavirus** (circular, supercoiled) and **Hepadna** (circular, incomplete).

4. Are icosahedral

   EXCEPT **Pox** (complex).

5. Replicate in the nucleus

   EXCEPT **Pox** (carries own DNA-dependent RNA polymerase).

Naked DNA viruses are **PAP** = **P**arvo, **A**deno, **P**apova; enveloped DNA viruses are **HPH** = **H**epadna, **P**ox, **H**erpes.

You need to be **naked** for a **PAP** smear.

HIGH-YIELD FACTS

Microbiology

RNA viruses

Viral Family	Envelope	RNA Structure	Capsid Symmetry	Medical Importance

Picornaviruses	No	SS + linear	Icosahedral	**P**oliovirus—polio-Salk/Sabin vaccines—IPV/OPV
				Echovirus—aseptic meningitis
				Rhinovirus—"common cold"
				Coxsackievirus—aseptic meningitis
				   herpangina—febrile pharyngitis
				   hand, foot, and mouth disease
				   myocarditis
				Hepatitis A—acute viral hepatitis *Micro1.29*

Caliciviruses	No	SS + linear	Icosahedral	Hepatitis E Norwalk virus—viral gastroenteritis
Reoviruses	No	DS linear Segmented	Icosahedral (double)	Reovirus—Colorado tick fever Rotavirus—#1 cause of fatal diarrhea in children
Flaviviruses	Yes	SS + linear	Icosahedral	Hepatitis C *Micro1.31* Yellow fever *Micro2.78* Dengue *Micro1.96* St. Louis encephalitis *Micro2.99*
Togaviruses	Yes	SS + linear	Icosahedral	Rubella (German measles) *Micro2.47* Eastern equine encephalitis Western equine encephalitis
Retroviruses	Yes	SS + linear	Icosahedral	Have reverse transcriptase HIV—AIDS HTLV—T-cell leukemia *Micro2.8*
Orthomyxoviruses	Yes	SS – linear Segmented	Helical	Influenza virus *Micro2.11*

Paramyxoviruses	Yes	SS – linear
		Nonsegmented
			Helical	**PaRaM**yxovirus:
				   Parainfluenza—croup *Micro1.80*
				   RSV—bronchiolitis in babies; Rx—ribavirin
				     Micro1.51
				   Measles *Micro2.23*
				   Mumps *Micro2.26*

Rhabdoviruses	Yes	SS – linear	Helical	Rabies *Micro2.41*
Filoviruses	Yes	SS – linear	Helical	Ebola/Marburg hemorrhagic fever—often fatal! *Micro1.97*
Coronaviruses	Yes	SS + linear	Helical	Coronavirus—"common cold"
Arenaviruses	Yes	SS – circular	Helical	LCV—lymphocytic choriomeningitis Meningitis—spread by mice
Bunyaviruses	Yes	SS – circular	Helical	California encephalitis Sandfly/Rift Valley fevers Crimea-Congo hemorrhagic fever *Micro1.95* Hantavirus—hemorrhagic fever, pneumonia
Deltavirus	Yes	SS – circular	Helical	Hepatitis D

SS, single-stranded; DS, double-stranded; +, + polarity; –, – polarity

(Adapted, with permission, from Levinson W, Jawetz E. *Medical Microbiology and Immunology: Examination and Board Review*, 6th ed. New York: McGraw-Hill, 2000:182.)

HIGH-YIELD FACTS

Microbiology

Naked viral genome infectivity	Naked nucleic acids of most dsDNA (except poxviruses and HBV) and (+) strand ssRNA (≈ mRNA) viruses are infectious. Naked nucleic acids of (−) strand ssRNA and dsRNA viruses are not infectious.	Viral nucleic acids with the same structure as host nucleic acids are infective alone; others require special enzymes (contained in intact virion).
	Naked (nonenveloped) RNA viruses include **C**alicivirus, **P**icornavirus, and **R**eovirus.	**Naked CPR.**

Enveloped viruses	Generally, enveloped viruses acquire their envelopes from plasma membrane when they exit from cell. Exceptions are herpesviruses, which acquire envelopes from nuclear membrane.

Virus ploidy	All viruses are haploid (with one copy of DNA or RNA) except retroviruses, which have 2 identical ssRNA molecules (≈ diploid).

Viral replication

DNA viruses	All replicate in the nucleus (except poxvirus).
RNA viruses	All replicate in the cytoplasm (except influenza virus and retroviruses).

Viral vaccines	Live attenuated vaccines induce humoral and cell-mediated immunity but have reverted to virulence on rare occasions. Killed vaccines induce only humoral immunity but are stable.	Dangerous to give live vaccines to immunocompromised patients or their close contacts.
	Live attenuated—measles, mumps, rubella, Sabin polio, VZV, yellow fever.	MMR = measles, mumps, rubella.
	Killed—rabies, influenza, hepatitis A, and Salk polio vaccines.	Sal**K** = **K**illed.
	Recombinant—HBV (antigen = recombinant HBsAg).	

Viral genetics

Recombination	Exchange of genes between 2 chromosomes by crossing over within regions of significant base sequence homology.
Reassortment	When viruses with segmented genomes (e.g., influenza virus) exchange segments. High-frequency recombination. Cause of worldwide pandemics.
Complementation	When 1 of 2 viruses that infect the cell has a mutation that results in a nonfunctional protein. The nonmutated virus "complements" the mutated one by making a functional protein that serves both viruses.
Phenotypic mixing	Genome of virus A can be coated with the surface proteins of virus B. Type B protein coat determines the infectivity of the phenotypically mixed virus. However, the progeny from this infection has a type A coat and is encoded by its type A genetic material.

Viral pathogens

Structure	Viruses
DNA enveloped viruses	Herpesviruses (herpes simplex virus types 1 and 2, varicella-zoster virus, cytomegalovirus, Epstein-Barr virus), hepatitis B virus, smallpox virus
DNA nucleocapsid viruses	Adenovirus, papillomaviruses, parvovirus
RNA enveloped viruses	Influenza virus, parainfluenza virus, respiratory syncytial virus, measles virus, mumps virus, rubella virus, rabies virus, human T-cell leukemia virus, human immunodeficiency virus
RNA nucleocapsid viruses	Enteroviruses (poliovirus, coxsackievirus, echovirus, hepatitis A virus), rhinovirus, reovirus

Slow virus infections

UCV *Micro2.97*

Virus exists in patient for months to years before it manifests as clinical disease. SSPE (late sequela of measles), PML (reactivation of JC virus) in immunocompromised patients, especially AIDS.

Segmented viruses

All are RNA viruses. They include **B**unyaviruses, **O**rthomyxoviruses (influenza viruses), **A**renaviruses, and **R**eoviruses. Influenza virus consists of 8 segments of negative-stranded RNA. These segments can undergo reassortment, causing antigenic shifts that lead to worldwide epidemics of the flu.

BOAR.

Picornavirus

Includes poliovirus, rhinovirus, coxsackievirus, echovirus, hepatitis A virus. RNA is translated into 1 large polypeptide that is cleaved by proteases into many small proteins. Can cause aseptic (viral) meningitis (except rhinovirus and hep A virus).

Pico**RNA**virus = small **RNA** virus.

Rhinovirus

UCV *Micro1.20*

Nonenveloped RNA virus. Cause of common cold— > 100 serologic types.

Rhino has a runny nose.

Rotavirus

UCV *Micro1.37*

Rotavirus, the most important global cause of infantile gastroenteritis, is a segmented dsRNA virus (a reovirus). Major cause of acute diarrhea in the United States during winter.

ROTA = Right Out The Anus.

Paramyxoviruses

Paramyxoviruses include those that cause parainfluenza (croup), mumps, and measles as well as RSV, which causes respiratory tract infection (bronchiolitis, pneumonia) in infants. Paramyxoviruses cause disease in children. All paramyxoviruses have 1 serotype except parainfluenza virus, which has 4.

Mumps virus

UCV *Micro2.26*

A paramyxovirus with 1 serotype.

Symptoms: aseptic **M**eningitis, **O**rchitis (inflammation of testes), and **P**arotitis. Can cause sterility (especially after puberty).

Mumps gives you **b**umps (parotitis).

MOP.

HIGH-YIELD FACTS

Microbiology

Measles virus

A paramyxovirus that causes measles. Koplik spots (bluish-gray spots on buccal mucosa) are diagnostic. SSPE, encephalitis (1 in 2000), or giant cell pneumonia (rarely, in immunosuppressed) are possible sequelae.

3 C's of measles:
  Cough
  Coryza
  Conjunctivitis
Also look for **K**oplik spots.

UCV *Micro2.23*

Influenza viruses

Enveloped, single-stranded RNA viruses with segmented genome. Contain hemagglutinin and neuraminidase antigens. Responsible for worldwide influenza epidemics; patients at risk for fatal bacterial superinfection. Rapid genetic changes.

Killed viral vaccine is major mode of protection; reformulated vaccine offered each fall to elderly, health-care workers, etc.

Genetic shift — Reassortment of viral genome (such as when human flu A virus recombines with swine flu A virus).

Genetic drift — Minor changes based on random mutation.

Amantadine and rimantadine are approved for use against influenza A (especially prophylaxis) but are not useful against influenza B or C.
Zanamivir (a neuraminidase inhibitor) useful for both influenza A and B.

UCV *Micro2.11*

Rabies virus

Negri bodies are characteristic cytoplasmic inclusions in neurons infected by rabies virus. Has bullet-shaped capsid. Rabies has long incubation period (weeks to 3 months). Causes fatal encephalitis with seizures and hydrophobia.
More commonly from bat, raccoon, and skunk bites than from dog bites in the United States.

Travels to the CNS by migrating in a retrograde fashion up nerve axons.

UCV *Micro2.41*

Arboviruses

Transmitted by arthropods (mosquitoes, ticks). Classic examples are dengue fever (also known as break-bone fever) and yellow fever. A variant of dengue fever in Southeast Asia is hemorrhagic shock syndrome.

ARBOvirus—**AR**thropod-**BO**rne virus including flavivirus, togavirus, and bunyavirus.

Yellow fever

Caused by flavivirus, an arbovirus transmitted by *Aedes* mosquitos. Virus has a monkey or human reservoir.
Symptoms: high fever, black vomitus, and jaundice. Councilman bodies (acidophilic inclusions) may be seen in liver.

Flavi = yellow.

UCV *Micro2.78*

Herpesviruses

Virus	Diseases	Route of transmission	
HSV-1	Gingivostomatitis, keratoconjunctivitis, temporal lobe encephalitis, herpes labialis *Micro2.89*	Respiratory secretions, saliva	Get herpes in a **CHEV**rolet: CMV
HSV-2	Herpes genitalis, neonatal herpes *Micro1.100*	Sexual contact, perinatal	HSV
VZV	Varicella-zoster (shingles), encephalitis, pneumonia *Micro1.101, 2.74*	Respiratory secretions	EBV VZV
EBV	Infectious mononucleosis, Burkitt's lymphoma *Micro2.10*	Respiratory secretions, saliva	
CMV	Congenital infection, mononucleosis, pneumonia *Micro1.75, 76, 77*	Congenital, transfusion, sexual contact, saliva, urine, transplant	
HHV-8	Kaposi's sarcoma (HIV patients)	Sexual contact	

UCV

Mononucleosis

Caused by EBV, a herpesvirus. Characterized by fever, hepatosplenomegaly, pharyngitis, and lymphadenopathy (especially posterior auricular nodes).

Peak incidence 15–20 years old. Positive heterophil Ab test. Abnormal circulating cytotoxic T cells (atypical lymphocytes).

Most common during peak kissing years ("kissing disease").

Monospot test—heterophil antibodies detected by agglutination of sheep RBCs.

UCV *Micro2.10*

Tzanck test

A smear of an opened skin vesicle to detect multinucleated giant cells. Used to assay for HSV-1, HSV-2, and VZV.

Tzanck heavens I do not have herpes.

Hepatitis transmission

HAV (RNA picornavirus) is transmitted primarily by fecal-oral route. Short incubation (3 weeks). No carriers. *Micro1.29*

Hep **A: A**symptomatic (usually).

HBV (DNA hepadnavirus) is transmitted primarily by parenteral, sexual, and maternal-fetal routes. Long incubation (3 months). Carriers. Reverse transcription occurs; however, the virion enzyme is a DNA-dependent DNA polymerase. *Micro1.30*

Hep **B: B**lood borne.

HCV (RNA flavivirus) is transmitted primarily via blood and resembles HBV in its course and severity. Carriers. Common cause of IV drug use hepatitis in the United States. *Micro1.31*

Hep **C: C**hronic, **C**irrhosis, **C**arcinoma, **C**arriers.

HDV (delta agent) is a defective virus that requires HBsAg as its envelope. Carriers.

Hep **D: D**efective, **D**ependent on HBV.

HEV (RNA calicivirus) is transmitted enterically and causes water-borne epidemics. Resembles HAV in course, severity, incubation. High mortality rate in pregnant women.

Hep **E: E**nteric, **E**xpectant mothers, **E**pidemics.

A and E by fecal-oral route: "The **vowels** hit your **bowels.**"

Both HBV and HCV predispose a patient to chronic active hepatitis, cirrhosis, and hepatocellular carcinoma.

UCV

Hepatitis serologic markers

IgM HAVAb	IgM antibody to HAV; best test to detect active hepatitis A.
HBsAg	Antigen found on surface of HBV; continued presence indicates carrier state.
HBsAb	Antibody to HBsAg; **provides immunity** to hepatitis B.
HBcAg	Antigen associated with core of HBV.
HBcAb	Antibody to HBcAg; positive during **window period.** IgM HBcAb is an indicator of recent disease.
HBeAg	A second, different antigenic determinant in the HBV core. Important indicator of transmissibility. (**BE**ware!)
HBeAb	Antibody to e antigen; indicates low transmissibility.

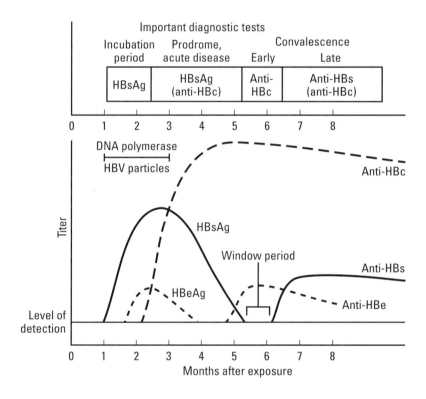

Test	Acute Disease	Window Phase	Complete Recovery	Chronic Carrier
HBsAg	+	−	−	+
HBsAb	−	−	+	−[b]
HBcAb	+[a]	+	+	+

[a]IgM in acute stage; IgG in chronic or recovered stage.

[b]Patient has surface antibody but available antibody is bound to HBsAg.

HIV

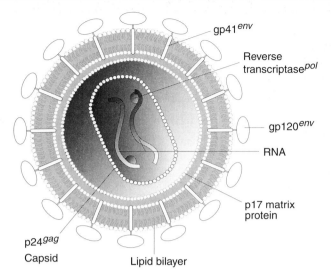

gp41^{env}

Reverse transcriptase^{pol}

gp120^{env}

RNA

p17 matrix protein

p24^{gag}
Capsid

Lipid bilayer

Diploid genome (2 molecules of RNA).

p24 = rectangular nucleocapsid protein.

gp41 and gp120 = envelope proteins.

Reverse transcriptase synthesizes dsDNA from RNA. DsDNA integrates into host genome.

(Adapted, with permission, from Levinson W, Jawetz E. *Medical Microbiology and Immunology: Examination and Board Review,* 6th ed. New York: McGraw-Hill, 2000:272.)

HIV diagnosis	Presumptive diagnosis made with ELISA (sensitive, high false-positive rate and low threshold, RULE OUT test); positive results are then confirmed with Western blot assay (specific, high false-negative rate and high threshold, RULE IN test). HIV PCR/viral load tests are increasing in popularity; they allow physician to monitor the effect of drug therapy on viral load. ELISA/Western blot tests look for antibodies to viral proteins; these tests are often falsely negative in the first 1–2 months of HIV infection.

Time course of HIV infection

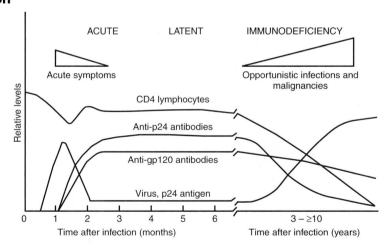

(Adapted, with permission, from Levinson W, Jawetz E. *Medical Microbiology and Immunology: Examination and Board Review,* 6th ed. New York: McGraw-Hill, 2000:276.)

Opportunistic infections in AIDS

Bacterial	Tuberculosis, *Mycobacterium avium–intracellulare* complex. <small>Micro2.68</small>
Viral	Herpes simplex, varicella-zoster virus, cytomegalovirus, progressive multifocal leukoencephalopathy (JC virus). <small>Micro1.76, 77, 100, 101, 2.97</small>
Fungal	Thrush (*Candida albicans*), cryptococcosis (cryptococcal meningitis), histoplasmosis, *Pneumocystis* pneumonia. <small>Micro1.69, 2.7, 2.36</small>
Protozoan	Toxoplasmosis, cryptosporidiosis. <small>Micro1.81, 2.65</small>

UCV

Prions

Infectious agents that do not contain RNA or DNA (consist only of proteins); diseases include Creutzfeldt-Jakob disease (CJD—rapid progressive dementia), kuru, scrapie (sheep), and "mad cow disease." Prions are associated with spongiform encephalopathy.

Normal flora: dominant

Skin—*Staphylococcus epidermidis*
Nose—*S. aureus*
Oropharynx—viridans streptococci
Dental plaque—*Streptococcus mutans*
Colon—*Bacteroides fragilis* > *E. coli*
Vagina—*Lactobacillus*, colonized by *E. coli* and group B strep.

Neonates delivered by cesarean section have no flora but are rapidly colonized after birth.

Common causes of pneumonia

Children (6 wks–18 yr) ➤	Adults (18–40 yr) ➤	Adults (40–65 yr) ➤	Elderly
Viruses (RSV)	*Mycoplasma*	*S. pneumoniae*	*S. pneumoniae*
Mycoplasma	*C. pneumoniae*	*H. influenzae*	Viruses
Chlamydia pneumoniae	*S. pneumoniae*	Anaerobes	Anaerobes
Streptococcus pneumoniae		Viruses	*H. influenzae*
		Mycoplasma	Gram-negative rods

Special groups:

Nosocomial (hospital acquired)	*Staphylococcus*, gram-negative rods
Immunocompromised	*Staphylococcus*, gram-negative rods, fungi, viruses, *Pneumocystis carinii*—with HIV
Aspiration	Anaerobes
Alcoholic/IV drug user	*S. pneumoniae*, *Klebsiella*, *Staphylococcus*
Postviral	*Staphylococcus*, *H. influenzae*
Neonate	Group B streptococci, *E. coli*
Atypical	*Mycoplasma*, *Legionella*, *Chlamydia*

Causes of meningitis

Newborn (0–6 mos) →	Children (6 mos–6 yrs) →	6–60 yrs →	60 yrs +
Group B streptococci	*Streptococcus pneumoniae*	**N. meningitidis**	***S. pneumoniae***
E. coli	*Neisseria meningitidis*	Enteroviruses	Gram-negative rods
Listeria	*Haemophilus influenzae B*	*S. pneumoniae*	*Listeria*
	Enteroviruses	HSV	

In HIV—*Cryptococcus*, CMV, toxoplasmosis (brain abscess), JC virus (PML).

Note: Incidence of *H. influenzae* meningitis has ↓ greatly with introduction of *H. influenzae* vaccine in last 10–15 years.

UCV *Micro2.18, 24, 79*

CSF findings in meningitis

	Pressure	Cell type	Protein	Sugar
Bacterial	↑	↑ PMNs	↑	↓
Fungal/TB	↑	↑ lymphocytes	↑	↓
Viral	normal/↑	↑ lymphocytes	normal	normal

Osteomyelitis

Most people—*Staphylococcus aureus*.
Sexually active—*Neisseria gonorrhoeae* (rare), septic arthritis more common.
Drug addicts—*Pseudomonas aeruginosa*.
Sickle cell—*Salmonella*.
Prosthetic replacement—*S. aureus* and *S. epidermidis*.
Vertebral—*Mycobacterium tuberculosis*.

Assume *S. aureus* if no other information.
Most osteomyelitis occurs in children.
Elevated ESR.

UCV *Micro2.109*

Urinary tract infections

Ambulatory—*E. coli* (50–80%), *Klebsiella* (8–10%).
Staphylococcus saprophyticus (10–30%) is the 2nd most common cause of UTI in young ambulatory women.
Hospital—*E. coli*, *Proteus*, *Klebsiella*, *Serratia*, *Pseudomonas*.
Epidemiology: women to men—10 to 1 (short urethra colonized by fecal flora).
Predisposing factors: flow obstruction, kidney surgery, catheterization, gynecologic abnormalities, diabetes, and pregnancy.

UTIs mostly caused by ascending infections. In males: babies with congenital defects; elderly with enlarged prostates.
UTI—dysuria, frequency, urgency, suprapubic pain.
Pyelonephritis—fever, chills, flank pain, and CVA tenderness.

UCV *Micro2.72, 73*

UTI bugs

Species	Features of the organism	
Serratia marcescens	Some strains produce a red pigment; often nosocomial and drug resistant.	SSEEK PP.
Staphylococcus saprophyticus	2nd leading cause of community-acquired UTI in sexually active women.	
Escherichia coli	Leading cause of UTI. Colonies show metallic sheen on EMB agar.	
Enterobacter cloacae	Often nosocomial and drug resistant.	
Klebsiella pneumoniae	Large mucoid capsule and viscous colonies.	
Proteus mirabilis	Motility causes "swarming" on agar; produces urease; associated with struvite stones.	
Pseudomonas aeruginosa	Blue-green pigment and fruity odor; usually nosocomial and drug resistant.	

Sexually transmitted diseases

Disease	Clinical features	Organism
Gonorrhea	Urethritis, cervicitis, PID, prostatitis, epididymitis, arthritis Micro1.91	*Neisseria gonorrhoeae*
1° syphilis	Painless chancre Micro2.59	*Treponema pallidum*
2° syphilis	Fever, lymphadenopathy, skin rashes, condylomata lata Micro2.60	
3° syphilis	Gummas, tabes dorsalis, general paresis, aortitis, Argyll-Robertson pupil	
Genital herpes	Painful penile, vulvar, or cervical ulcers Micro1.100	HSV-2
Chlamydia	Urethritis, cervicitis, conjunctivitis, Reiter's syndrome, PID Path3.92	*Chlamydia trachomatis* (D–K)
Lymphogranuloma venereum	Ulcers, lymphadenopathy, rectal strictures Micro2.21	*C. trachomatis* (L1–L3)
Trichomoniasis	Vaginitis	*Trichomonas vaginalis*
AIDS	Opportunistic infections, Kaposi's sarcoma, lymphoma	HIV
Condylomata acuminata	Genital warts, koilocytes	HPV 6 and 11
Hepatitis B	Jaundice Micro1.30	HBV
Chancroid	Painful genital ulcer	*Haemophilus ducreyi*

UCV

Pelvic inflammatory disease

Top bugs—*Chlamydia trachomatis* (subacute, often undiagnosed), *Neisseria gonorrhoeae* (acute, high fever). *C. trachomatis* is the most common STD in the United States (3–4 million cases per year). Cervical motion tenderness (chandelier sign), purulent cervical discharge. PID may include salpingitis, endometritis, hydrosalpinx, and tubo-ovarian abscess.

Salpingitis is a risk factor for ectopic pregnancy, infertility, chronic pelvic pain, and adhesions.
Other STDs include *Gardnerella* (clue cells) and *Trichomonas* (motile on wet prep).

UCV Micro2.104

HIGH-YIELD FACTS

Microbiology

Nosocomial infections

Risk factor	Pathogen	Notes
Newborn nursery	CMV, RSV	The 2 most common causes
Urinary catheterization	E. coli, Proteus mirabilis	of nosocomial infections are E. coli (UTI) and S. aureus (wound infection).
Respiratory therapy equipment	Pseudomonas aeruginosa	Presume Pseudomonas **AIR**uginosa when **AIR** or
Work in renal dialysis unit	HBV	burns are involved.
Hyperalimentation	Candida albicans	
Water aerosols	Legionella	Legionella when water source is involved.

Infections dangerous in pregnancy

ToRCHeS = Toxoplasma, Rubella, CMV, HSV/HIV, Syphilis.

Bug hints (if all else fails)

Pus, empyema, abscess—Staphylococcus aureus.

Pediatric infection—Haemophilus influenzae (including epiglottitis).

Pneumonia in CF, burn infection—Pseudomonas aeruginosa.

Branching rods in oral infection—Actinomyces israelii.

Traumatic open wound—Clostridium perfringens.

Surgical wound—S. aureus.

Dog or cat bite—Pasteurella multocida.

Currant jelly sputum—Klebsiella.

Sepsis/meningitis in newborn—Group B strep.

Antibody structure and function

Variable part of L and H chains recognizes antigens. Constant part of H chain of IgM and IgG fixes complement. Heavy chain contributes to F_c and F_{ab} fractions. Light chain contributes only to F_{ab} fraction.

F_c:

Constant

Carboxy terminal

Complement-binding
(IgG + IgM only)

Carbohydrate
side chains

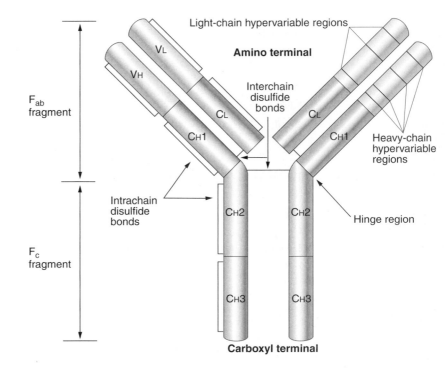

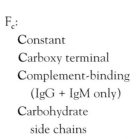

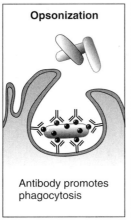

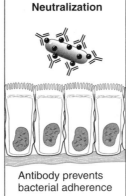

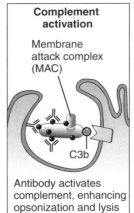

Opsonization	Neutralization	Complement activation
Antibody promotes phagocytosis	Antibody prevents bacterial adherence	Antibody activates complement, enhancing opsonization and lysis

Membrane attack complex (MAC)

C3b

Immunoglobulin isotypes

IgG	Main antibody in 2° response. Most abundant. Fixes complement, crosses the placenta, opsonizes bacteria, neutralizes bacterial toxins and viruses.
IgA	Prevents attachment of bacteria and viruses to mucous membranes, does not fix complement. Monomer or dimer. Found in secretions. Picks up secretory component from epithelial cells before secretion.
IgM	Produced in the 1° response to an antigen. Fixes complement but does not cross the placenta. Antigen receptor on the surface of B cells. Monomer or pentamer.
IgD	Unclear function. Found on the surface of many B cells and in serum.
IgE	Mediates immediate (type I) hypersensitivity by inducing the release of mediators from mast cells and basophils when exposed to allergen. Mediates immunity to worms. Lowest concentration in serum.

Ig epitopes

Allotype (polymorphism)—Ig epitope that differs among members of same species. Can be on light chain or heavy chain.

Isotype (IgG, IgA, etc.)—Ig epitope common to a single class of Ig (5 classes, determined by heavy chain).

Idiotype (specific for a given Ag)—Ig epitope determined by antigen-binding site.

Isotype = *iso* (same). Common to same class.

Idiotype = *idio* (unique). Hypervariable region is unique.

MHC I and II

MHC—major histocompatibility complex. Consists of 3 class I genes (A, B, C) and 3 class II genes (DP, DQ, DR). All nucleated cells have class I MHC proteins.

Antigen-presenting cells (e.g., macrophages and dendritic cells) also have class II MHC proteins.

Class II are the main determinants of organ rejection.

MHC I Ag loading occurs in RER (viral antigens).

MHC II Ag loading occurs in acidified endosome.

Class I—1 polypeptide, with β_2-microglobulin.

Class II—2 polypeptides, an α and a β chain.

Differentiation of B and T cells

Th1 cells (produce IL-2 and γ-interferon)—activate macrophages (increase killing efficiency of intracellular bacteria) and Tc cells.

Th2 cells (produce IL-4 and IL-5)—help B cells make Ab (B = 2nd letter of alphabet).

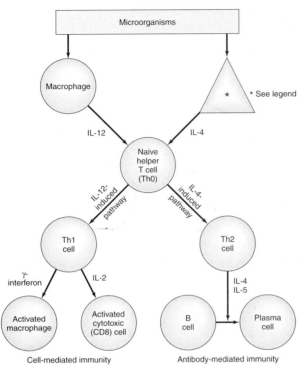

*The human cell that produces the IL-4 that induces naive helper T cells to become Th2 cells has not been identified.

(Adapted, with permission, from Levinson W, Jawetz E. *Medical Microbiology and Immunology: Examination and Board Review*, 6th ed. New York: McGraw-Hill, 2000:349.)

Major function of B cells and T cells

Antibody-mediated immunity (B cells)

Host defense against infection (opsonize bacteria, neutralize toxins and viruses)

Allergy (e.g., hay fever)

Autoimmunity

Cell-mediated immunity (T cells)

Host defense against infection (especially *Mycobacterium tuberculosis*, viruses, and fungi)

Allergy (e.g., poison oak)

Graft and tumor rejection

Regulation of antibody response (help and suppression)

(Adapted, with permission, from Levinson W, Jawetz E. *Medical Microbiology and Immunology: Examination and Board Review*, 6th ed. New York: McGraw-Hill, 2000:337.)

Adjuvant definition

Adjuvants are nonspecific stimulators of the immune response but are not immunogenic by themselves. Adjuvants are given with a weak immunogen to enhance response. Human vaccines contain aluminum hydroxide or lipid adjuvants.

Adjuvant—that which aids another.

T-cell glycoproteins

Helper T cells have CD4, which binds to class II MHC on antigen-presenting cells. Cytotoxic T cells have CD8, which binds to class I MHC on virus-infected cells.

Product of CD and MHC = 8. ($CD4 \times MHC$ **II** = **8** = $CD8 \times MHC$ **I**).

CD3 complex—cluster of polypeptides associated with a T-cell receptor. Important in signal transduction.

Antigen-presenting cells:
1. Macrophage
2. B cell
3. Dendritic cell

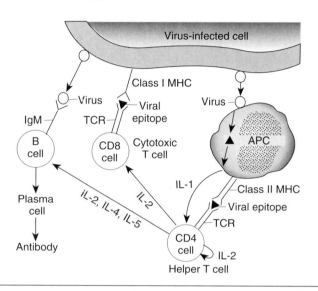

T-cell activation

Th activation:
1. Foreign body is phagocytosed by APC
2. Foreign antigen is presented on MHC II and recognized by TCR on Th cell
3. "Costimulatory signal" is given by interaction of B7 and CD28
4. Th cell activated to produce IL-2 and γ-interferon

Tc activation:
1. Endogenously synthesized (viral or self) proteins are presented on MHC I and recognized by TCR on Tc cell
2. IL-2 from Th cell activates Tc cell to kill virus-infected cell

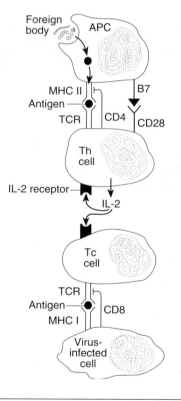

Anergy

Self-reactive T cells become nonreactive without costimulatory molecule.

B cells also become anergic through clonal deletion or clonal anergy, but tolerance is less complete than in T cells.

Important cytokines

IL-1	Secreted by macrophages. Stimulates T cells, B cells, neutrophils, fibroblasts, and epithelial cells to grow, differentiate, or synthesize specific products. An endogenous pyrogen.	**"Hot T-bone stEAk":** IL-1: fever **(hot)** IL-2: stimulates **T** cells IL-3: stimulates **bone** marrow
IL-2	Secreted by helper T cells. Stimulates growth of helper and cytotoxic T cells.	IL-4: stimulates Ig**E** production
IL-3	Secreted by activated T cells. Supports the growth and differentiation of bone marrow stem cells. Has a function similar to GM-CSF.	IL-5: stimulates Ig**A** production
IL-4	Secreted by helper T cells. Promotes growth of B cells. Enhances the synthesis of IgE and IgG.	
IL-5	Secreted by helper T cells. Promotes differentiation of B cells. Enhances the synthesis of IgA. Stimulates production and activation of eosinophils.	
IL-8	Major chemotactic factor for neutrophils.	
γ-interferon	Secreted by helper T cells. Stimulates macrophages.	
TNF-α	Secreted by macrophages. ↑ IL-2 receptor synthesis by helper T cells. ↑ B-cell proliferation. Attracts and activates neutrophils.	
TNF-β	Secreted by activated T lymphocytes. Functions similar to those of TNF-α.	

Acute phase response

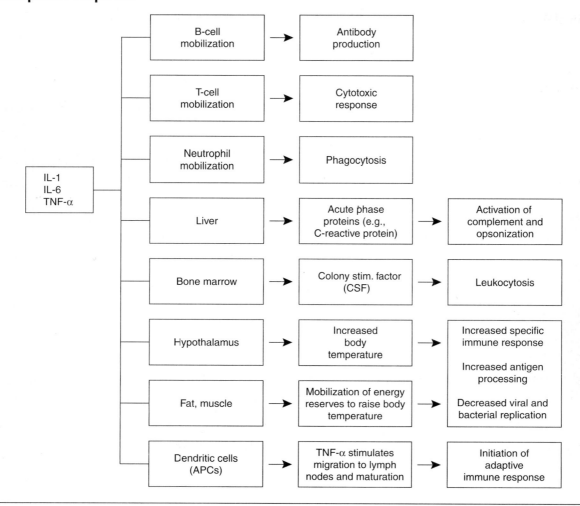

Complement

Complement defends against gram-negative bacteria. Activated by IgG or IgM in the **classic** pathway, and activated by toxins (including endotoxin), aggregated IgA, or other conditions in the alternate pathway.

GM makes **classic** cars.

C1, C2, C3, C4—viral neutralization.

C3b—opsonization.

C3a, C5a—anaphylaxis.

C5a—neutrophil chemotaxis.

C5b-9—cytolysis by membrane attack complex (MAC).

Deficiency of C1 esterase inhibitor leads to hereditary angioedema (overactive complement).

Deficiency of C3 leads to severe, recurrent pyogenic sinus and respiratory tract infections.

Deficiency of C6–C8 leads to *Neisseria* bacteremia.

Deficiency of decay-accelerating factor (DAF) leads to paroxysmal nocturnal hemoglobinuria (PNH).

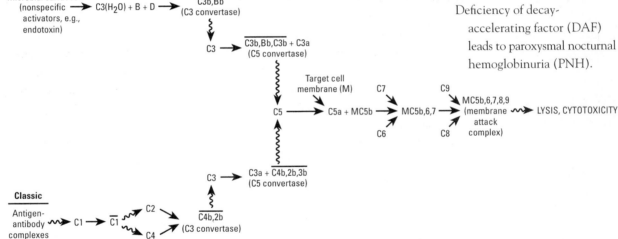

(Adapted, with permission, from Levinson W, Jawetz E. *Medical Microbiology and Immunology: Examination and Board Review*, 6th ed. New York: McGraw-Hill, 2000:381.)

UCV Micro2.3

Interferon mechanism

Interferons (α, β) are proteins that place uninfected cells in an antiviral state. Interferons induce the production of a 2nd protein that inhibits viral protein synthesis by degrading viral mRNA (but not host mRNA).

Interferes with viral protein synthesis by:

1. α- and β-interferons inhibit viral protein synthesis
2. γ-interferons increase MHC Class I and Class II expression and antigen presentation in all cells
3. Activates NK cells to kill virus-infected cells

Hypersensitivity

Type I

Mast cell or basophil

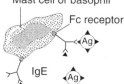

Anaphylactic and atopic—Ag cross-links IgE on presensitized mast cells and basophils, triggering release of vasoactive amines (i.e., histamine). Reaction develops rapidly after Ag exposure due to preformed Ab. Examples include anaphylaxis, asthma, local wheal and flare.

First and Fast (anaphylaxis). I, II, and III are all antibody mediated.

Type II

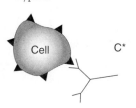

Cytotoxic—IgM, IgG bind to Ag on "enemy" cell, leading to lysis (by complement) or phagocytosis. Examples include autoimmune hemolytic anemia, Rh disease (erythroblastosis fetalis), Goodpasture's syndrome, rheumatic fever.

Cy-2-toxic.
Antibody and complement lead to membrane attack complex (MAC).

Type III

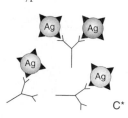

Immune complex—Ag-Ab complexes activate complement, which attracts neutrophils; neutrophils release lysosomal enzymes. Examples include PAN, immune complex GN, SLE, rheumatoid arthritis.

Imagine an immune complex as 3 things stuck together: Ag-Ab-complement.

Serum sickness—an immune complex disease (type III) in which Abs to the foreign proteins are produced (takes 5 days). Immune complexes form and are deposited in membranes, where they fix complement (leads to tissue damage). More common than Arthus reaction. *Path2.44*

Most serum sickness is now caused by drugs (not serum). Fever, urticaria, arthralgias, proteinuria, lymphadenopathy 5–10 days after Ag exposure.

Arthus reaction—a local subacute Ab-mediated hypersensitivity (type III) reaction. Intradermal injection of Ag induces antibodies, which form Ag-Ab complexes in the skin. Characterized by edema, necrosis, and activation of complement. Examples include hypersensitivity pneumonitis, thermophilic actinomycetes.

Ag-Ab complexes cause the Arthus reaction.

Type IV

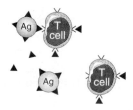

Delayed (cell-mediated) type—sensitized T lymphocytes encounter antigen and then release lymphokines (leads to macrophage activation). Examples include TB skin test, transplant rejection, contact dermatitis (e.g., poison ivy, poison oak). *Path1.32*

4th and last—delayed. Cell mediated; therefore, it is not transferable by serum.

ACID:
Anaphylactic and Atopic (type I)
Cytotoxic (type II)
Immune complex (type III)
Delayed (cell-mediated) (type IV)

C* = complement

Immune deficiencies

B-cell deficiencies

Bruton's agammaglobulinemia	X-linked recessive defect in a tyrosine-kinase gene associated with low levels of all classes of immunoglobulins. Associated with recurrent **B**acterial infections after 6 months of age, when levels of maternal IgG antibody decline. Occurs in **B**oys (X-linked). Micro2.6
Selective immunoglobulin deficiency	Deficiency in a specific class of immunoglobulins—possibly due to a defect in isotype switching. Selective IgA deficiency is the most common selective immunoglobulin deficiency. Presents with sinus and lung infections, milk allergies, and anaphylaxis to blood transfusions. Micro2.4

T-cell deficiencies

Thymic aplasia (DiGeorge syndrome)	Thymus and parathyroids fail to develop owing to failure of development of the 3rd and 4th pharyngeal pouches. Presents with **T**etany owing to hypocalcemia. Congenital defects of heart and great vessels. Recurrent viral, fungal, and protozoal infections. Anat.42
Chronic mucocutaneous candidiasis	T-cell dysfunction specifically against *Candida albicans*. Presents with skin and mucous membrane *Candida* infections.

B- and T-cell deficiencies

Severe combined immunodeficiency (SCID)	Defect in early stem-cell differentiation. Presents with recurrent viral, bacterial, fungal, and protozoal infections. May have multiple causes (e.g., failure to synthesize class II MHC antigens, defective IL-2 receptors, or adenosine deaminase deficiency). Micro2.5
Wiskott-Aldrich syndrome	X-linked defect in the ability to mount an IgM response to capsular polysaccharides of bacteria. Associated with elevated IgA levels, normal IgE levels, and low IgM levels. Triad of symptoms includes recurrent pyogenic infections, eczema, and thrombocytopenia.
Ataxia-telangiectasia	Defect in DNA repair enzymes with associated IgA deficiency. Presents with cerebellar problems (ataxia) and spider angiomas (telangiectasia).

Phagocytic deficiencies

Chronic granulomatous disease	Defect in phagocytosis of neutrophils owing to lack of NADPH oxidase activity or similar enzymes. Presents with marked susceptibility to opportunistic infections with bacteria, especially *S. aureus* and *E. coli*, and *Aspergillus*. Diagnosis confirmed with negative nitroblue tetrazolium dye reduction test. Micro2.2
Chédiak-Higashi disease	Autosomal-recessive. Defect in microtubular function and lysosomal emptying of phagocytic cells. Presents with recurrent pyogenic infections by staphylococci and streptococci. Micro1.45
Job's syndrome	Failure of γ-interferon production by helper T cells. Neutrophils fail to respond to chemotactic stimuli. Presents with recurrent "cold" (noninflamed) staphylococcal abscesses, eczema, and high levels of IgE.
Leukocyte adhesion deficiency syndrome	Defect in LFA-1 adhesion proteins on phagocytes. Presents early in life with severe pyogenic infections.
Hyper-IgM syndrome	Defect in CD40 ligand on CD4 T helper cells leads to inability to class switch. Presents early in life with severe pyogenic infections. High levels of IgM, very low levels of IgG, IgA, and IgE.
IL-12 receptor deficiency	Presents with disseminated mycobacterial infections.

Passive vs. active immunity

Active	Induced after exposure to foreign antigens. Slow onset. Long-lasting protection (memory).	After exposure to **T**etanus toxin, **B**otulinum toxin, **H**BV, or **R**abies, patients are given preformed antibodies (passive)—**T**o **B**e **H**ealed **R**apidly.
Passive	Based on receiving preformed antibodies from another host. Rapid onset. Short life span of antibodies.	

Antigen variation

Classic examples:
    Bacteria—*Salmonella* (two flagellar variants), *Borrelia* (relapsing fever), *Neisseria gonorrhoeae* (pilus protein).
    Virus—influenza (major = shift, minor = drift).
    Parasites—trypanosomes (programmed rearrangement).

Some mechanisms for variation include DNA rearrangement and RNA segment rearrangement (e.g., influenza major shift).

Autoantibodies

Autoantibody	Associated disorder
Antinuclear antibodies (ANA)	Systemic lupus
Anti-dsDNA, anti-Smith	Specific for systemic lupus
Anti-histone	Drug-induced lupus
Anti-IgG (rheumatoid factor)	Rheumatoid arthritis
Anti-neutrophil	Vasculitis
Anti-centromere	Scleroderma (CREST)
Anti-Scl-70	Scleroderma (diffuse)
Anti-mitochondria	1° biliary cirrhosis
Anti-gliadin	Celiac disease
Anti–basement membrane	Goodpasture's syndrome
Anti–epithelial cell	Pemphigus vulgaris
Anti-microsomal	Hashimoto's thyroiditis

Transplant rejection

Hyperacute rejection	Antibody mediated due to the presence of preformed anti-donor antibodies in the transplant recipient. Occurs within minutes after transplantation.
Acute rejection	Cell mediated due to cytotoxic T lymphocytes reacting against foreign MHCs. Occurs weeks after transplantation. Reversible with immunosuppressants such as cyclosporin and OKT3.
Chronic rejection	Antibody-mediated vascular damage (fibrinoid necrosis); occurs months to years after transplantation. Irreversible.
Graft-versus-host disease	Grafted immunocompetent T cells proliferate in the irradiated immunocompromised host and reject cells with "foreign" proteins, resulting in severe organ dysfunction. Major symptoms include a maculopapular rash, jaundice, hepatosplenomegaly, and diarrhea.

Pathology

"The beginning of health is to know the disease."
—Spanish proverb

Questions dealing with this discipline are difficult to prepare for because of the sheer volume of material. Review the basic principles and hallmark characteristics of the key diseases. Given the increasingly clinical orientation of Step 1, it is no longer enough to know only the "trigger word" associations of certain diseases (e.g., café-au-lait macules and neurofibromatosis); you must also know the clinical descriptions of these findings.

Given the clinical slant of the USMLE Step 1, it is also important to review the classic presenting signs and symptoms of diseases as well as their associated laboratory findings. Delve into the signs, symptoms, and pathophysiology of the major diseases having a high prevalence in the United States (e.g., alcoholism, diabetes, hypertension, heart failure, ischemic heart disease, infectious disease). Be prepared to think one step beyond the simple diagnosis to treatment or complications.

The examination includes a number of color photomicrographs and photographs of gross specimens that are presented in the setting of a brief clinical history. However, read the question and the choices carefully before looking at the illustration, because the history will help you identify the pathologic process. Flip through an illustrated pathology textbook, color atlases, and appropriate Web sites in order to look at the pictures in the days before the exam. Pay attention to potential clues such as age, sex, ethnicity, occupation, recent activities and exposures, and specialized lab tests.

High-Yield Clinical Vignettes

High-Yield Images

High-Yield Topics

Congenital

Neoplastic

Hematologic

Gastrointestinal

Respiratory

Neurologic

Rheumatic/Autoimmune

Endocrine/Reproductive

Cardiovascular

Renal

Alcoholism

Findings

Glossy Photos

These abstracted case vignettes are designed to demonstrate the thought processes necessary to answer multistep clinical reasoning questions.

Vignette	Question	Answer
Woman with previous cesarean section has a scar in her lower uterus close to the opening of the os.	What is she at increased risk for?	Placenta previa.
35-year-old man has high blood pressure in arms and low pressure in legs.	What is the diagnosis?	Coarctation of the aorta.
Woman presents with diffuse goiter and hyperthyroidism.	What are the expected values of TSH and thyroid hormones?	Low TSH and high thyroid hormones.
Patient exhibits an extended expiratory phase.	What is the disease process?	Obstructive lung disease.
Woman presents with headache, visual disturbance, galactorrhea, and amenorrhea.	What is the diagnosis?	Prolactinoma.
		UCV Path1.59
Baby has foul-smelling stool and recurrent pulmonary infections.	What is the diagnosis, and what test is used?	Cystic fibrosis; chloride sweat test.
Obese woman presents with hirsutism and increased levels of serum testosterone.	What is the diagnosis?	Polycystic ovarian syndrome.
Man presents with pain and swelling of the knees, subcutaneous nodules around the joints and Achilles tendon, and exquisite pain in the metatarsophalangeal joint of his right big toe. Biopsy shows needle-like crystals.	What is the diagnosis?	Gouty arthritis.
48-year-old female with progressive lethargy and extreme sensitivity to cold temperatures.	What is the diagnosis?	Hypothyroidism.
		UCV Path1.57
Patient with elevated serum cortisol levels undergoes a dexamethasone suppression test. 1 mg of dexamethasone does not decrease cortisol levels; 8 mg does.	What is the diagnosis?	Pituitary tumor.
During a game, a young football player collapses and dies immediately.	What type of cardiac disease?	Hypertrophic cardiomyopathy.
		UCV Path1.16

Vignette	Question	Answer
Child has been anemic since birth.	Splenectomy would result in increased hematocrit in what disease?	Spherocytosis.
43-year-old man experiences dizziness and tinnitus. CT shows enlarged internal acoustic meatus.	What is the diagnosis?	Schwannoma.
Child exhibits weakness and enlarged calves.	What is the disease, and how is it inherited?	Duchenne's muscular dystrophy, X-linked recessive.
25-year-old female presents with sudden uniocular vision loss and slightly slurred speech. She has a history of weakness and paresthesias that have resolved.	What is the diagnosis?	MS.
Teenager presents with nephritic syndrome and hearing loss.	What is his disease?	Alport's syndrome.
Tall, thin male teenager has abrupt-onset dyspnea and left-sided chest pain. There is hyperresonant percussion on the affected side, and breath sounds are diminished.	What is the diagnosis?	Pneumothorax.
Young man is concerned about his wife's inability to conceive and her recurrent URIs. She has dextrocardia.	Which of her proteins is defective?	Dynein (Kartagener's).
55-year-old man who is a smoker and a heavy drinker presents with a new cough and flu-like symptoms. Gram stain shows no organisms; silver stain of sputum shows gram-negative rods.	What is the diagnosis?	*Legionella* pneumonia.
Patient has a stroke after incurring multiple long bone fractures in MVA trauma.	What caused the infarct?	Fat emboli.
25-year-old woman presents with a low-grade fever, a rash across her nose that gets worse when she is out in the sun, and widespread edema.	You are concerned about what disease?	SLE.

Vignette	Question	Answer
50-year-old man complains of diarrhea; on physical exam his face is plethoric and a heart murmur is detected.	What is the diagnosis?	Carcinoid syndrome.
Elderly woman presents with a headache and jaw pain. Labs show elevated ESR.	What is the diagnosis?	Temporal arteritis.
Pregnant woman at 16 weeks of gestation presents with an atypically large abdomen.	What abnormality might be seen on blood test, and what is the disorder?	High hCG; hydatidiform mole.
80-year-old man presents with a systolic crescendo-decrescendo murmur.	What is the most likely cause?	Aortic stenosis. UCV *Path1.3*
Woman of short stature presents with shortened 4th and 5th metacarpals.	What endocrine disorder comes to mind?	Albright's hereditary osteodystrophy, or pseudohypoparathyroidism.
After a stressful life event, 30-year-old man has diarrhea and blood per rectum; intestinal biopsy shows transmural inflammation.	What is the diagnosis?	Crohn's.
Young man presents with mental deterioration and tremors. He has brown pigmentation in a ring around the periphery of his cornea and altered LFTs.	What treatment should he receive?	Penicillamine for Wilson's disease.
Patient presents with fatigue, and blood tests show a macrocytic, megaloblastic anemia.	What is the danger of giving folate alone?	Masks signs of neural damage with vitamin B_{12} deficiency.
10-year-old child "spaces out" in class (e.g., stops talking midsentence and then continues as if nothing had happened). During spells, there is slight quivering of lips.	What is the diagnosis?	Absence seizure.

All of these images are high yield and should be carefully studied. Many of these images are represented in the Pathology glossy insert.

- Gross photograph of abdominal aorta with aneurysm → most likely a consequence of what process? → atherosclerosis.
- Gross photograph of hydatidiform mole ("bunch of grapes") → high levels of what substance are present? → hCG.
- Gross photograph of section of small intestine of weight lifter with focal hemorrhages → what is the process responsible for this? → strangulation of a hernia.
- Chest x-ray shows collapse of middle lobe of right lung and mass in right bronchus; patient has history of recurrent pneumonias → what is the diagnosis? → bronchogenic carcinoma.
- Middle-aged woman with intermittent syncope has a mass removed from the right atrium → H&E shows wispy, mucus-like tissue → what is the diagnosis? → myxoma.
- Chest x-ray shows pneumothorax → what are the clinical findings? → pleuritic chest pain and shortness of breath.
- 1-year-old baby presents with big red splotch on face that blanches on palpation. He is developmentally normal and has no neurologic symptoms → what is the likely course of this lesion? → regression (vs. the port-wine stain of Sturge-Weber).
- Gross photograph of lung shows peripheral lesion with caseous necrosis → what is the diagnosis? → TB. *Reactivation in upper lobe.*
- H&E of lung biopsy from plumber shows elongated structures with clubbed ends in tissue → what is the diagnosis? increased risk for what? → asbestosis; malignant mesothelioma.
- H&E of glomerulus → multiple mesangial nodules → lesion is indicative of what disease? → diabetes mellitus. *Nodular glomerulosclerosis.*
- H&E of granuloma → what is activated? → macrophages.
- Karyotype with three 21 chromosomes → what features would patient have? → flat facies, simian crease, epicanthal folds.
- Gross photograph of polycystic kidneys in adult male → what is the mode of inheritance? → autosomal dominant. *IF in baby then think recessive.*
- Patient with anemia, hypercalcemia, and bone pain (on palpation) bone marrow biopsy shows slide packed with plasma cells (with large, round, off-center nucleus) → what is the diagnosis? → multiple myeloma.

Type 2 diabetes → Amyloid in Pancreas due to exhaustion of Islets trying to keep up with hyperglycemia.

Congenital

1. Maternal complications of birth (e.g., Sheehan's syndrome, puerperal infection).
2. Failure to thrive: common causes.
3. Causes of kernicterus (hemolytic disease of the newborn).

Neoplasia

1. Bone and cartilage tumors (e.g., osteosarcoma, giant cell tumor, Ewing's sarcoma).
2. Clinical features of lymphomas (Burkitt's and other non-Hodgkin's lymphomas).
3. Risk factors for common carcinomas (e.g., lung, breast).
4. Chemical carcinogens (e.g., vinyl chloride, nitrosamines, aflatoxin) and mechanisms of carcinogenesis (e.g., initiator vs. promoter).
5. Malignancies associated with pneumoconioses (e.g., asbestosis, silicosis).
6. AIDS-associated neoplasms (Kaposi's sarcoma, B-cell lymphoma).
7. Pituitary tumors (e.g., prolactinoma) and other sellar lesions (e.g., craniopharyngioma).
8. Tumors of the mouth, pharynx, and larynx (e.g., vocal cord tumors in smokers).
9. Modes of spread of certain cancers (e.g., renal cell carcinoma, stomach carcinoma).
10. Clinical features of leukemias (e.g., demographics, pathology, prognosis).

[handwritten margin note: AIDS ↓ ↘ B-cell lymph. / Kaposi]

Nervous System

1. Hydrocephalus: types (e.g., communicating, obstructive), sequelae.
2. CNS manifestations of viral infections (e.g., HIV, HSV).
3. Spinal muscular atrophies (e.g., Werdnig-Hoffmann disease, ALS).
4. Histopathologic changes of common degenerative diseases (e.g., Alzheimer's, Parkinson's).

Rheumatic/Autoimmune

1. Transplant rejection (hyperacute, acute, chronic).
2. Psoriasis and sarcoidosis: skin/joint involvement.
3. Autoantibodies (e.g., antimicrosomal) and disease associations.

Vascular/Hematology

1. Common hematologic diseases (e.g., thrombocytopenia, clotting factor deficiencies, lymphoma, leukemia).
2. Valvular heart disease (e.g., mitral stenosis, mitral regurgitation, aortic stenosis, aortic regurgitation, tricuspid regurgitation), including clinical presentation, associated murmurs, and cardiac catheterization results.
3. Thoracic and abdominal aortic aneurysms: similarities and differences.
4. Polycythemia: primary (polycythemia vera) and secondary causes (e.g., hypoxia), clinical manifestations (e.g., pruritus, fatigue).

[vertical side text: HIGH-YIELD FACTS / Pathology]

General

1. Common clinical features of AIDS (e.g., CNS, pulmonary, GI, dermatologic manifestations).
2. Dermatologic manifestations of systemic disease (e.g., neoplasia, inflammatory bowel disease, meningococcemia, systemic lupus erythematosus).
3. Geriatric pathology: diseases common in the elderly, normal physiologic changes with age.
4. Renal failure: acute versus chronic, features of uremia.
5. Acid-base disturbances, including renal tubular acidosis.
6. Wound repair.
7. Dehydration (e.g., hyponatremic vs. isotonic vs. hypernatremic), including appropriate treatment.
8. Menstrual disorders (e.g., amenorrhea, abnormal uterine bleeding).
9. Cell injury and death.
10. Malabsorption (e.g., celiac sprue, bacterial overgrowth, disaccharidase deficiency).

Common congenital malformations

1. Heart defects (congenital rubella)
2. Hypospadias
3. Cleft lip with or without cleft palate
4. Congenital hip dislocation
5. Spina bifida ✓
6. Anencephaly ✓
7. Pyloric stenosis (associated with polyhydramnios); projectile vomiting

Neural tube defects (spina bifida and anencephaly) are associated with ↑ levels of AFP (in the amniotic fluid and maternal serum). Their incidence is ↓ with maternal folate ingestion during pregnancy.

Congenital heart disease ✓

R-to-L shunts (early cyanosis)— "blue babies"

1. **T**etralogy of Fallot (most common cause of early cyanosis)
2. **T**ransposition of great vessels
3. **T**runcus arteriosus

The 3 T's:
Tetralogy
Transposition
Truncus
Children may squat to ↑ venous return.

L-to-R shunts (late cyanosis)— "blue kids"

1. **V**SD (most common congenital cardiac anomaly)
2. **A**SD (loud S1, wide fixed split S2)
3. **P**DA (close with indomethacin)

Frequency—VSD > ASD > PDA.
↑ pulmonary resistance due to arteriolar thickening.
→ progressive pulmonary hypertension; R → L shunt (Eisenmenger's).

Eisenmenger's syndrome ←

Uncorrected VSD, ASD, or PDA leads to progressive pulmonary hypertension. As pulmonary resistance ↑, the shunt changes from L → R to R → L, which causes late cyanosis (clubbing and polycythemia).

UCV *Path1.14*

Tetralogy of Fallot

1. **P**ulmonary stenosis ✓
2. **R**VH ←
3. **O**verriding aorta (overrides the VSD) —
4. **V**SD ✓

This leads to early cyanosis from a R-to-L shunt across the VSD. On x-ray, boot-shaped heart due to RVH. Patients suffer "cyanotic spells."

The cause of tetralogy of Fallot is anterosuperior displacement of the infundibular septum.

UCV *Anat.7*

PROVe.

(Adapted, with permission, from Chandrasoma P. *Concise Pathology*, 3rd ed. Stamford, CT: Appleton & Lange, 1997:345.)

① Pulmonary artery stenosis ✓
② Right ventricle Hypertrophy ←
③ Overriding aorta ✓
④ VSD ✓

Transposition of great vessels

Aorta leaves RV (anterior) and pulmonary trunk leaves LV (posterior) → separation of systemic and pulmonary circulations. Not compatible with life unless a shunt is present to allow adequate mixing of blood (e.g., VSD, PDA, or patent foramen ovale).

Due to failure of the aorticopulmonary septum to spiral.

Without surgical correction, most infants die within the 1st months of life. Common congenital heart disease in offspring of diabetic mothers.

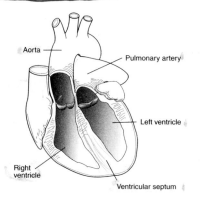

Aorta
Pulmonary artery
Left ventricle
Right ventricle
Ventricular septum

(Adapted, with permission, from Way LW (ed). *Current Surgical Diagnosis and Treatment,* 10th ed. Stamford, CT: Appleton & Lange, 1994:405.)

Coarctation of aorta

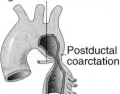

Ligamentum arteriosum
Postductal coarctation
Descending aorta

Infantile type—aortic stenosis proximal to insertion of ductus arteriosus (preductal).

Adult type—stenosis is distal to ductus arteriosus (postductal). Associated with notching of the ribs, hypertension in upper extremities, weak pulses in lower extremities.

UCV *Anat.4*

Male-to-female ratio 3:1.
Check femoral pulses on physical exam.
INfantile: **IN** close to the heart. (Associated with Turner's syndrome.) A**D**ult: **D**istal to **D**uctus.

Patent ductus arteriosus

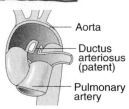

Aorta
Ductus arteriosus (patent)
Pulmonary artery

In fetal period, shunt is R to L (normal). In neonatal period, lung resistance ↓ and shunt becomes L to R with subsequent RV hypertrophy and failure (abnormal). Associated with a continuous, "machine-like" murmur. Patency is maintained by PGE synthesis and low oxygen tension.

UCV *Anat.6*

Indomethacin is used to close a PDA. PGE is used to keep a PDA open, which may be necessary to sustain life in conditions such as transposition of the great vessels.

Autosomal trisomies

Down syndrome (trisomy 21), 1:700	Most common chromosomal disorder and cause of congenital mental retardation. Findings: mental retardation, flat facial profile, prominent epicanthal folds, simian crease, duodenal atresia, congenital heart disease (most common malformation is septum primum–type ASD due to endocardial cushion defects), Alzheimer's disease in affected individuals > 35 years old, ↑ risk of ALL. 95% of cases due to meiotic nondisjunction of homologous chromosomes; associated with advanced maternal age (from 1:1500 in women < 20 to 1:25 in women > 45). 4% of cases due to robertsonian translocation, and 1% of cases due to Down mosaicism (no maternal association).	Drinking age (21). ↓ levels of AFP.
Edwards' syndrome (trisomy 18), 1:8000	Findings: severe mental retardation, rocker bottom feet, low-set ears, micrognathia, congenital heart disease, clenched hands (flexion of fingers), prominent occiput. Death usually occurs within 1 year of birth.	Election age (18).
Patau's syndrome (trisomy 13), 1:6000	Findings: severe mental retardation, microphthalmia, microcephaly, cleft lip/palate, abnormal forebrain structures, polydactyly, congenital heart disease. Death usually occurs within 1 year of birth.	Puberty (13).

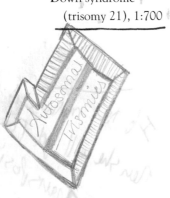

UCV *Path2.11*

Genetic gender disorders

Klinefelter's syndrome [male] (XXY), 1:850 *Bio.60*	Testicular atrophy, eunuchoid body shape, tall, long extremities, gynecomastia, female hair distribution. Presence of inactivated X chromosome (Barr body).	One of the most common causes of hypogonadism in males.
Turner's syndrome [female] (XO), 1:3000 *Path3.57*	Short stature, ovarian dysgenesis, webbing of neck, coarctation of the aorta, most common cause of primary amenorrhea. No Barr body.	"Hugs and kisses" (XO) from Tina **Turner** (female).
Double Y males [male] (XYY), 1:1000	Phenotypically normal, very tall, severe acne, antisocial behavior (seen in 1–2% of XYY males).	Observed with ↑ frequency among inmates of penal institutions.

UCV

Duchenne's and Becker's muscular dystrophies

Duchenne's muscular dystrophy is an X-linked recessive muscular disease featuring a deleted dystrophin gene, leading to accelerated muscle breakdown. Onset before 5 years of age. Weakness begins in pelvic girdle muscles and progresses superiorly. Pseudohypertrophy of calf muscles due to fibrofatty replacement of muscle; cardiac myopathy. The use of Gowers' maneuver, requiring assistance of the upper extremities to stand up, is characteristic (indicates proximal lower limb weakness).

Becker's muscular dystrophy is due to dystrophin gene mutations (not deletions) and is less severe. Diagnosis by muscle biopsy. ↑ serum CPK.

Duchenne's = Deleted Dystrophin.

UCV *Bio.85*

Handwritten note: ↓ levels of AFP.

Pseudohermaphroditism

	Disagreement between the phenotypic (external genitalia) and gonadal (testes vs. ovaries) sex.	Gender identity is based on external genitalia and sex of upbringing.
Female pseudo-hermaphrodite (XX)	Ovaries present, but external genitalia are virilized or ambiguous. Due to excessive and inappropriate exposure to androgenic steroids during early gestation (i.e., congenital adrenal hyperplasia or exogenous administration of androgens during pregnancy).	
Male pseudo-hermaphrodite (XY)	Testes present, but external genitalia are female or ambiguous. Most common form is testicular feminization (androgen insensitivity), which results from a mutation in the androgen receptor gene (X-linked recessive); blind-end vagina.	

True hermaphrodite (46,XX or 47,XXY)	Both ovary and testicular tissue present; ambiguous genitalia.	

(46XX), (47,XYY)

Testicular feminization syndrome (46,XY)	Defect in DHT receptor resulting in normal-appearing female; female external genitalia with rudimentary vagina; uterus and uterine tubes generally absent; develops testes (often found in labia majora; surgically removed to prevent malignancy). Levels of testosterone, estrogen, and LH are all high.	
5α-reductase deficiency	Unable to convert testosterone to DHT. Ambiguous genitalia until puberty, when ↑ testosterone causes masculinization of genitalia. Testosterone/estrogen levels are normal; LH is normal or ↑.	
Cri-du-chat syndrome	Congenital deletion of short arm of chromosome 5 (46,XX or XY, 5p–). Findings: microcephaly, severe mental retardation, high-pitched crying/mewing, epicanthal folds, cardiac abnormalities.	*Cri du chat* = cry of the cat.
Fragile X syndrome	X-linked defect affecting the methylation and expression of the *FMR1* gene. The 2nd most common cause of genetic mental retardation (the most common cause is Down syndrome). Associated with macro-orchidism (enlarged testes), long face with a large jaw, large everted ears, and autism.	Triplet repeat disorder (CGG_n) that may show genetic anticipation. Fragile **X** = e**X**tra large testes, jaw, ears.

5 α reductase deficiency.

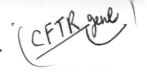
(handwritten: CFTR gene)

Cystic fibrosis	Autosomal-recessive defect in CFTR gene on chromosome 7. Defective Cl⁻ channel → secretion of abnormally thick mucus that plugs lungs, pancreas, and liver → recurrent pulmonary infections (*Pseudomonas* species and *Staphylococcus aureus*), chronic bronchitis, bronchiectasis, pancreatic insufficiency (malabsorption and steatorrhea), meconium ileus in newborns. ↑ concentration of Cl⁻ ions in sweat test is diagnostic.	Infertility in males. Fat-soluble vitamin deficiencies (A, D, E, K). Can present as failure to thrive in infancy. Most common lethal genetic disease of Caucasians.

(handwritten: 90% of cases are due to mutations in APKD1)

Autosomal-dominant diseases

Adult polycystic kidney disease *Path2.49*	**Always bilateral,** massive enlargement of kidneys due to multiple large cysts. Patients present with pain, hematuria, hypertension, progressive renal failure. 90% of cases are due to mutation in APKD1 (chromosome 16). Associated with polycystic liver disease, berry aneurysms, mitral valve prolapse. Juvenile form is recessive.
Familial hypercholesterolemia (type IIA)	Elevated LDL owing to defective or absent LDL receptor. Heterozygotes (1 in 500) have cholesterol ≈ 300 mg/dL. Homozygotes (very rare) have cholesterol ≈ 700+ mg/dL, severe atherosclerotic disease early in life, and tendon xanthomas (classically in the Achilles tendon); myocardial infarction may develop before age 20.
Marfan's syndrome *Path2.12*	Fibrillin gene mutation → connective tissue disorders. Skeletal abnormalities—tall with long extremities, hyperextensive joints, and long, tapering fingers and toes. Cardiovascular—cystic medial necrosis of aorta → aortic incompetence and dissecting aortic aneurysms. Floppy mitral valve. Ocular—subluxation of lenses.
Von Recklinghausen's disease (NFT1)	Findings: café-au-lait spots, neural tumors, Lisch nodules (pigmented iris hamartomas). Also marked by skeletal disorders (e.g., scoliosis) and ↑ tumor susceptibility. On long arm of chromosome 17; 17 letters in von Recklinghausen.
Von Hippel–Lindau disease *Path3.35*	Findings: hemangioblastomas of retina/cerebellum/medulla; about half of affected individuals develop multiple bilateral renal cell carcinomas and other tumors. Associated with deletion of VHL gene (tumor suppressor) on chromosome 3 (3p). Von Hippel–Lindau = 3 words for chromosome **3.**
Huntington's disease	Findings: depression, progressive dementia, choreiform movements, caudate atrophy, and ↓ levels of GABA and acetylcholine in the brain. Symptoms manifest in affected individuals between the ages of 20 and 50. Gene located on chromosome **4;** triplet repeat disorder. "Hunting **4** food."
Familial **A**denomatous **P**olyposis *Path1.83*	Colon becomes covered with adenomatous polyps after puberty. Features: deletion on chromosome **F**ive; **A**utosomal-dominant inheritance; **P**ositively will get colon cancer (100% without resection).
Hereditary spherocytosis	Spheroid erythrocytes; hemolytic anemia; increased MCHC. Splenectomy is curative.

(handwritten: Fibrillin gene mutation)

(handwritten: ddcc)

Autosomal-recessive diseases	Cystic fibrosis, albinism, α_1-antitrypsin deficiency, phenylketonuria, thalassemias, sickle cell anemias, glycogen storage diseases, mucopolysaccharidoses (except Hunter's), sphingolipidoses (except Fabry's), infant polycystic kidney disease, hemochromatosis.
X-linked recessive disorders	Fragile X, Duchenne's muscular dystrophy, hemophilia A and B, Fabry's, G6PD deficiency, Hunter's syndrome, ocular albinism, Lesch-Nyhan syndrome, Bruton's agammaglobulinemia, Wiskott-Aldrich syndrome. Female carriers of X-linked recessive disorders are rarely affected because of random inactivation of X chromosomes in each cell.
Neural tube defects	Associated with low folic acid intake during pregnancy. Elevated AFP in amniotic fluid. Spina bifida occulta—failure of bony spinal canal to close, but no structural herniation. Usually seen at lower vertebral levels. Meningocele—meninges herniate through spinal canal defect. ✓ Meningomyelocele—meninges and spinal cord herniate through spinal canal defect.

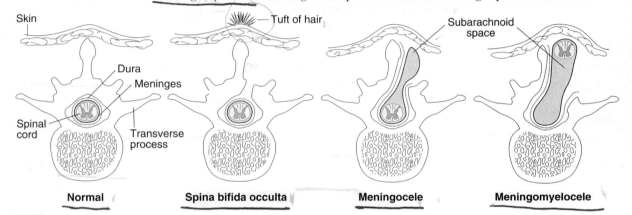

| | Normal | Spina bifida occulta | Meningocele | Meningomyelocele |

UCV *Anat.71*

Fetal alcohol syndrome	Newborns of mothers who consumed significant amounts of alcohol (teratogen) during pregnancy (highest risk at 3–8 weeks) have a higher incidence of congenital abnormalities, including pre- and postnatal developmental retardation, microcephaly, facial abnormalities, limb dislocation, and heart and lung fistulas. Mechanism may include inhibition of cell migration. The number one cause of congenital malformations in the United States.

UCV *Pharm.65*

highest Risk is at 3-8 weeks

Neoplastic progression

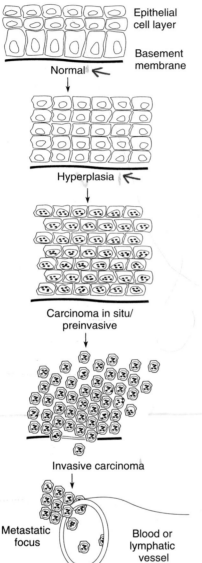

Epithelial cell layer

Basement membrane

Normal

- Normal cells with basal → apical differentiation

Hyperplasia

- Cells have increased in number—**hyperplasia**
- Abnormal proliferation of cells with loss of size, shape, and orientation—**dysplasia**

In situ Carcinoma

Carcinoma in situ/ preinvasive

- **In situ carcinoma**
- Neoplastic cells have not invaded basement membrane
- High nuclear/cytoplasmic ratio and clumped chromatin
- Neoplastic cells encompass entire thickness

Invasive carcinoma

- Cells have invaded basement membrane using **collagenases** and **hydrolases**
- Will metastasize if they reach a blood or lymphatic vessel

Metastatic focus

Blood or lymphatic vessel

Metastasis—spread to distant organ
- Must survive immune attack
- "Seed and soil" theory of metastasis
  - Seed = tumor embolus
  - Soil = target organ—liver, lungs, bone, brain...

(Adapted, with permission, from McPhee SJ et al. *Pathophysiology of Disease: An Introduction to Clinical Medicine,* 3rd ed. New York: McGraw-Hill, 2000:84.)

Collagenases and Hydrolases

HIGH-YIELD FACTS

Pathology

-plasia definitions

Hyperplasia— ↑ in number of cells (reversible).

Metaplasia—1 adult cell type is replaced by another (reversible). Often 2° to irritation and/or environmental exposure (e.g., squamous metaplasia in trachea and bronchi of smokers).

Dysplasia—abnormal growth with loss of cellular orientation, shape, and size in comparison to normal tissue maturation, commonly preneoplastic (reversible).

Anaplasia—abnormal cells lacking differentiation; like primitive cells of same tissue, often equated with undifferentiated malignant neoplasms. Tumor giant cells may be formed.

Neoplasia—a clonal proliferation of cells that is uncontrolled and excessive.

What you see in the Esophagus?

Tumor grade vs. stage

Grade	Histologic appearance of tumor. Usually graded I–IV based on degree of differentiation and number of mitoses per high-power field; character of tumor itself.	Stage has more prognostic value than grade. TNM staging system: **T** = size of **T**umor **N** = **N**ode involvement **M** = **M**etastases
Stage	Based on site and size of 1° lesion, spread to regional lymph nodes, presence of metastases; spread of tumor in a specific patient.	

Tumor nomenclature

Cell type	Benign	Malignant
Epithelium	Adenoma, papilloma	Adenocarcinoma, papillary carcinoma
Mesenchyme		
Blood cells		Leukemia, lymphoma
Blood vessels	Hemangioma	Angiosarcoma
Smooth muscle	Leiomyoma	Leiomyosarcoma
Skeletal muscle	Rhabdomyoma	Rhabdomyosarcoma
Bone	Osteoma	Osteosarcoma
Fat	Lipoma	Liposarcoma
> 1 cell type	Mature teratoma	Immature teratoma

The term **carcinoma** implies epithelial origin, whereas **sarcoma** denotes mesenchymal origin. Both terms imply malignancy.

Diseases associated with neoplasms	Condition	Neoplasm
	1. **Down** syndrome	1. Acute Lymphoblastic Leukemia—"We will **ALL** go **DOWN** together"
	2. Xeroderma pigmentosum	2. Squamous cell and basal cell carcinomas of skin
	3. Chronic atrophic gastritis, pernicious anemia, postsurgical gastric remnants	3. Gastric adenocarcinoma
	4. Tuberous sclerosis (facial angiofibroma, seizures, mental retardation)	4. Astrocytoma and cardiac rhabdomyoma
	5. Actinic keratosis	5. Squamous cell carcinoma of skin
	6. Barrett's esophagus (chronic GI reflux)	6. Esophageal adenocarcinoma
	7. Plummer-Vinson syndrome (atrophic glossitis, esophageal webs, anemia; all due to iron deficiency)	7. Squamous cell carcinoma of esophagus
	8. Cirrhosis (alcoholic, hepatitis B or C)	8. Hepatocellular carcinoma
	9. Ulcerative colitis	9. Colonic adenocarcinoma
	10. Paget's disease of bone	10. 2° osteosarcoma and fibrosarcoma
	11. Immunodeficiency states	11. Malignant lymphomas
	12. AIDS	12. Aggressive malignant lymphomas (non-Hodgkin's) and Kaposi's sarcoma
	13. Autoimmune diseases (e.g., Hashimoto's thyroiditis, myasthenia gravis)	13. Benign and malignant thymomas
	14. Acanthosis nigricans (hyperpigmentation and epidermal thickening)	14. Visceral malignancy (stomach, lung, breast, uterus)
	15. Dysplastic nevus	15. Malignant melanoma

Oncogenes

Gain of function.

Gene	Associated tumor
c-myc	Burkitt's lymphoma
bcl-2	Follicular and undifferentiated lymphomas (inhibits apoptosis)
erb-B2	Breast, ovarian, and gastric carcinomas
ras	Colon carcinoma

Tumor suppressor genes

Loss of function; both alleles must be lost for expression of disease.

Gene	Chromosome	Associated tumor
Rb	13q	Retinoblastoma, osteosarcoma
BRCA1 and 2	17q, 13q	Breast and ovarian cancer
p53	17p	Most human cancers, Li-Fraumeni syndrome

HIGH-YIELD FACTS

Pathology

Tumor markers

PSA (prostatic acid phosphatase)	Prostatic carcinoma.	Tumor markers should not be used as the primary tool for cancer diagnosis. They may be used to confirm diagnosis, to monitor for tumor recurrence, and to monitor response to therapy.
CEA	Carcinoembryonic antigen. Very nonspecific but produced by ~ 70% of colorectal and pancreatic cancers; also produced by gastric and breast carcinomas.	
AFP	Normally made by fetus. Hepatocellular carcinomas. ✓ Nonseminomatous germ cell tumors of the testis (e.g., yolk sac tumor). ✓	
β-hCG	Hydatidiform moles, Choriocarcinomas, and Gestational trophoblastic tumors.	
CA-125	Ovarian, malignant epithelial tumors.	
S-100	Melanoma, neural tumors, astrocytomas.	
Alkaline phosphatase	Metastases to bone, obstructive biliary disease, Paget's disease of bone.	

Oncogenic viruses

Virus	Associated cancer
HTLV-1	Adult T-cell leukemia
HBV, HCV	Hepatocellular carcinoma
EBV	Burkitt's lymphoma, nasopharyngeal carcinoma
HPV	Cervical carcinoma (16, 18), penile/anal carcinoma
HHV-8 (Kaposi's sarcoma–associated herpesvirus)	Kaposi's sarcoma

Chemical carcinogens

Toxin	Affected organ
Aflatoxins, vinyl chloride	Liver
Nitrosamines	Esophagus, stomach
Asbestos	Lung (mesothelioma and bronchogenic carcinoma)
Arsenic	Skin (squamous cell)
CCl_4	Liver (centrilobular necrosis, fatty change)
Naphthalene (aniline) dyes	Bladder (transitional cell carcinoma)

used as food preservatives

C-myc = Burkitt's lymphoma
erb-B2 = gastric, ovarian & breast.

Local effects of tumors

Local effect	Cause
Mass	Tissue lump or tumor.
Nonhealing ulcer	Destruction of epithelial surfaces (e.g., stomach, colon, mouth, bronchus).
Hemorrhage	From ulcerated area or eroded vessel.
Pain	Any site with sensory nerve endings. Tumors in brain are initially painless.
Seizures	Tumor mass in brain.
Obstruction	Of bronchus → pneumonia.
	Of biliary tree → jaundice.
	Of left colon → constipation.
Perforation	Of ulcer in viscera → peritonitis, free air.
Bone destruction	Pathologic fracture, collapse of bone.
Inflammation	Of serosal surface → pleural effusion, pericardial effusion, ascites.
Space-occupying lesion	Raised intracranial pressure with brain neoplasms. Anemia due to bone marrow replacement.
Localized loss of sensory or motor function	Compression or destruction of nerve (e.g., recurrent laryngeal nerve by lung or thyroid cancer, with hoarseness).
Edema	Venous or lymphatic obstruction.

Prostatic adenocarcinoma

Common in men over age 50. Arises most often from the posterior lobe (peripheral zone) of the prostate gland and is most frequently diagnosed by digital rectal examination (hard nodule) and prostate biopsy. Prostatic acid phosphatase and prostate-specific antigen (PSA) are useful tumor markers. Osteoblastic metastases in bone may develop in late stages, as indicated by an ↑ in serum alkaline phosphatase and PSA.

UCV *Path2.63*

[handwritten: Double epithelial layer surrounded single gland]
[handwritten: Glands Back to Back]
[handwritten: BnPH occurs around periurethral area (starts Anteriorly).]
[handwritten: PAP]

Skin cancer

Squamous cell carcinoma	Very common. Associated with excessive exposure to sunlight and arsenic exposure. Commonly appear on hands and face. Locally invasive, but rarely metastasizes. Histopathology: keratin "pearls."	Actinic keratosis is a precursor to squamous cell carcinoma. *Path1.29*
Basal cell carcinoma	Most common in sun-exposed areas of body. Locally invasive, but almost never metastasizes. Gross pathology: pearly papules. *Path1.31*	Basal cell tumors have "palisading" nuclei.
Melanoma	Common tumor with significant risk of metastasis. Associated with sunlight exposure; fair-skinned persons are at ↑ risk. Incidence ↑. **Depth** of tumor correlates with risk of metastasis. *Path1.40*	Dysplastic nevus is a precursor to melanoma.

UCV

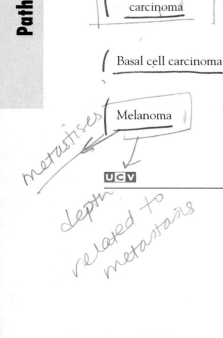
[handwritten: metastises]
[handwritten: depth related to metastasis]

[handwritten: Dysplastic Nevus is a precursor to melanoma.]

Primary bone tumors

Benign

Osteochondroma (exostosis) — Most common benign bone tumor. Usually in men younger than age 25. Commonly originates from long metaphysis. Malignant transformation to chondrosarcoma is rare. May be a hamartoma rather than a true neoplasm.

Giant cell tumor — Occurs most commonly at epiphyseal end of long bones. Peak incidence 20–40 years old. Locally aggressive benign tumor often around the distal femur, proximal tibial region. Characteristic "double bubble" or "soap bubble" appearance on x-ray. Spindle-shaped cells with multinucleated giant cells.

Malignant

Osteosarcoma (osteogenic carcinoma) — Most common 1° malignant tumor of bone. Peak incidence in men 10–20 years old. Commonly found in the metaphysis of long bones. Predisposing factors include Paget's disease of bone, bone infarcts, radiation, and familial retinoblastoma. Codman's triangle (from elevation of periosteum) on x-ray.

Ewing's sarcoma — Anaplastic small cell malignant tumor. Most common in boys < 15. Extremely aggressive with early mets, but responsive to chemotherapy. Characteristic "onion-skin" appearance in bone. Commonly appears in diaphysis of long bones, pelvis, scapula, and ribs. 11;22 translocation.

Chondrosarcoma — Malignant cartilaginous tumor. Most common in men aged 30–60. Usually located in pelvis, spine, scapula, humerus, tibia, or femur. May be of 1° origin or from osteochondroma.

Ewing's Sarcoma = occurs mostly
in boys less than 15 years
of age.

PAP

familial Retinoblastoma

Actinic Keratosis = is a precursor to SCC4

Primary brain tumors

Clinical presentation due to mass effects (e.g., seizures, dementia, focal lesions); 1° brain tumors rarely undergo metastasis. The majority of adult tumors are supratentorial, while the majority of childhood tumors are infratentorial.

Adult peak incidence

A. Glioblastoma multiforme (grade IV astrocytoma)
Most common 1° brain tumor. Prognosis grave; < 1 year life expectancy. Found in cerebral hemispheres. Can cross corpus callosum ("butterfly glioma").
"Pseudopalisading" tumor cells border central areas of necrosis and hemorrhage.

B. Meningioma
2nd most common 1° brain tumor. Most often occurs in convexities of hemispheres and parasagittal region. Arises from arachnoid cells external to brain. Resectable.
Psammoma bodies—spindle cells concentrically arranged in a whorled pattern.

C. Schwannoma
3rd most common 1° brain tumor. Schwann cell origin; often localized to 8th nerve → acoustic schwannoma. Bilateral schwannoma found in NF2.
Antoni A—compact palisading nuclei. Antoni B—loose pattern.

D. Oligodendroglioma
Relatively rare, slow growing, benign. Most often in frontal lobes.
"Fried egg" appearance of cells in tumor. Often calcified.

E. Pituitary adenoma
Prolactin secreting is most common form. Bitemporal hemianopia (due to pressure on optic chiasm) and hypopituitarism are sequelae.
Derived from Rathke's pouch.

Childhood peak incidence

F. Low-grade astrocytoma (pilocytic astrocytoma)
Diffusely infiltrating glioma. In children, most often found in posterior fossa. Benign; good prognosis.
Rosenthal fibers.

G. Medulloblastoma
Highly malignant cerebellar tumor. A form of primitive neuroectodermal tumor (PNET). Can compress 4th ventricle, causing hydrocephalus.
Rosettes or perivascular pseudorosette pattern of cells. Radiosensitive.

H. Ependymoma
Ependymal cell tumors most commonly found in 4th ventricle. Can cause hydrocephalus.
Characteristic perivascular rosettes. Rod-shaped blepharoblasts (basal ciliary bodies) found near nucleus.

I. Hemangioblastoma
Most often cerebellar; associated with von Hippel–Lindau syndrome when found with retinoblastoma.
Foamy cells and high vascularity are characteristic. Can produce EPO → 2° polycythemia.

J. Craniopharyngioma
Benign childhood tumor, confused with pituitary adenoma (can also cause bitemporal hemianopia). Calcification is common.
Derived from remnants of Rathke's pouch. Most common childhood supratentorial tumor.

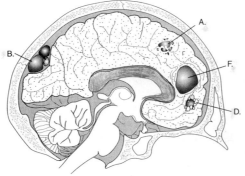

Supratentorial

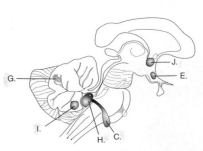

Infratentorial

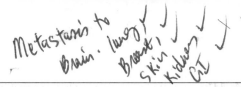
Metastasis to Brain: lung, Breast, Skin, Kidney, GI (handwritten)

Metastasis to brain	1° tumors that metastasize to brain—Lung, Breast, Skin (melanoma), Kidney (renal cell carcinoma), GI. Overall, approximately 50% of brain tumors are from metastases.	Lots of Bad Stuff Kills Glia.

UCV *Path3.21*

Metastasis to liver	The liver and lung are the most common sites of metastasis after the regional lymph nodes. 1° tumors that metastasize to the liver—Colon > Stomach > Pancreas > Breast > Lung.	Metastases >> 1° liver tumors. Cancer Sometimes Penetrates Benign Liver.

Metastasis to bone	These 1° tumors metastasize to bone—Breast, Lung, Thyroid, Testes, Kidney, Prostate. Metastases from breast and prostate are most common. Metastatic bone tumors are far more common than 1° bone tumors.	"BLT with a Kosher Pickle." Lung = Lytic. Prostate = blastic. Breast = Both lytic and blastic.

From Breast and Prostate most common metas. (handwritten)

Paraneoplastic effects of tumors

Neoplasm	Causes	Effect	
Small cell lung carcinoma	ACTH or ACTH-like peptide	Cushing's syndrome	ACTH
Small cell lung carcinoma and intracranial neoplasms	ADH or ANP	SIADH	ADH/ANP
Squamous cell lung carcinoma, renal cell carcinoma, breast carcinoma, multiple myeloma, and bone metastasis (lysed bone)	PTH-related peptide, TGF-α, TNF-α, IL-2	Hypercalcemia	PTH
Renal cell carcinoma	Erythropoietin	Polycythemia	EPO
Thymoma, bronchogenic carcinoma	Antibodies against presynaptic Ca²⁺ channels at NMJ	Lambert-Eaton syndrome	Ab: Ca²⁺
Various neoplasms	Hyperuricemia due to excess nucleic acid turnover (i.e., cytotoxic therapy)	Gout	Hyperuricemia

(handwritten annotations: "Small" bracket next to Cushing's/SIADH; "Squamous" bracket next to Hypercalcemia)

PATHOLOGY—HEMATOLOGIC

Cancer epidemiology

	Male	Female	
Incidence	Prostate (32%)	Breast (32%)	Deaths from lung cancer have plateaued in males but continue to ↑ in females.
	Lung (16%)	Lung (13%)	
	Colon and rectum (12%)	Colon and rectum (13%)	Cancer is the 2nd leading cause of death in the United States (heart disease is 1st).
Mortality	Lung (33%)	Lung (23%)	
	Prostate (13%)	Breast (18%)	

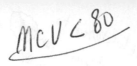

MCV < 80

Anemia

Type	Etiology
Microcytic, hypochromic (MCV < 80)	Iron deficiency— ↑ TIBC, ↓ ferritin, ↓ serum iron _Bio.76_
	Thalassemias
	Lead poisoning
Macrocytic (MCV > 100)	Megaloblastic—vitamin B_{12}/folate deficiency
	Drugs that block DNA synthesis (e.g., sulfa drugs, AZT)
	Marked reticulocytosis
Normocytic, normochromic	Hemorrhage
	Enzyme defects (e.g., G6PD deficiency, PK deficiency)
	RBC membrane defects (e.g., hereditary spherocytosis)
	Bone marrow disorders (e.g., aplastic anemia, leukemia)
	Hemoglobinopathies (e.g., sickle cell disease)
	Autoimmune hemolytic anemia
	Anemia of chronic disease— ↓ TIBC, ↑ ferritin, ↓ serum iron, ↑ storage iron in marrow macrophages

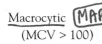
LITtle

MARS

Anything that destroys RBC.

Body lies to store Iron

Vitamin B_{12} and folate deficiencies are associated with hypersegmented PMNs. Unlike folate deficiency, vitamin B_{12} deficiency is associated with neurologic problems.
↓ serum haptoglobin and ↑ serum LDH indicate RBC hemolysis. Direct Coombs' test is used to distinguish between immune- vs. non-immune-mediated RBC hemolysis.

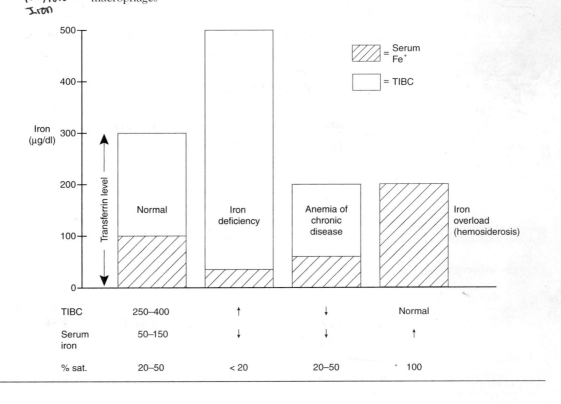

	Normal	Iron deficiency	Anemia of chronic disease	Iron overload (hemosiderosis)
TIBC	250–400	↑	↓	Normal
Serum iron	50–150	↓	↓	↑
% sat.	20–50	< 20	20–50	100

UCV

Aplastic anemia

Pancytopenia characterized by severe anemia, neutropenia, and thrombocytopenia caused by failure or destruction of multipotent myeloid stem cells, with inadequate production or release of differentiated cell lines.

Causes	Radiation, benzene, chloramphenicol, alkylating agents, antimetabolites, viral agents (HCV, CMV, EBV, herpes zoster-varicella, parvo B19), Fanconi's anemia, idiopathic (immune-mediated, 1° stem-cell defect).
Symptoms	Fatigue, malaise, pallor, purpura, mucosal bleeding, petechiae, infection.
Pathologic features	Pancytopenia with normal cell morphology; hypocellular bone marrow with fatty infiltration.
Treatment	Withdrawal of offending agent, allogenic bone marrow transplantation, RBC and platelet transfusion, G-CSF or GM-CSF.

UCV Path2.15

Fatigue = Anemia
Purpura = Thrombocytic prob.

Hereditary spherocytosis

Intrinsic, extravascular hemolysis due to spectrin defect. RBCs are small and round with no central pallor → less membrane → ↑ MCHC (normal Hgb and MCV). Osmotic fragility test used to confirm. Associated with gallstones, splenomegaly, anemia, and jaundice. Distinguish from warm antibody hemolysis by direct Coombs' test. Hereditary spherocytosis is Coombs negative.

Blood dyscrasias

Sickle cell anemia	HbS mutation is a single amino acid replacement in β chain (substitution of normal glutamic acid with valine). Low O$_2$ or dehydration precipitates sickling. Heterozygotes (sickle cell trait) are relatively malaria resistant (balanced polymorphism). Complications in homozygotes (sickle cell disease) include aplastic crisis (due to B19 parvovirus infection), autosplenectomy, ↑ risk of encapsulated organism infection, Salmonella osteomyelitis, painful crisis (vaso-occlusive), and splenic sequestration crisis.	8% of African-Americans carry the HbS trait; 0.2% have the disease. Sickled cells are crescent-shaped RBCs.
	HbC defect is a different β chain mutation; patients with HbC or HbSC (1 of each mutant gene) have milder disease than do HbSS patients. New therapies for sickle cell anemia include hydroxyurea (↑ HbF) and bone marrow transplantation. *Path2.36*	
α-thalassemia	There are 4 α-globin genes. In α-thalassemia, the α-globin chain is underproduced (as a function of number of bad genes, 1–4). There is no compensatory increase of any other chains. HbH (β$_4$-tetramers, lacks 3 α-globin genes). Hb Barts (γ$_4$-tetramers, lacks all 4 α-globin genes) results in hydrops fetalis and intrauterine fetal death.	Thalassemia is prevalent in Mediterranean populations (*thalassa* = sea). Think of thalaSEAmia.
β-thalassemia	In β-thalassemia minor (heterozygote), the β chain is underproduced; in β-thalassemia major (homozygote), the β chain is absent. In both cases, fetal hemoglobin production is compensatorily increased but is inadequate. HbS/β-thalassemia heterozygote has mild to moderate disease. *Path2.37*	β-thalassemia major results in severe anemia requiring blood transfusions. Cardiac failure due to 2° hemochromatosis.

UCV

HbS

High yield facts @ Pathology

DIC

Activation of coagulation cascade leading to microthrombi and global consumption of platelets, fibrin, and coagulation factors.

Causes
Obstetric complications (most common cause), gram-negative sepsis, transfusion, trauma, malignancy, acute pancreatitis, nephrotic syndrome.

Lab findings
↑ PT, ↑ PTT, ↑ fibrin split products (D dimers), ↓ platelet count.

UCV *Path2.22*

Bleeding disorders

Platelet abnormalities (microhemorrhage)
- Mucous membrane bleeding
- Petechiae
- Purpura
- Prolonged bleeding time

[handwritten: ITP (Ab: platelet, ↑ mk) / TTP (schistocytes, drugs) / DIC (↑ fibrin split products)]

Causes include ITP (antiplatelet antibodies and ↑ megakaryocytes), TTP (schistocytes), drugs, and DIC (↑ fibrin split products).

[handwritten: PBH]

Coagulation factor defects (macrohemorrhage)
- Hemarthroses (bleeding into joints)
- Easy bruising
- Prolonged PT and/or aPTT

[handwritten: HA: 8 / HB: 9 / VWD: VWF]

Coagulopathies include hemophilia A (factor VIII deficiency), hemophilia B (factor IX deficiency), and von Willebrand's disease (deficiency of von Willebrand's antigen), the most common bleeding disorder.

[handwritten: SEVEN]

PT (extrinsic) *[handwritten: 2, 5, 7, 10]*
PTT (intrinsic) *[handwritten: All except 7 + 13.]*

Factors II, V, VII, and X.
All factors except VII and XIII.

Hemorrhagic disorders

Disorder	Platelet count	Bleeding time	PT	PTT
Qualitative platelet defects[a]	—	↑	—	—
Vascular bleeding	—	↑	—	—
Thrombocytopenia	↓	↑	—	—
Hemophilia A (factor VIII deficiency)	—	—	—	↑
Hemophilia B (factor IX deficiency)	—	—	—	↑
Von Willebrand's disease	—	↑	—	↑
Disseminated intravascular coagulation	↓	↑	↑	↑

[a]Bernard-Soulier disease = defect of platelet adhesion; Glanzmann's thrombasthenia = defect of platelet aggregation.

Lymphomas—Hodgkin's and NHL

Hodgkin's	NHL
Presence of Reed-Sternberg (RS) cells	NHL associated with HIV and immunosuppression
Localized, single group of nodes; extranodal rare; contiguous spread	Multiple, peripheral nodes; extranodal involvement common; noncontiguous spread
Constitutional signs/symptoms—low-grade fever, night sweats, weight loss	Majority involve B cells (except lymphoblastic T-cell origin)
Mediastinal lymphadenopathy	No hypergammaglobulinemia (cf. multiple myeloma, where excess B cells are in resting stage)
50% of cases associated with EBV; bimodal distribution: young and old; more common in men except nodular sclerosis type	Fewer constitutional signs/symptoms
Good prognosis = ↑ lymphocytes, ↓ RS	Peak incidence 20–40 years old

Hodgkin's

Type	RS	Lymphocytes	Prognosis	Comments
NS (65–75%)	+	+++	Excellent	Most common; collagen banding; women > men; primarily young adults
MC (25%)	++++	+++	Intermediate	Numerous RS cells
LP (6%)	+	++++	Excellent	< 35-year-old male
LD (rare)	*	+	Poor	Older males with disseminated disease

*RS high relative to lymphocytes

NHL

Type	Occurs in	Cell type	Genetics	Comments
Small lymphocytic lymphoma	Adults	B cells		Clinically presents like CLL; low grade
Follicular lymphoma (small cleaved cell)	Adults	B cells	t(14;18) bcl-2 expression	Most common (adult) Difficult to cure; indolent course; bcl-2 is involved in apoptosis
Diffuse large cell	Usually older adults, but 20% occur in children	80% B cells 20% T cells (mature)		Aggressive but up to 50% are curable
Lymphoblastic lymphoma	Children most often	T cells (immature)		Most common in children; commonly presents with ALL and mediastinal mass; very aggressive T-cell lymphoma
Burkitt's lymphoma	Children most often	B cells	t(8;14) c-myc gene moves next to heavy-chain Ig gene(14)	High-grade "starry-sky" appearance; associated with EBV; endemic in Africa

Leukemias

[handwritten: Anemia. infection. Hemorrhage.]

General considerations— ↑ number of circulating leukocytes in blood; bone marrow infiltrates of leukemic cells; marrow failure can cause anemia (↓ RBCs), infections (↓ WBCs), and hemorrhage (↓ platelets); leukemic cell infiltrates in liver, spleen, and lymph nodes are common.

[handwritten: t(15;17) M3]

ALL *[handwritten: children]* — Children; lymphoblasts; most responsive to therapy.

AML *[handwritten: Auer rods, Adults]* — Auer rods (myeloblasts); adults.

CLL *[handwritten: Adults smudge Warm Ab]* — Older adults; lymphadenopathy; hepatosplenomegaly; few symptoms; indolent course; ↑ smudge cells in peripheral blood smear; warm Ab autoimmune hemolytic anemia; very similar to SLL (small lymphocytic lymphoma).

CML *[handwritten: 9:22]* — Most commonly associated with Philadelphia chromosome (t[9;22], *bcr-abl*); myeloid stem cell proliferation; may accelerate to AML ("blast crisis").

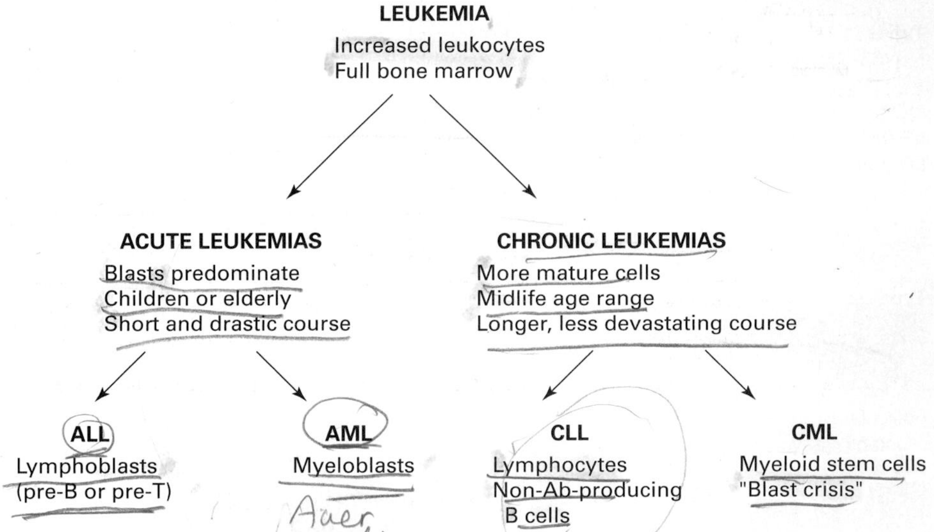

LEUKEMIA
Increased leukocytes
Full bone marrow

ACUTE LEUKEMIAS
Blasts predominate
Children or elderly
Short and drastic course

CHRONIC LEUKEMIAS
More mature cells
Midlife age range
Longer, less devastating course

ALL
Lymphoblasts
(pre-B or pre-T)

AML
Myeloblasts
[handwritten: Auer rods.]

CLL
Lymphocytes
Non-Ab-producing
B cells

CML
Myeloid stem cells
"Blast crisis"

UCV *Path2.13, 14, 19, 20*

Chromosomal translocations

Translocation	Associated disorder
t(9;22) (Philadelphia chromosome)	CML (*bcr-abl* hybrid)
t(8;14)	Burkitt's lymphoma (c-*myc* activation)
t(14;18)	Follicular lymphomas (*bcl-2* activation)
t(15;17)	M3 type of AML (responsive to all-*trans* retinoic acid)
t(11;22) *[handwritten: – Tallest]*	Ewing's sarcoma
t(11;14)	Mantle cell lymphoma

Lymphomas and leukemias

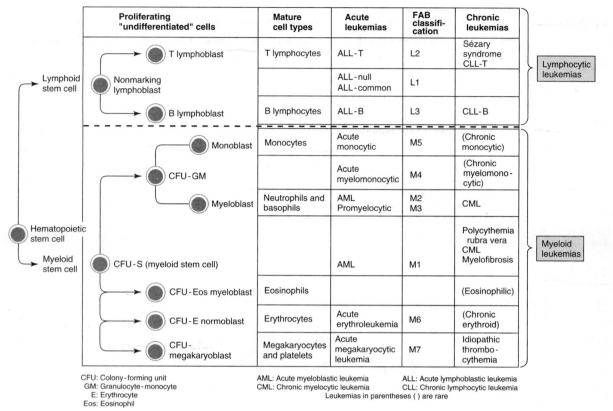

	Proliferating "undifferentiated" cells		Mature cell types	Acute leukemias	FAB classification	Chronic leukemias	
Lymphoid stem cell	Nonmarking lymphoblast	T lymphoblast	T lymphocytes	ALL-T	L2	Sézary syndrome CLL-T	Lymphocytic leukemias
				ALL-null ALL-common	L1		
		B lymphoblast	B lymphocytes	ALL-B	L3	CLL-B	
		Monoblast	Monocytes	Acute monocytic	M5	(Chronic monocytic)	Myeloid leukemias
	CFU-GM			Acute myelomonocytic	M4	(Chronic myelomono-cytic)	
		Myeloblast	Neutrophils and basophils	AML Promyelocytic	M2 M3	CML	
	CFU-S (myeloid stem cell)			AML	M1	Polycythemia rubra vera CML Myelofibrosis	
	CFU-Eos myeloblast		Eosinophils			(Eosinophilic)	
	CFU-E normoblast		Erythrocytes	Acute erythroleukemia	M6	(Chronic erythroid)	
	CFU-megakaryoblast		Megakaryocytes and platelets	Acute megakaryocytic leukemia	M7	Idiopathic thrombo-cythemia	

CFU: Colony-forming unit
GM: Granulocyte-monocyte
E: Erythrocyte
Eos: Eosinophil

AML: Acute myeloblastic leukemia
CML: Chronic myelocytic leukemia

ALL: Acute lymphoblastic leukemia
CLL: Chronic lymphocytic leukemia

Leukemias in parentheses ( ) are rare

(Adapted, with permission, from Chandrasoma P, Taylor CE. *Concise Pathology,* 3rd ed. Stamford, CT: Appleton & Lange, 1998:410.)

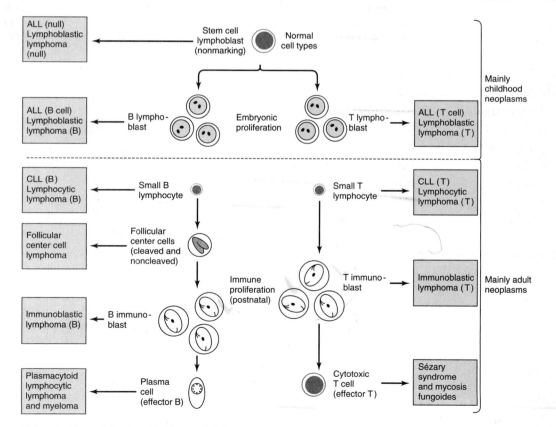

(Adapted, with permission, from Chandrasoma P, Taylor CE. *Concise Pathology,* 2nd ed. Norwalk, CT: Appleton & Lange, 1994.)

Multiple myeloma

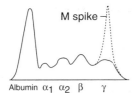

M spike

Albumin α_1 α_2 β γ

Monoclonal plasma cell ("fried-egg" appearance) cancer that arises in the marrow and produces large amounts of IgG (55%) or IgA (25%). Most common 1° tumor arising within bone in adults. Destructive bone lesions and consequent hypercalcemia. Renal insufficiency, ↑ susceptibility to infection, and anemia. Associated with 1° amyloidosis and punched-out lytic bone lesions on x-ray. Characterized by monoclonal immunoglobulin spike (M protein) on serum protein electrophoresis and Ig light chains in urine (Bence Jones protein). Blood smear shows RBCs stacked like poker chips (rouleau formation). Compare with Waldenström's macroglobinemia → M spike = IgM; no lytic lesions.

UCV *Path2.31*   (Adapted, with permission, from Stobo J. *The Principles and Practice of Medicine*, 23rd ed. Stamford, CT: Appleton and Lange, 1996:806.)

PATHOLOGY—GASTROINTESTINAL

Achalasia

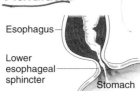

Esophagus

Lower esophageal sphincter

Stomach

Failure of relaxation of lower esophageal sphincter due to loss of myenteric (Auerbach's) plexus. Causes progressive dysphagia. Barium swallow shows dilated esophagus with an area of distal stenosis. Associated with an ↑ risk of esophageal carcinoma.

A-chalasia = absence of relaxation.
2° achalasia may arise from Chagas' disease.
"Bird beak" on barium swallow.

UCV *Path1.75*

Barrett's esophagus

Glandular (columnar epithelial) metaplasia—replacement of stratified squamous epithelium with gastric (columnar) epithelium in the distal esophagus.

BARRett's = Becomes Adenocarcinoma, Results from Reflux.

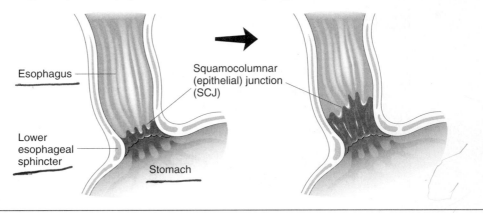

Esophagus

Squamocolumnar (epithelial) junction (SCJ)

Lower esophageal sphincter

Stomach

UCV *Path1.77*

Esophageal cancer

Risk factors for esophageal cancer are:
Achalasia ✔
Barrett's esophagus ✔
Corrosive esophagitis/Cigarettes ✔
Diverticuli
Esophageal web/EtOH
Familial

ABCDEF.
Usually squamous cell carcinoma (Barrett's is an exception).

UCV *Path2.5*

Congenital pyloric stenosis

Hypertrophy of the pylorus causes obstruction. Palpable mass in epigastric region and projectile vomiting at ≈ 2 weeks of age. Treatment is surgical incision.

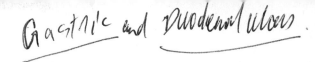

Gastric and Duodenal ulcers

Chronic gastritis → Gastric carcinoma

Type A (fundal)	Autoimmune disorder characterized by **A**utoantibodies to parietal cells, pernicious **A**nemia, and **A**chlorhydria.	Type **A** = 4 **A**'s.
Type B (antral)	Caused by *H. pylori* infection.	Type **B** = a **B**ug, *H. pylori*. Both carry ↑ risk of gastric carcinoma.

UCV Path1.81

Peptic ulcer disease (2x in smokers)

Gastric ulcer (70% HP)	Pain **G**reater with meals—weight loss. *H. pylori* infection in 70%; NSAID use also implicated. Due to ↓ mucosal protection against gastric acid.
Duodenal ulcer (100% HP)	Pain **D**ecreases with meals—weight gain. Almost 100% have *H. pylori* infection. → (Metronidazole, Bismuth salt, Amoxicillin/tetracyclin) Due to ↑ gastric acid secretion or ↓ mucosal protection. Hypertrophy of Brunner's glands.

Gastric ulcers → Pain increases with meals.

Pain decreases with ulcers.

Tend to have clean, "punched-out" margins unlike the raised/irregular margins of carcinoma. Potential complications include bleeding, penetration, perforation, and obstruction (not intrinsically precancerous). *H. pylori* infection can be treated with "BAM" ← "triple therapy" (metronidazole, bismuth salicylate, and either amoxicillin or tetracycline) with or without a proton pump inhibitor. Incidence of peptic ulcer disease is twice as great in smokers.

UCV Anat.21

Inflammatory bowel disease

	Crohn's disease	Ulcerative colitis
Possible etiology	Infectious.	Autoimmune.
Location	May involve any portion of the GI tract, usually the terminal ileum, small intestine, and colon. **Skip** lesions, rectal sparing.	*Colitis* = colon inflammation. Continuous lesions with rectal involvement.
Gross morphology	Transmural inflammation. **Cobblestone** mucosa, creeping **fat,** bowel wall thickening ("string sign" on x-ray), linear ulcers, fissures.	Mucosal inflammation. Friable mucosal pseudopolyps with freely hanging mesentery.
Microscopic morphology	Noncaseating granulomas.	Crypt abscesses and ulcers.
Complications	Strictures, fistulas, perianal disease, malabsorption–nutritional depletion.	Severe stenosis, toxic megacolon, **colorectal carcinoma.**
Extraintestinal manifestations	Migratory polyarthritis, erythema nodosum.	Pyoderma gangrenosum, sclerosing cholangitis.

crypts, colorectal carcinoma, sclerosing cholangitis

UCV Path1.84, 102

For **Crohn's,** think of a **fat** old **crone skipping** down a **cobblestone** road.

For Ulcerative colitis, think crypts, carcinoma, cholangitis.

Crypt abscesses and ulcers are Ulcerative colitis.

HIGH-YIELD FACTS

Pathology

Diverticular disease

Diverticulum
Blind pouch leading off the alimentary tract, lined by mucosa, muscularis, and serosa, that communicates with the lumen of the gut. Most diverticula (esophagus, stomach, duodenum, colon) are acquired and are termed "false" in that they lack or have an attenuated muscularis propria.

Diverticulosis
— *sigmoid colon.*
The prevalence of diverticulosis (many diverticula) in patients over age 60 approaches 50%. Caused by ↑ intraluminal pressure and focal weakness in the colonic wall. Most frequently involves the sigmoid colon. Associated with low-fiber diets. Most often asymptomatic or associated with vague discomfort.

Diverticulitis
Inflammation of diverticula classically causing LLQ pain. May be complicated by perforation, peritonitis, abscess formation, or bowel stenosis.

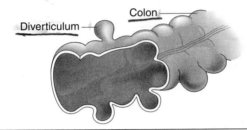

UCV *Path1.85*

Intussusception and volvulus

Intussusception—"telescoping" of 1 bowel segment into distal segment; can compromise blood supply.

*re*Volvulus—twisting of portion of bowel around its mesentery; can lead to obstruction.

Stomach cancer

Almost always adenocarcinoma. Early aggressive local spread and node/liver mets. Associated with dietary nitrosamines, achlorhydria, chronic gastritis. Termed **linitis plastica** when diffusely infiltrative (thickened, rigid appearance).

Virchow's node—involvement of supraclavicular node by mets from stomach.
Krukenberg's tumor—bilateral mets to ovaries. Abundant mucus, "signet-ring" cells.

Hirschsprung's disease

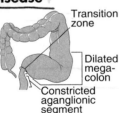

Transition zone

Dilated mega-colon

Constricted aganglionic segment

Congenital megacolon characterized by lack of enteric nervous plexus in segment (Auerbach's and Meissner's plexuses) on intestinal biopsy. Due to failure of neural crest cell migration. Presents as chronic constipation early in life. Dilated portion of the colon proximal to the aganglionic segment, resulting in a "transition zone."

Think of a giant spring that has **sprung** in the colon.

UCV *Anat.19*

Colorectal cancer risk factors

Villous adenomas
Risk factors for carcinoma of colon—colorectal villous adenomas, chronic inflammatory bowel disease, low-fiber diet, ↑ age, familial adenomatous polyposis (FAP), hereditary nonpolyposis colorectal cancer (HNPCC), personal and family history of colon cancer. Peutz-Jeghers is not a risk factor. Screen patients > 50 years old with stool occult blood test.

UCV *Path2.4*

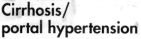

(Fetor Hepaticus) *(handwritten)*

Cirrhosis/portal hypertension

Hematemesis *(handwritten)*
Melena *(handwritten)*

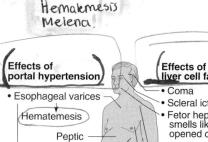

Effects of portal hypertension
- Esophageal varices
  - (Hematemesis)
  - Peptic ulcer
- Melena
- Splenomegaly
- Caput medusae
- Ascites
- Testicular atrophy
- Hemorrhoids

Effects of liver cell failure
- Coma
- Scleral icterus
- Fetor hepaticus (breath smells like a freshly opened corpse)
- Spider nevi
- Gynecomastia
- Jaundice
- Loss of sexual hair ✓
- Liver "flap" = asterixis (coarse hand tremor)
- Bleeding tendency (decreased prothrombin)
- Anemia
- Ankle edema ✓

(Adapted, with permission, from Chandrasoma P, Taylor CE. *Concise Pathology*, 3rd ed. Stamford, CT: Appleton & Lange, 1998:654.)

UCV *Anat.22, Path1.91*

Cirrho (Greek) = tawny yellow. Diffuse fibrosis of liver, destroys normal architecture. Nodular regeneration. Micronodular—nodules < 3 mm, uniform size. Due to metabolic insult (e.g., alcohol). Macronodular—nodules > 3 mm, varied size. Usually due to significant liver injury leading to hepatic necrosis (e.g., postinfectious or drug-induced hepatitis). ↑ risk of hepatocellular carcinoma.

Alcoholic hepatitis

AST > ALT *(handwritten)*
1.5 *(handwritten)*

Swollen and necrotic hepatocytes, neutrophil infiltration, Mallory bodies (hyaline), fatty change, and sclerosis around central vein. SGOT (AST) to SGPT (ALT) ratio is usually > 1.5.

A Scotch and **T**onic:
AST elevated (> ALT) with alcoholic hepatitis.

UCV *Path1.93*

Budd-Chiari syndrome

(IVC Hepatic veins) *(handwritten)*

Occlusion of IVC or hepatic veins with centrilobular congestion and necrosis, leading to congestive liver disease (hepatomegaly, ascites, abdominal pain, and eventual liver failure). Associated with polycythemia vera, pregnancy, hepatocellular carcinoma.

UCV *Path1.78*

Wilson's disease

Ceruloplasmin *(handwritten)*

Due to failure of copper to enter circulation in the form of ceruloplasmin. Leads to copper accumulation, especially in liver, brain, cornea. Also known as hepatolenticular degeneration.
Wilson's disease is characterized by:

Asterixis
Basal ganglia degeneration (parkinsonian symptoms)
Ceruloplasmin ↓, **C**irrhosis, **C**orneal deposits (Kayser-Fleischer rings), **C**opper accumulation, **C**arcinoma (hepatocellular), **C**horeiform movements
Dementia

Treat with penicillamine.

ABCD. PARK *(handwritten)*

UCV *Bio.41*

Hemochromatosis

↑ iron deposition in many organs. Classic triad of micronodular pigment cirrhosis, "bronze" diabetes, skin pigmentation. Results in CHF and an ↑ risk of hepatocellular carcinoma. Disease may be a 1° (autosomal-recessive) disorder or 2° to chronic transfusion therapy. ↑ ferritin, ↑ transferrin saturation.

Total body iron may reach 50 g, enough to set off metal detectors at airports.
Treat with repeated phlebotomy, deferoxamine.

UCV *Path1.90*

HIGH-YIELD FACTS

Pathology

Jaundice

Normally, liver cells conjugate bilirubin and excrete it into bile, where it is converted by bacteria to urobilinogen (some of which is reabsorbed). Some urobilinogen is also formed directly from heme metabolism. Termed unconjugated (indirect) bilirubin before conjugation and conjugated (direct) after. Conjugated is soluble (can enter urine).

→ From intestine

Jaundice type	Hyperbilirubinemia	Urine bilirubin	Urine urobilinogen
Hepatocellular Hepatic	Conjugated/unconjugated	↑	Normal/↓
Obstructive posthepatic	Conjugated	↑	↓
Hemolytic prehepatic	Unconjugated	Absent (acholuria) since uncon is insoluble.	↑ in Hemolytic Jaundice. Since ↑ production and excretion is ↑ (since no obstruction)

Hereditary hyperbilirubinemias

↑ unconjugated

Gilbert's syndrome — Mildly ↓ UDP-glucuronyl transferase. Asymptomatic, but unconjugated bilirubin is elevated without overt hemolysis. Associated with stress.   *Bio.40*

Gilbert's may represent a milder form.

Crigler-Najjar syndrome, type I — Absent UDP-glucuronyl transferase. Presents early in life; patients die within a few years.   *Bio.38*

Findings: jaundice, kernicterus (bilirubin deposition in brain), ↑ unconjugated bilirubin.

Treatment: plasmapheresis and phototherapy.

Crigler-Najjar type I is a severe disease. Type II is less severe and responds to phenobarbital.

↑ conjugated

Dubin-Johnson syndrome — Black liver — Conjugated hyperbilirubinemia due to defective liver excretion. Grossly black liver.   *Bio.39*

Rotor's syndrome is similar but less severe and does not cause black liver.

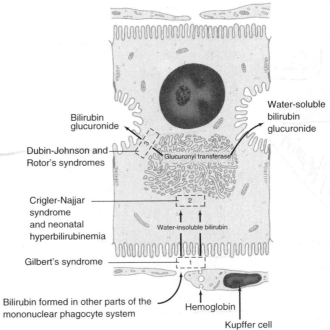

Bilirubin glucuronide

Water-soluble bilirubin glucuronide

Dubin-Johnson and Rotor's syndromes

Glucuronyl transferase

Crigler-Najjar syndrome and neonatal hyperbilirubinemia

Water-insoluble bilirubin

Gilbert's syndrome

Bilirubin formed in other parts of the mononuclear phagocyte system

Hemoglobin

Kupffer cell

(Adapted, with permission, from Junqueira LC, Carneiro J, Kelley RO. *Basic Histology*, 9th ed. Stamford, CT: Appleton & Lange, 1999.)

UCV

Bile prob → cholesterol prob. → shit load probs

Biliary cirrhosis

Primary	Autoimmune disorder with antimitochondrial antibodies; severe obstructive jaundice, itching, hypercholesterolemia (xanthoma).
Secondary	Due to extrahepatic biliary obstruction. ↑ in pressure in intrahepatic ducts → injury/fibrosis. Often complicated by ascending cholangitis (bacterial infection), bile stasis, and "bile lakes."

Hepatocellular carcinoma

UCV *Path1.94*

Also called hepatoma. Most common 1° malignant tumor of the liver in adults. ↑ incidence of hepatocellular carcinoma is associated with hepatitis B and C, Wilson's disease, hemochromatosis, α_1-antitrypsin deficiency, alcoholic cirrhosis, and carcinogens (e.g., aflatoxin B1).

Hepatocellular carcinoma, like renal cell carcinoma, is commonly spread by hematogenous dissemination.
Elevated AFP. ✓

Reye's syndrome

UCV *Pharm.32*

Rare, often fatal childhood hepatoencephalopathy. Findings: fatty liver (microvesicular fatty change), hypoglycemia, coma. Associated with viral infection (especially VZV and influenza B) and salicylates; thus, aspirin is no longer recommended for children (use acetaminophen, with caution).

"Don't give your baby a baby aspirin."

Gallstones

Cystic duct
Hepatic duct
Stone in the common bile duct
Fibrosed gallbladder with gallstones
Pancreatic duct

Form when solubilizing bile acids and lecithin are overwhelmed by ↑ cholesterol and/or bilirubin.
Three types of stones:
1. Cholesterol stones (radiolucent with 10–20% opaque due to calcifications)—associated with obesity, Crohn's disease, cystic fibrosis, advanced age, clofibrate, estrogens, multiparity, rapid weight loss, and Native American origin.
2. Mixed stones (radiolucent)—have both cholesterol and pigment components. Most common type.
3. Pigment stones (radiopaque)—seen in patients with chronic RBC hemolysis, alcoholic cirrhosis, advanced age, and biliary infection.
Diagnose with ultrasound. Treat with cholecystectomy.

Risk factors (4 F's):
1. Female
2. Fat → ↑ cholesterol → ↑ stones
3. Fertile
4. Forty
May present with Charcot's triad of epigastric/RUQ pain, fever, jaundice.

Acute pancreatitis

hypocalcemia

UCV *Path1.97*

Causes: Gallstones, Ethanol, Trauma, Steroids, Mumps, Autoimmune disease, Scorpion sting, Hyperlipidemia, Drugs.
✗ Clinical presentation: epigastric abdominal pain radiating to back.
Labs: elevated amylase, lipase (higher specificity).
Can lead to DIC, ARDS, diffuse fat necrosis, hypocalcemia, and pseudocyst formation.
✗ Chronic pancreatitis is strongly associated with alcoholism.

GET SMASHeD.
ddI can cause a fatal pancreatitis!

Pancreatic adenocarcinoma

Prognosis averages 6 months or less; very aggressive; usually already metastasized at presentation; tumors more common in pancreatic head (obstructive jaundice).

Often presents with:

1. Abdominal pain radiating to back ✓
2. Weight loss ✓
3. Anorexia ✓
4. Migratory thrombophlebitis (Trousseau's syndrome) ✓
5. Pancreatic duct obstruction (malabsorption with palpable gallbladder)

UCV *Path2.10*

(Reid index > 50%)

PATHOLOGY—RESPIRATORY

(Obstructive lung disease (COPD))

Obstruction of air flow, resulting in air trapping in the lungs. PFTs— ↓ FEV_1/FVC ratio (hallmark).

Types:

1. **Chronic Bronchitis** ("Blue Bloater")—productive cough for ≥ 3 consecutive months in 2 or more years. Hypertrophy of mucus-secreting glands in the bronchioles (Reid index > 50%). Leading cause is smoking. Findings: wheezing, crackles, cyanosis. *Path2.80*

destruction of Lung parenchyma

2. **Emphysema** ("pink puffer")—enlargement of air spaces and ↓ recoil resulting from destruction of alveolar walls. Caused by smoking (centriacinar emphysema) and α_1-antitrypsin deficiency (panacinar emphysema and liver cirrhosis) → ↑ elastase activity. Findings: dyspnea, ↓ breath sounds, tachycardia, ↓ I/E ratio. *Path2.81*

↓ Breath sound ↑ HR (Tachycardia) Emphysema

3. **Asthma**—bronchial hyperresponsiveness causes reversible bronchoconstriction. Can be triggered by viral URIs, allergens, and stress. Findings: cough, wheezing, dyspnea, tachypnea, hypoxemia, ↓ I/E ratio, pulsus paradoxus. *Path2.76*

4. **Bronchiectasis**—chronic necrotizing infection of bronchi → dilated airways, purulent sputum, recurrent infections, hemoptysis. Associated with bronchial obstruction, cystic fibrosis, poor ciliary motility.

UCV

Restrictive lung disease

Restricted lung expansion causes ↓ lung volumes (↓ VC and TLC). PFTs—FEV_1/FVC ratio > 80%.

Types:

1. Poor breathing mechanics (extrapulmonary):
   a. Poor muscular effort—polio, myasthenia gravis.
   b. Poor apparatus—scoliosis.
2. Poor lung expansion (pulmonary):
   a. Defective alveolar filling—pneumonia, ARDS, pulmonary edema. *Bio.97, Path2.52*
   b. Interstitial fibrosis—causes ↑ recoil (↓ compliance), thereby limiting alveolar expansion. Complications include cor pulmonale. Can be seen in diffuse interstitial pulmonary fibrosis and bleomycin toxicity. Symptoms include gradual progressive dyspnea and cough. *Path2.84*

UCV

HIGH-YIELD FACTS

Pathology

Lung—physical findings

AIR   SOLID

Abnormality	Breath Sounds	Resonance	Fremitus	Tracheal Deviation
Bronchial obstruction	Absent over area	↓	↓	Toward side of lesion
Pleural effusion	↓ over effusion	Dullness	↓	—
Pneumonia (lobar)	May have bronchial breath sounds over lesion	Dullness	↑	—
Pneumothorax	↓	Hyperresonant	Absent	Away from side of lesion

Obstructive vs. restrictive lung disease

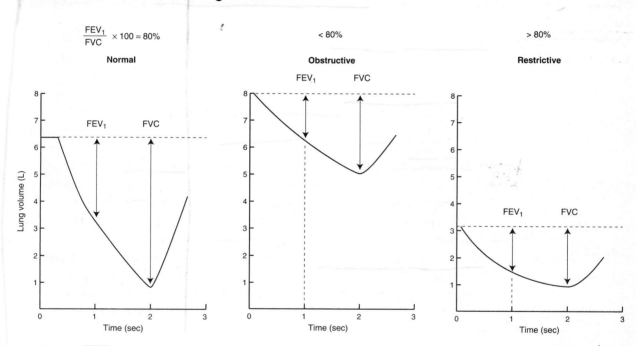

$$\frac{FEV_1}{FVC} \times 100 = 80\%$$

Normal   < 80%   > 80%

Obstructive   Restrictive

Note: Obstructive lung volumes > normal (↑ TLC, ↑ FRC, ↑ RV); restrictive lung volumes < normal. In both obstructive and restrictive, FEV_1 and FVC are reduced, but in obstructive, FEV_1 is more dramatically reduced, resulting in a ↓ FEV_1/FVC ratio.

Asbestosis

Diffuse pulmonary interstitial fibrosis caused by inhaled asbestos fibers. ↑ risk of pleural mesothelioma and bronchogenic carcinoma. Long latency. Ferruginous bodies in lung (asbestos fibers coated with hemosiderin). Ivory-white pleural plaques.

Asbestosis and smoking greatly ↑ risk of bronchogenic cancer (smoking not additive with mesothelioma). Seen in shipbuilders and plumbers.

Asbestosis causes pleural mesothelioma Bronchogenic Carcinoma. Largocarcinoma.

HIGH-YIELD FACTS

Pathology

Neonatal respiratory distress syndrome

Surfactant deficiency leading to ↑ surface tension, resulting in alveolar collapse. Surfactant is made by type II pneumocytes most abundantly after 35th week of gestation. The lecithin-to-sphingomyelin ratio in the amniotic fluid, a measure of lung maturity, is usually < 1.5 in neonatal respiratory distress syndrome.

Surfactant—dipalmitoyl phosphatidylcholine.

Treatment: maternal steroids before birth; artificial surfactant for infant.

UCV Bio.91

Kartagener's syndrome

Immotile cilia due to a dynein arm defect. Results in sterility (sperm also immotile), bronchiectasis, and recurrent sinusitis (bacteria and particles not pushed out); associated with situs inversus (e.g., dextrocardia).

UCV Bio.59

Lung cancer

Bronchogenic carcinoma	Tumors that arise centrally: 1. Squamous cell carcinoma—clear link to Smoking; ectopic PTH-related peptide production 2. Small cell carcinoma—clear link to Smoking; associated with ectopic hormone production (ADH, ACTH); may lead to Lambert-Eaton syndrome Tumors that arise peripherally: 1. Adenocarcinoma (most common) 2. Bronchioalveolar carcinoma (thought not to be related to smoking) 3. Large cell carcinoma—undifferentiated	Lung cancer is the leading cause of cancer death. Presentation: cough, hemoptysis, bronchial obstruction, wheezing, pneumonic "coin" lesion on x-ray. **SPHERE** of complications: Superior vena caval syndrome Pancoast's tumor Horner's syndrome Endocrine (paraneoplastic)
Carcinoid tumor	Can cause carcinoid syndrome.	Recurrent laryngeal symptoms (hoarseness)
Metastases	Very common. Brain (epilepsy), bone (pathologic fracture), and liver (jaundice, hepatomegaly).	Effusions (pleural or pericardial)

UCV Path2.85

Pneumonia

3

Type	Organism(s)	Characteristics
Lobar	Pneumococcus most frequently	Intra-alveolar exudate → consolidation; may involve entire lung.
Bronchopneumonia	*Staphylococcus aureus, H. flu, Klebsiella, S. pyogenes*	Acute inflammatory infiltrates from bronchioles into adjacent alveoli; patchy distribution involving ≥ 1 lobes.
Interstitial (atypical) pneumonia	Viruses (RSV, adenoviruses), *Mycoplasma, Legionella*	Diffuse patchy inflammation localized to interstitial areas at alveolar walls; distribution involving ≥ 1 lobes.

Pancoast's tumor

Carcinoma that occurs in apex of lung and may affect cervical sympathetic plexus, causing Horner's syndrome.

Horner's syndrome—ptosis, miosis, anhidrosis.

PAM-HORNY

(Cerebral cortex) Huntington disease
↑q/loss GABAergic neurons · Atrophy of caudate nucleus

Degenerative diseases

Cerebral cortex	**Alzheimer's disease**—most common cause of dementia in the elderly. Associated with senile plaques (β-amyloid core) and neurofibrillary tangles (abnormally phosphorylated tau protein). Familial form (10%) associated with genes on chromosomes 1, 14, 19 (Apo-E4 allele), and 21 (p-App gene).	Multi-infarct dementia is the 2nd most common cause of dementia in the elderly.
	Pick's disease—associated with Pick bodies (intracytoplasmic inclusion bodies) and is specific for the frontal and temporal lobes.	
Basal ganglia and brain stem	**Huntington's disease**—autosomal-dominant inheritance, chorea, dementia. Atrophy of caudate nucleus (loss of GABAergic neurons). *Path3.15*	Chromosome 4—expansion of CAG repeats.
	Parkinson's disease—associated with Lewy bodies and depigmentation of the substantia nigra (loss of dopaminergic neurons). Rare cases have been linked to exposure to MPTP, a contaminant in illicit street drugs. *Anat.68*	**TRAP** = **T**remor (at rest), cogwheel **R**igidity, **A**kinesia, and **P**ostural instability (you are **TRAP**ped in your body).
Spinocerebellar	**Olivopontocerebellar atrophy; Friedreich's ataxia.** *Path3.11*	
Motor neuron	**Amyotrophic lateral sclerosis (ALS)**—associated with **both** lower and upper motor neuron signs. *Path3.1*	Commonly known as Lou Gehrig's disease.
	Werdnig-Hoffmann disease—presents at birth as a "floppy baby"; tongue fasciculations.	
	Polio—lower motor neuron signs.	

UCV

Opportunistic CNS infections in AIDS

2 common organisms that target the brain:
1. *Toxoplasma* → diffuse (intracerebral) calcifications
2. *Cryptococcus* → periventricular calcifications

Toxoplasma and Cryptococcus

Intracranial hemorrhage

Epidural hematoma ✓	Rupture of middle meningeal artery, often 2° to fracture of temporal bone. Lucid interval.	CT shows "biconcave disk" not crossing suture lines.
Subdural hematoma ✓	Rupture of bridging veins. Venous bleeding (less pressure) with delayed onset of symptoms. Seen in elderly individuals, alcoholics, blunt trauma.	Crescent-shaped hemorrhage that crosses suture lines.
Subarachnoid hemorrhage ✓	Rupture of an aneurysm (usually berry aneurysm) or an AVM. Patients complain of "worst headache of my life." Bloody or xanthochromic spinal tap.	
Parenchymal hematoma	Caused by hypertension, amyloid angiopathy, diabetes mellitus, and tumor.	

UCV *Path3.10, 31, 32*

PATHOLOGY—NEUROLOGIC (continued)

Berry aneurysms

EDAM

UCV *Path3.5*

Berry aneurysms occur at the bifurcations in the circle of Willis. Most common site is bifurcation of the anterior communicating artery. Rupture (most common complication) leads to hemorrhagic stroke/subarachnoid hemorrhage. Associated with adult polycystic kidney disease, Ehlers-Danlos syndrome, and Marfan's syndrome.

Demyelinating and dysmyelinating diseases

UCV

1. **Multiple sclerosis (MS)**—↑ prevalence with greater distance from the equator; periventricular plaques, preservation of axons, loss of oligodendrocytes, reactive astrocytic gliosis; ↑ protein (IgG) in CSF. Many patients have a relapsing-remitting course. Patients can present with optic neuritis (sudden loss of vision), MLF syndrome (internuclear ophthalmoplegia), hemiparesis, hemisensory symptoms, or bladder/bowel incontinence.   *Path3.23*
2. **Progressive multifocal leukoencephalopathy (PML)**—associated with JC virus and seen in 2–4% of AIDS patients (reactivation of latent viral infection).   *Micro2.97*
3. **Postinfectious encephalomyelitis.**
4. **Metachromatic leukodystrophy** (a sphingolipidosis).   *Bio.64*
5. **Guillain-Barré syndrome** (see below).

Classic triad of **MS** is a **SIN:**
   Scanning speech ✓
   Intention tremor ✓
   Nystagmus ✓

Guillain-Barré syndrome (acute idiopathic polyneuritis)

UCV *Path3.13*

Inflammation and demyelination of peripheral nerves and motor fibers of ventral roots (sensory effect less severe than motor), causing symmetric ascending muscle weakness beginning in distal lower extremities. Facial diplegia in 50% of cases. Autonomic function may be severely affected (e.g., cardiac irregularities, hypertension, or hypotension).

Findings: elevated CSF protein with normal cell count ("albumino-cytologic dissociation"). Elevated protein → papilledema.

Associated with infections (e.g., herpesvirus or *Campylobacter jejuni* infection), inoculations, and stress, but no definitive link to pathogens.

Poliomyelitis

Caused by poliovirus, which is transmitted by the fecal-oral route. Replicates in the oropharynx and small intestine before spreading through the bloodstream to the CNS, where it leads to the destruction of cells in the anterior horn of the spinal cord, leading in turn to LMN destruction.

Symptoms — Malaise, headache, fever, nausea, abdominal pain, sore throat. Signs of LMN lesions—muscle weakness and atrophy, fasciculations, fibrillation, and hyporeflexia.

Findings — CSF with lymphocytic pleocytosis with slight elevation of protein. Virus recovered from stool or throat.

Seizures

Partial seizures—1 area of the brain.

1. Simple partial (awareness intact)—motor, sensory, autonomic, psychic
2. Complex partial (impaired awareness)

Generalized seizures—diffuse.

1. Absence—blank stare (petit mal)
2. Myoclonic—quick, repetitive jerks
3. Tonic-clonic—alternating stiffening and movement (grand mal)
4. Tonic—stiffening
5. Atonic—"drop" seizures

Epilepsy is a disorder of recurrent seizures (febrile seizures are not epilepsy). Partial seizures can secondarily generalize.

Causes of seizures by age:
Children—genetic, infection, trauma, congenital, metabolic.
Adults—tumors, trauma, stroke, infection.
Elderly—stroke, tumor, trauma, metabolic, infection.

Broca's vs. Wernicke's aphasia

Broca's is nonfluent aphasia with intact comprehension (expressive aphasia). Wernicke's is fluent aphasia with impaired comprehension (receptive aphasia).
Broca's area—inferior frontal gyrus.
Wernicke's area—superior temporal gyrus.

Broca's is **Bro**ken speech; Wernicke's is **W**ordy but makes no sense.

Wernicke's = "What?"

UCV *Path3.2*

Horner's syndrome

Sympathectomy of face (lesion above T1):

1. Ptosis (slight drooping of eyelid)
2. Anhidrosis (absence of sweating) and flushing (rubor) of affected side of face
3. Miosis (pupil constriction)

Associated with Pancoast's tumor.

PAM is horny.

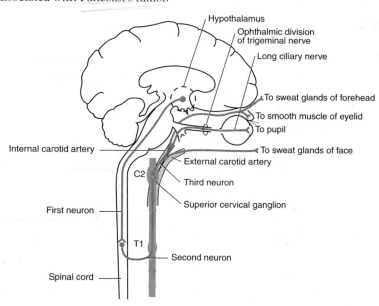

(Adapted, with permission, from Simon RP et al. *Clinical Neurology,* 4th ed. Stamford, CT: Appleton & Lange, 1999:146.)

The 3-neuron oculosympathetic pathway above projects from the hypothalamus to the intermediolateral column of the spinal cord, then to the superior cervical (sympathetic) ganglion, and finally to the pupil, the smooth muscle of the eyelids, and the sweat glands of the forehead and face. Interruption of these pathways results in Horner's syndrome.

Syringomyelia

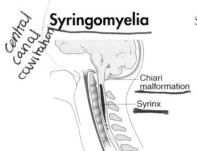

(handwritten: Central canal cavitation)

Softening and cavitation around central canal of spinal cord. Crossing fibers of spinothalamic tract are damaged. Bilateral loss of pain and temperature sensation in upper extremities with preservation of touch sensation.

Syrinx (Greek) = tube, as in syringe.
Often presents in patients with Arnold-Chiari malformation.
Most common at C8–T1.

(handwritten: Bilateral loss of pain and temp in upper extremities. but touch in there.)

UCV Path3.33

Tabes dorsalis

Degeneration of dorsal columns and dorsal roots due to 3° syphilis, resulting in impaired proprioception and locomotor ataxia. Associated with Charcot's joints, shooting (lightning) pain, Argyll Robertson pupils, and absence of deep tendon reflexes.

PATHOLOGY—RHEUMATIC/AUTOIMMUNE

Osteoarthritis

(handwritten: End of day pain)

✓ Mechanical—wear and tear of joints leads to destruction of articular cartilage, subchondral bone formation, sclerosis, osteophytes, eburnation, Heberden's nodes (DIP), and Bouchard's nodes (PIP).
Common in older patients.
Classic presentation—pain in weight-bearing joints after use (e.g., at the end of the day), improving with rest. No systemic symptoms.

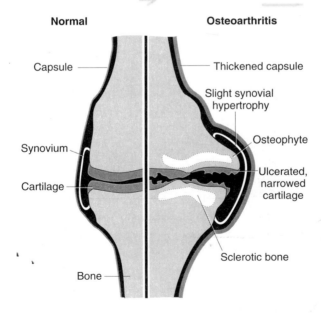

Normal	Osteoarthritis
Capsule	Thickened capsule
	Slight synovial hypertrophy
	Osteophyte
Synovium	
Cartilage	Ulcerated, narrowed cartilage
	Sclerotic bone
Bone	

(Adapted, with permission, from Stobo J. *The Principles and Practice of Medicine,* 23rd ed. Stamford, CT: Appleton & Lange, 1996:241.)

UCV Path3.73

Rheumatoid arthritis

(handwritten: morning stiffness; Female >)

✓ Autoimmune—inflammatory disorder affecting synovial joints, with pannus formation in joints (MCP, PIP), subcutaneous rheumatoid nodules, ulnar deviation, subluxation.
Common in females. 80% of RA patients have positive rheumatoid factor (anti-IgG Ab).
Classic presentation—morning stiffness improving with use, symmetric joint involvement, and systemic symptoms (fever, fatigue, pleuritis, pericarditis).

UCV Path3.93

(side margin: HIGH-YIELD FACTS / Pathology)

Gout

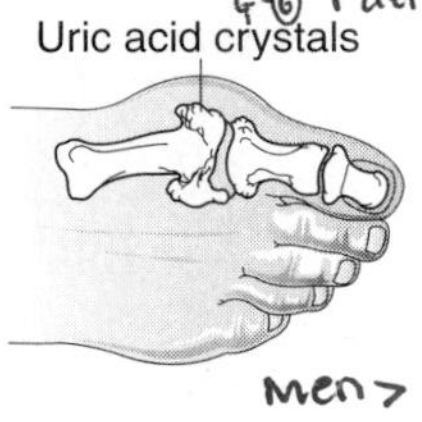

[handwritten: Lesch-Nyhan, PRPP excess, ↑ uric acid, G-6-P deficiency]

Uric acid crystals

[handwritten: men >]

UCV Bio.95

Precipitation of monosodium urate crystals into joints due to hyperuricemia, which can be caused by Lesch-Nyhan syndrome, PRPP excess, ↓ excretion of uric acid, or glucose-6-phosphatase deficiency. Also associated with the use of thiazide diuretics, which competitively inhibit the secretion of uric acid. Asymmetric joint distribution. Favored manifestation is painful MTP joint in the big toe (podagra). Tophus formation (often on external ear or Achilles tendon). Crystals are needle shaped and negatively birefringent. Treatment is allopurinol, probenecid, colchicine, and NSAIDs. More common in men.

[handwritten right margin: TOE]

Pseudogout

UCV Path3.90

Caused by deposition of calcium pyrophosphate crystals within the joint space. Forms basophilic, rhomboid crystals (as opposed to the negatively birefringent, needle-shaped crystals in gout). Usually affects large joints (classically the knee). > 50 years old; both sexes affected equally. No treatment.

[handwritten right margin: knee]

Celiac sprue

UCV Path1.80

Autoimmune-mediated intolerance of gliadin (wheat) leading to steatorrhea. Associated with people of northern European descent. Findings include blunting of villi, lymphocytes in the lamina propria, and abnormal D-xylose test. Associated with dermatitis herpetiformis. 10–15% lead to malignancy (most often B-cell lymphoma).

Systemic lupus erythematosus

[handwritten: Female >]

[handwritten: Anti-Smith Ab]
[handwritten: Anti-ds DNA]
[handwritten: Very specific for SLE.]

UCV Path2.59, 3.95

90% are female and between ages 14 and 45. Symptoms are fever, fatigue, weight loss, joint pain, malar rash, and photosensitivity. May also occur with pleuritis, pericarditis, nonbacterial verrucous endocarditis, Raynaud's phenomenon. **Wire loop** lesions in kidney with immune complex deposition (with nephrotic syndrome); death from renal failure and infections. False positives on syphilis tests (RPR/VDRL). Lab tests detect presence of:

1. Antinuclear antibodies (ANA)—sensitive, but not specific for SLE
2. Antibodies to double-stranded DNA (anti-dsDNA)—very specific
3. Anti-Smith antibodies (anti-Sm)—very specific

SLE causes LSE (Libman-Sacks Endocarditis)—valvular vegetations found on **both** sides of valve (mitral valve stenosis) and do not embolize.

Most common and severe in black females.

Drugs that can produce an SLE-like syndrome that is commonly reversible—**HIPP**: **H**ydralazine, **I**NH, **P**henytoin, **P**rocainamide. Antihistone antibody.

Pharm.77

Associated with thymoma.

Sarcoidosis

[handwritten: GRAIN]

UCV Path2.92

Characterized by immune-mediated, widespread noncaseating granulomas and elevated serum ACE levels. Common in black females.

Associated with restrictive lung disease, bilateral hilar lymphadenopathy, erythema nodosum, Bell's palsy, epithelial granulomas containing microscopic Schaumann and asteroid bodies, uveoparotitis, and hypercalcemia (due to elevated conversion of vitamin D to its active form in epithelioid macrophages).

GRAIN:

Gammaglobulinemia
Rheumatoid arthritis
ACE increase
Interstitial fibrosis
Noncaseating granulomas

HIGH-YIELD FACTS

Pathology

Ankylosing spondylitis	Chronic inflammatory disease of spine and large joints, sacroiliitis, uveitis, and aortic regurgitation. Commonly affects males (10–30 years old). 90% of cases are associated with B27 (gene that codes for HLA MHC-I).	
Reiter's syndrome AUC UCV Path3.92	A seronegative spondyloarthropathy. HLA-B27 link. Classic triad: 1. Urethritis 2. Conjunctivitis and anterior uveitis 3. Arthritis Has a strong predilection for **males.**	"Can't see (anterior uveitis/conjunctivitis), can't pee (urethritis), can't climb a tree (arthritis)." Post-GI or chlamydia infections.
Sjögren's syndrome UCV Path3.94	Classic triad—dry eyes (conjunctivitis, xerophthalmia), dry mouth (dysphagia, xerostomia), arthritis. Parotid enlargement, increased risk of B-cell lymphoma. Predominantly affects **females** between 40 and 60 years of age.	Associated with rheumatoid arthritis. Sicca syndrome—dry eyes, dry mouth, nasal and vaginal dryness, chronic bronchitis, reflux esophagitis.
Scleroderma (progressive systemic sclerosis—PSS) UCV Path3.89	Excessive fibrosis and collagen deposition throughout the body. 75% female. Commonly sclerosis of skin but also of cardiovascular and GI systems and kidney. 2 major categories: 1. Diffuse scleroderma—widespread skin involvement, rapid progression, early visceral involvement. Associated with anti-Scl-70 antibody. 2. **CREST** syndrome—**C**alcinosis, **R**aynaud's phenomenon, **E**sophageal dysmotility, **S**clerodactyly, and **T**elangiectasia. Limited skin involvement, often confined to fingers and face. More benign clinical course. Associated with anticentromere antibody.	
Goodpasture's syndrome UCV Path2.56	Findings: pulmonary hemorrhages, renal lesions, hemoptysis, hematuria, anemia, crescentic glomerulonephritis. Anti–glomerular basement membrane antibodies produce linear staining on immunofluorescence.	There are 2 Good Pastures for this disease: Glomerulus and Pulmonary. Also a type II hypersensitivity disease. Most common in men 20–40 years.

PATHOLOGY—ENDOCRINE/REPRODUCTIVE

Cushing's syndrome	↑ cortisol due to a variety of causes. Etiologies include: 1. Cushing's disease (1° pituitary adenoma); ↑ ACTH 2. 1° adrenal (hyperplasia/neoplasia); ↓ ACTH 3. Ectopic ACTH production (e.g., small cell lung cancer); ↑ ACTH 4. Iatrogenic; ↓ ACTH The clinical picture includes hypertension, weight gain, moon facies, truncal obesity, buffalo hump, hyperglycemia (insulin resistance), skin changes (thinning, striae), osteoporosis, and immune suppression.

Hyperaldosteronism

Primary (Conn's syndrome)	Caused by an aldosterone-secreting tumor, resulting in hypertension, hypokalemia, metabolic alkalosis, and **low** plasma renin.
Secondary	Due to renal artery stenosis, chronic renal failure, CHF, cirrhosis, or nephrotic syndrome. Kidney perception of low intravascular volume results in an overactive renin-angiotensin system. Therefore, it is associated with **high** plasma renin.

Treatment includes spironolactone, a diuretic that works by acting as an aldosterone antagonist.

UCV *Bio.11*

Addison's disease

1° deficiency of aldosterone and cortisol due to adrenal atrophy, causing hypotension (hyponatremic volume contraction) and skin hyperpigmentation ($\uparrow$ ACTH $\rightarrow$ MSH activity). Characterized by **A**drenal **A**trophy and **A**bsence of hormone production; involves **A**ll 3 cortical divisions. Distinguish from 2° insufficiency, which has no skin hyperpigmentation ($\downarrow$ pituitary ACTH production).

UCV *Bio.4*

Tumors of the adrenal medulla

Pheochromocytoma	The most common tumor of the adrenal medulla in adults. Derived from chromaffin cells (arise from neural crest).
Neuroblastoma	The most common tumor of the adrenal medulla in children, but it can occur anywhere along the sympathetic chain.

Pheochromocytomas may be associated with neurofibromatosis, MEN type II, and MEN type III.

Pheochromocytoma

Most of these neoplasms secrete a combination of norepinephrine and epinephrine. Urinary VMA levels and plasma catecholamines are elevated. Associated with MEN type II and type III. Treated with alpha antagonists, especially phenoxybenzamine, a nonselective, **irreversible** alpha blocker.
Episodic hyperadrenergic symptoms **(5 P's):**
  Pressure (elevated blood pressure)
  Pain (headache)
  Perspiration
  Palpitations
  Pallor/diaphoresis

Rule of 10's:
  10% malignant
  10% bilateral
  10% extra-adrenal
  10% calcify
  10% kids
  10% familial

UCV *Bio.26*

Multiple endocrine neoplasias (MEN)

MEN type I (Wermer's syndrome)—pancreas (e.g., ZE syndrome, insulinomas, VIPomas), parathyroid, and pituitary tumors.
MEN type II (Sipple's syndrome)—medullary carcinoma of the thyroid, pheochromocytoma, parathyroid tumor or adenoma.
MEN type III (formerly MEN IIb)—medullary carcinoma of the thyroid, pheochromocytoma, and oral and intestinal ganglioneuromatosis (mucosal neuromas).

MEN I = 3 "**P**" organs (**P**ancreas, **P**ituitary, and **P**arathyroid).
All MEN syndromes have autosomal-dominant inheritance.

HIGH-YIELD FACTS

Pathology

Hypothyroidism and hyperthyroidism

Hypothyroidism	Cold intolerance, hypoactivity, weight gain, fatigue, lethargy, ↓ appetite, constipation, weakness, ↓ reflexes, myxedema (facial/periorbital), dry, cool skin, and coarse, brittle hair. *Path1.57*	↑ TSH (sensitive test for 1° hypothyroidism), ↓ total T_4, ↓ free T_4, ↓ T_3 uptake. Riedel's thyroiditis—thyroid replaced by fibrous tissue (hypothyroid).
Hyperthyroidism	Heat intolerance, hyperactivity, weight loss, chest pain/palpitations, arrhythmias, diarrhea, ↑ reflexes, warm, moist skin, and fine hair. *Path1.54*	↓ TSH (if 1°), ↑ total T_4, ↑ free T_4, ↑ T_3 uptake.
Graves' disease	An autoimmune hyperthyroidism with thyroid-stimulating/TSH receptor antibodies. Ophthalmopathy (proptosis, EOM swelling), pretibial myxedema, diffuse goiter. *Bio.14*	

Hashimoto's thyroiditis	Autoimmune disorder resulting in hypothyroidism. Slow course; moderately enlarged, nontender thyroid. Lymphocytic infiltrate with germinal centers. Antimicrosomal antibodies.	
Subacute thyroiditis (de Quervain's)	Self-limited hypothyroidism often following a flu-like illness. Elevated ESR, jaw pain, and early inflammation.	May be hyperthyroid early in course.
Thyroid cancer	1. Papillary carcinoma—most common, good prognosis, "ground-glass" nuclei, psammoma bodies. 2. Follicular carcinoma—poor prognosis, uniform follicles. 3. Medullary carcinoma—from parafollicular "C cells"; produces calcitonin, sheets of cells in amyloid stroma. MEN II/III. 4. Undifferentiated/anaplastic—older patients, horrible prognosis.	
Cretinism	Endemic cretinism occurs wherever endemic goiter is prevalent (lack of dietary iodine); sporadic cretinism is caused by defect in T_4 formation or developmental failure in thyroid formation. Findings: pot-bellied, pale, puffy-faced child with protruding umbilicus and protuberant tongue. *Path1.56*	Cretin means Christ-like (French *chrétien*). Those affected were considered so mentally retarded as to be incapable of sinning. Still common in China.

Cretinism = can be due to defect in T4 formation.

Diabetes mellitus

Acute manifestations   Polydipsia, polyuria, polyphagia, weight loss, DKA (type 1), hyperosmolar coma (type 2), unopposed secretion of GH and epinephrine (exacerbating hyperglycemia).

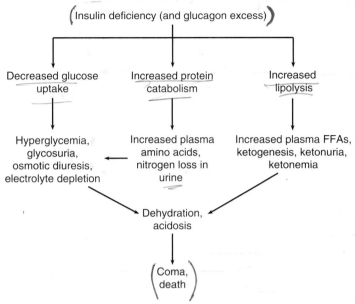

Chronic manifestations   Nonenzymatic glycosylation:

1. Small vessel disease (diffuse thickening of BM), retinopathy (hemorrhage, exudates, microaneurysms), nephropathy (nodular sclerosis, progressive proteinuria, chronic renal failure, arteriosclerosis leading to HTN)
2. Large vessel atherosclerosis, coronary artery disease, peripheral vascular occlusive disease and gangrene, cerebrovascular disease
3. Neuropathy (motor, sensory, and autonomic degeneration)
4. Cataracts, glaucoma (sorbitol accumulation)

Tests   Fasting serum glucose, glucose tolerance test, HbA_{1c} (measures long-term diabetic control)

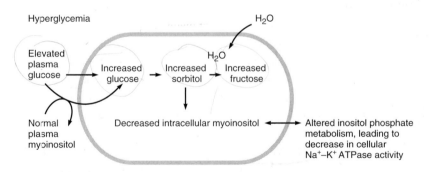

(Adapted, with permission, from Wyngaarden JB, Smith LH Jr, Bennett JC (eds). *Cecil Textbook of Medicine*, 19th ed. Philadelphia: W. B. Saunders, 1992.)

In the sorbitol pathway shown above, hyperglycemia increases intracellular sorbitol, which in turn is associated with depletion of intracellular myoinositol levels. Hyperglycemia may also ↓ myoinositol directly by inhibiting its uptake.

UCV *Path1.51, 52*

TYPE I = is Juvenile (onset.)

Type 1 vs. type 2 diabetes mellitus

Variable	Type 1—juvenile onset (IDDM)	Type 2—adult onset (NIDDM)
Incidence	15%	85%
Insulin necessary in treatment	Always	Sometimes
Age (exceptions commonly occur)	< 30	> 40
Association with obesity	No	Yes
Genetic predisposition	Weak, polygenic	Strong, polygenic
Association with HLA system	Yes (HLA-DR 3 and 4)	No
Glucose intolerance	Severe	Mild to moderate
Ketoacidosis	Common	Rare
β cell numbers in the islets	↓	Variable
Serum insulin level	↓	Variable
Classic symptoms of polyuria, polydipsia, thirst, weight loss	Common	Sometimes
Theorized cause	Viral or immune destruction of β cells	↑ resistance to insulin

Diabetic ketoacidosis	One of the most important complications of type 1 diabetes. Usually due to an increase in insulin requirements from an increase in stress (e.g., infection). Excess fat breakdown and ↑ ketogenesis from the ↑ in free fatty acids, which are then made into ketone bodies.	
Signs/symptoms	Kussmaul respirations (rapid/deep breathing), hyperthermia, nausea/vomiting, abdominal pain, psychosis/dementia, dehydration. Fruity breath odor.	
Labs	Hyperglycemia, ↑ H$^+$, ↓HCO$_3^-$ (anion gap metabolic acidosis), ↑ blood ketone levels, leukocytosis.	
Complications	Life-threatening mucormycosis, *Rhizopus* infection, cerebral edema, cardiac arrhythmias, heart failure.	
Treatment	Fluids, insulin, and potassium; glucose if necessary to prevent hypoglycemia.	

GIVE TOGETHER

Diabetes insipidus	Characterized by intensive thirst and polyuria together with an inability to concentrate urine with fluid restriction owing to lack of ADH (central DI) or to a lack of renal response to ADH (nephrogenic DI). Caused by lithium or demeclocycline.
Findings	Urine specific gravity < 1.006; serum osmolality > 290 mOsm/L.
Treatment	Adequate fluid intake. For central DI—intranasal desmopressin (ADH analog). For nephrogenic DI—hydrochlorothiazide, indomethacin, or amiloride.

UCV *Bio.7*

SIADH

too much ADH is being secreted.

UCV *Bio.30*

Syndrome of inappropriate antidiuretic hormone secretion: 1. Excessive water retention 2. Hyponatremia 3. Serum hypo-osmolarity with urine osmolarity > serum osmolarity Very low serum sodium levels can lead to seizures (correct slowly).	Causes include: 1. Ectopic ADH (small cell lung cancer) 2. CNS disorders/head trauma 3. Pulmonary disease 4. Drugs

HIGH-YIELD FACTS

Pathology

Hyperparathyroidism

Primary

Usually an adenoma. Hypercalcemia, hypercalciuria, hypophosphatemia, elevated PTH.

[handwritten: ↓ phosphate ↑ Ca²⁺]

Osteitis fibrosa cystica (von Recklinghausen's syndrome)—cystic bone spaces filled with non-neoplastic fibrous tissue.

Secondary

2° hyperplasia due to ↓ serum Ca²⁺, most often in chronic renal disease. Hypocalcemia, hyperphosphatemia, ↑ PTH.

Renal osteodystrophy—bone lesions due to 2° hyperparathyroidism due in turn to renal disease.

Hypoparathyroidism

Hypocalcemia, tetany. Due to accidental surgical excision (thyroid surgery) or DiGeorge's syndrome.

Pseudohypoparathyroidism—autosomal-recessive kidney unresponsiveness to PTH. Hypocalcemia, shortened 4th/5th digits, short stature.

Carcinoid syndrome!

Rare syndrome caused by carcinoid tumors (neuroendocrine cells), especially those of the small bowel; the tumors secrete high levels of serotonin (5HT) that does not get metabolized by the liver due to liver metastases. Results in recurrent **diarrhea, cutaneous flushing, asthmatic wheezing,** and **right-sided valvular disease.** Most common tumor of appendix. ↑ 5-HIAA in urine.

[handwritten: 1 Diarrhea, 2 Cut. flushing, 3 Asthmatic wheezing, 4 Right-sided valvular disease]

Rule of 1/3s:
1/3 metastasize
1/3 present with 2nd malignancy
1/3 multiple
Treat with octreotide.

UCV Bio.37

Zollinger-Ellison syndrome

Gastrin-secreting tumor that is usually located in the pancreas. Causes recurrent ulcers. May be associated with MEN syndrome type I.

UCV Path1.103

Osteoporosis!

Reduction of bone mass in spite of normal bone mineralization.

Affects whites > blacks > Asians.

Type I

Postmenopausal (10–15 years after menopause); ↑ bone resorption due to ↓ estrogen levels. Treated with estrogen replacement.

Vertebral crush fractures—acute back pain, loss of height, kyphosis.

Type II

Senile osteoporosis—affects men and women > 70 years.

Distal radius (Colles') fractures, vertebral wedge fractures.

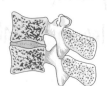
Mild compression fracture

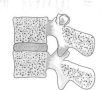
Normal vertebra

UCV Path3.85

Distention Hypertrophy of bladder Hydronephrosis

HIGH-YIELD FACTS

Pathology

Benign prostatic hyperplasia

Common in men over age 50. May be due to an age-related increase in estradiol with possible sensitization of the prostate to the growth-promoting effects of DHT. Characterized by a nodular enlargement of the periurethral (lateral and middle) lobes of the prostate gland, compressing the urethra into a vertical slit. Often presents with ↑ frequency of urination, nocturia, difficulty starting and stopping the stream of urine, and dysuria. May lead to distention and hypertrophy of the bladder, hydronephrosis, and urinary tract infections. Not considered a premalignant lesion.

UCV *Path2.52*

Hydatidiform mole

A pathologic ovum ("empty egg"—ovum with no DNA) resulting in cystic swelling of chorionic villi and proliferation of chorionic epithelium (trophoblast). Most common precursor of choriocarcinoma. High β-hCG. "Honeycombed uterus," "cluster of grapes" appearance. Genotype of a **complete** mole is 46,XX and is **completely** paternal in origin (no maternal chromosomes); no associated fetus. **PART**ial mole is made up of 3 or more **PARTS** (triploid or tetraploid).

UCV *Path3.51*

Mg sulfate Diazepam

Pregnancy-induced hypertension (preeclampsia-eclampsia)

Preeclampsia is the triad of hypertension, proteinuria, and edema; eclampsia is the addition of seizures to the triad. Affects 7% of pregnant women from 20 weeks' gestation to 6 weeks postpartum. ↑ incidence in patients with preexisting hypertension, diabetes, chronic renal disease, and autoimmune disorders. Can be associated with HELLP syndrome (**H**emolysis, **E**levated LFTs, **L**ow **P**latelets).

Clinical features

Headache, blurred vision, abdominal pain, edema of face and extremities, altered mentation, hyperreflexia; lab findings may include thrombocytopenia, hyperuricemia.

Treatment

Delivery of fetus as soon as viable. Otherwise bed rest, salt restriction, and monitoring and treatment of hypertension. For eclampsia, a medical emergency, IV magnesium sulfate and diazepam.

UCV *Path3.67*

Pregnancy complications

1. Abruptio placentae—premature separation of placenta. **Painful** uterine bleeding (usually during 3rd trimester). Fetal death. May be associated with DIC.
2. Placenta accreta—defective decidual layer allows placenta to attach directly to myometrium. Predisposed by prior C-section or inflammation. May have massive hemorrhage after delivery.
3. Placenta previa—attachment of placenta to lower uterine segment. May occlude cervical os. **Painless** bleeding in any trimester.
4. Ectopic pregnancy—most often in fallopian tubes, predisposed by salpingitis (PID).

Placenta previa = when the placenta attaches to lower uterine segment.

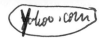

Uterine pathology

Endometriosis — *menstrual pain, bleeding* — Non-neoplastic endometrial glands/stroma in abnormal locations outside the uterus. Characterized by cyclic bleeding (menstrual type) from ectopic endometrial tissue resulting in blood-filled, "chocolate cysts." Ovary is most common site. Clinically manifest by severe menstrual-related pain. Often results in infertility.

Adenomyosis — Endometriosis within the myometrium.

Endometrial hyperplasia — *vaginal bleeding* — Abnormal endometrial gland proliferation usually caused by excess estrogen stimulation. ↑ risk for endometrial carcinoma. Most commonly manifest clinically by vaginal bleeding.

Endometrial carcinoma — *vaginal bleeding* — Most common gynecologic malignancy. Peak age 55–65 years old. Clinically presents with vaginal bleeding. Typically preceded by endometrial hyperplasia. Risk factors include prolonged estrogen use (compare with carcinomas of cervix), obesity, diabetes, and HTN.

Leiomyoma *most common* — *↑ preg, ↓ menopause* — Most common of all tumors in females. Often presents with multiple tumors. ↑ incidence in blacks. Malignant transformation is rare. Estrogen sensitive—tumor size ↑ with pregnancy and ↓ with menopause. Does not progress to leiomyosarcoma (leiomyomas are de novo).

Leiomyosarcoma — Bulky tumor with areas of necrosis and hemorrhage, typically arising de novo (not from leiomyoma). ↑ incidence in blacks. Highly aggressive tumor with tendency to recur. May protrude from cervix and bleed.

Polycystic ovarian syndrome (Stein-Leventhal syndrome)

↑LH due to peripheral estrogen production leads to anovulation. Manifest clinically by amenorrhea, infertility, obesity, and hirsutism. Treat with weight loss, OCPs, gonadotropin analogs, or surgery.

Ovarian cysts

1. Follicular cyst—distention of unruptured graafian follicle. May be associated with hyperestrinism and endometrial hyperplasia.
2. Corpus luteum cyst—hemorrhage into persistent corpus luteum. Menstrual irregularity.
3. Theca-lutein cyst—often bilateral/multiple. Due to gonadotropin stimulation. Associated with choriocarcinoma and moles.

Ovarian germ cell tumors

1. Dysgerminoma—analogous to male seminoma.
2. Yolk sac tumor—similar to testicular form; produces α-fetoprotein.
3. Choriocarcinoma—like testicular version. Increased hCG.
4. Teratoma—constitutes 90% of germ cell tumors of ovary. All 3 germ layers. Mature teratoma ("dermoid cyst") is benign. Struma ovarii—monodermal, composed only of thyroid tissue.

Ovarian non–germ cell tumors

1. Serous cystadenoma—20% of ovarian tumors. Frequently bilateral, lined with fallopian tube–like epithelium. Benign.
2. Serous cystadenocarcinoma—50% ovarian tumors, malignant.
3. Mucinous cystadenoma—multilocular cyst lined by mucus-secreting epithelium. Benign.
4. Mucinous cystadenocarcinoma—malignant. Pseudomyxoma peritonei—intraperitoneal accumulation of mucinous material.
5. Brenner tumor—benign tumor that resembles **B**ladder epithelium.
6. Ovarian fibroma—bundles of spindle-shaped fibroblasts. Meigs' syndrome—triad of ovarian fibroma, ascites, and hydrothorax.
7. Granulosa cell tumor—secretes estrogen → precocious puberty (kids). Can cause endometrial hyperplasia or carcinoma in adults. Call-Exner bodies—small follicles filled with eosinophilic secretions.

Breast disease

Type	Characteristics
Fibrocystic disease	Presents with diffuse breast pain and multiple lesions, often bilateral. Biopsy shows fibrocystic elements. Usually does not indicate ↑ risk of carcinoma. Histologic types: 1. Cystic—fluid filled. 2. Epithelial hyperplasia—↑ in number of epithelial cell layers in terminal duct lobule. ↑ **risk of carcinoma** with atypical cells. Occurs > 30 years. 3. Fibrosis—hyperplasia of breast stroma. 4. Sclerosing—increased acini and intralobular fibrosis.
Benign tumors	Cystosarcoma phyllodes—large, bulky mass of connective tissue and cysts. Breast surface has "leaflike" appearance. Fibroadenoma—most common tumor < 25 years. Small, mobile, firm mass with sharp edges. ↑ size and tenderness with pregnancy. Intraductal papilloma—tumor of lactiferous ducts; presents with nipple discharge.
Malignant tumors (carcinoma)	Common postmenopause. Arise from mammary duct epithelium or lobular glands. Histologic types: 1. Comedocarcinoma—cheesy consistency of tumor tissue due to central necrosis. 2. Infiltrating ductal—most common carcinoma. Firm, fibrous mass. 3. Inflammatory—lymphatic involvement; poor prognosis. 4. Paget's disease—eczematous patches on nipple. Paget cells—large cells with clear halo; suggest underlying ductal cancer. 5. Infiltrating lobular—often multiple/bilateral. Clusters of cells fill intralobular ductules. 6. Medullary—cellular with scant stroma and lymphocytic infiltrate.
Risk factors	Gender, age, early 1st menarche (< 12 years old), delayed 1st pregnancy (> 30 years old), late menopause (> 50 years old), family history of 1st-degree relative with breast cancer at a young age. Risk is NOT increased by fibroadenoma or nonhyperplastic cysts.

Handwritten annotation: You will get Pain + multiple lesions + often Bilateral.

PATHOLOGY—CARDIOVASCULAR

Hypertension

Risk factors	↑ age, obesity, diabetes, smoking, genetics, black > white > Asian.
Features	90% of HTN is primary (essential) and related to ↑ CO or ↑ TPR; remaining 10% mostly 2° to renal disease.
Predisposes to	Coronary heart disease, cerebrovascular accidents, CHF, renal failure, and aortic dissection.
Pathology	Hyaline thickening and atherosclerosis.

Atherosclerosis

	Disease of elastic arteries and large and medium-sized muscular arteries.
Risk factors	Smoking, hypertension, diabetes mellitus, hyperlipidemia, family history.
Progression	Fatty streaks → proliferative plaque → complex atheromas.
Complications	Aneurysms, ischemia, infarcts, peripheral vascular disease, thrombus, emboli.
Location	Abdominal aorta > coronary artery > popliteal artery > carotid artery.
Symptoms	Angina, claudication, but can be asymptomatic.

UCV *Path1.4*

Ischemic heart disease

Possible manifestations:

1. **Angina** (CAD narrowing > 75%):
   a. Stable—mostly 2° to atherosclerosis (retrosternal chest pain with exertion)
   b. Prinzmetal's variant—occurs at rest 2° to coronary artery spasm
   c. Unstable/crescendo—thrombosis in a branch (worsening chest pain)
2. **Myocardial infarction**—most often occurs in CAD involving the left anterior descending artery
3. **Sudden cardiac death**—death from cardiac causes within 1 hour of onset of symptoms, most commonly due to a lethal arrhythmia
4. **Chronic ischemic heart disease**—progressive onset of congestive heart failure over many years due to chronic ischemic myocardial damage

LAD

Infarcts: red vs. pale

Red (hemorrhagic) infarcts occur in loose tissues with collaterals, such as lungs, intestine, or following reperfusion.

Pale infarcts occur in solid tissues with single blood supply, such as brain, heart, kidney, and spleen.

REd = **RE**perfusion.

Evolution of MI

Coronary artery occlusion: LAD > RCA > circumflex.

Symptoms: severe retrosternal pain, pain in left arm and/or jaw, shortness of breath, fatigue, adrenergic symptoms.

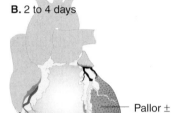

A. First day

Occluded artery

Infarct

Pallor

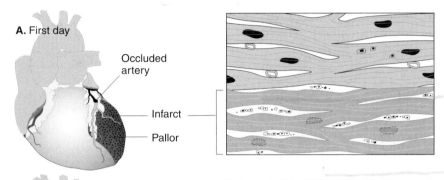

Coagulative necrosis leads to release of contents of necrotic cells into bloodstream with the beginning of neutrophil emigration

B. 2 to 4 days

Pallor ± hyperemia

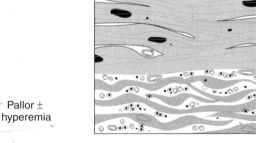

Tissue surrounding infarct shows acute inflammation

Dilated vessels (hyperemia)

Neutrophil emigration

Muscle shows extensive coagulative necrosis

C. 5 to 10 days

Hyperemic border; central yellow-brown softening— maximally yellow and soft by 10 days

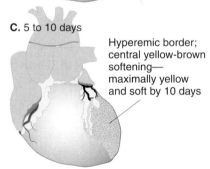

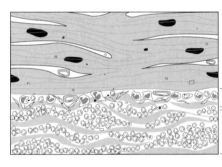

Outer zone (ingrowth of granulation tissue)

Macrophages

Neutrophils

D. 7 weeks

Recanalized artery

Gray-white

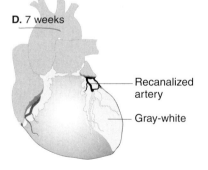

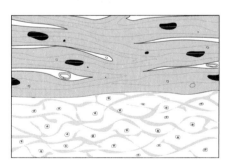

Contracted scar complete

UCV *Path1.7*   (Adapted, with permission, from Chandrasoma P. *Pathology Notes.* Norwalk, CT: Appleton & Lange, 1991:244.)

HIGH-YIELD FACTS

Pathology

Diagnosis of MI	In the first 6 hours, ECG is the gold standard.

Cardiac troponin I is used within the first 4 hours up to 7–10 days; more specific than other protein markers.

CK-MB is test of choice in the first 24 hours post-MI.

LDH$_1$ (former test of choice) is also elevated from 2 to 7 days post-MI.

AST is nonspecific and can be found in cardiac, liver, and skeletal muscle cells.

ECG changes can include ST elevation (transmural ischemia) and Q waves (transmural infarct).

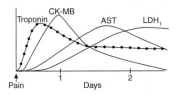

MI complications

1. Cardiac arrhythmia (90%); highest rise 2 days postinfarct
2. LV failure and pulmonary edema (60%)
3. Thromboembolism—mural thrombus
4. Cardiogenic shock (large infarct—high risk of mortality)
5. Rupture of ventricular free wall, interventricular septum, papillary muscle (4–10 days post-MI), cardiac tamponade
6. Fibrinous pericarditis—friction rub (3–5 days post-MI)
7. Dressler's syndrome—autoimmune phenomenon resulting in fibrinous pericarditis (several weeks post-MI)

Cardiomyopathies

Dilated (congestive) cardiomyopathy	Most common cardiomyopathy (90% of cases). Etiologies include chronic **A**lcohol abuse, **B**eriberi, postviral myocarditis by **C**oxsackievirus B, chronic **C**ocaine use, **D**oxorubicin toxicity, peripartum cardiomyopathy. Heart dilates and looks like a balloon on chest x-ray.	Systolic dysfunction ensues. **ABCD:** Alcohol Beriberi (wet) Coxsackievirus B, Cocaine, Chagas' disease Doxorubicin Diastolic dysfunction ensues.
Path1.13		
Hypertrophic cardiomyopathy (formerly IHSS)	Hypertrophy often asymmetric and involving the intraventricular septum. 50% of cases are familial and are inherited as an AD trait. Cause of sudden death in young athletes. Walls of LV are thickened and chamber becomes banana shaped on echocardiogram.	
Path1.16		
Restrictive/obliterative cardiomyopathy	Major causes include sarcoidosis, amyloidosis, scleroderma, hemochromatosis, endocardial fibroelastosis, and endomyocardial fibrosis (Löffler's).	

Heart murmurs

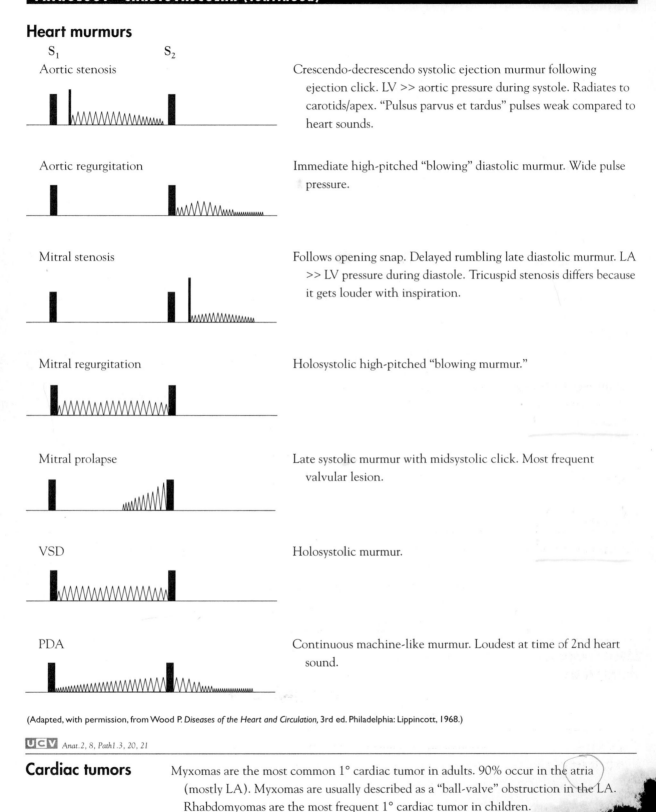

S_1 S_2

Aortic stenosis

Crescendo-decrescendo systolic ejection murmur following ejection click. LV >> aortic pressure during systole. Radiates to carotids/apex. "Pulsus parvus et tardus" pulses weak compared to heart sounds.

Aortic regurgitation

Immediate high-pitched "blowing" diastolic murmur. Wide pulse pressure.

Mitral stenosis

Follows opening snap. Delayed rumbling late diastolic murmur. LA >> LV pressure during diastole. Tricuspid stenosis differs because it gets louder with inspiration.

Mitral regurgitation

Holosystolic high-pitched "blowing murmur."

Mitral prolapse

Late systolic murmur with midsystolic click. Most frequent valvular lesion.

VSD

Holosystolic murmur.

PDA

Continuous machine-like murmur. Loudest at time of 2nd heart sound.

(Adapted, with permission, from Wood P. *Diseases of the Heart and Circulation*, 3rd ed. Philadelphia: Lippincott, 1968.)

UCV *Anat.2, 8, Path1.3, 20, 21*

Cardiac tumors

Myxomas are the most common 1° cardiac tumor in adults. 90% occur in the atria (mostly LA). Myxomas are usually described as a "ball-valve" obstruction in the LA. Rhabdomyomas are the most frequent 1° cardiac tumor in children.
Metastases most common heart tumor.

UCV *Path1.6*

Myxomas   Vis   Rhabdomyo.

Adults   280   children

CHF

Abnormality	Cause
Ankle, sacral edema	RV failure → ↑ venous pressure → fluid transudation.
Hepatomegaly (nutmeg liver)	↑ central venous pressure → ↑ resistance to portal flow. Rarely, leads to "cardiac cirrhosis."
Pulmonary congestion	LV failure → ↑ pulmonary venous pressure → pulmonary venous distention and transudation of fluid. Presence of hemosiderin-laden macrophages ("heart failure" cells).
Dyspnea on exertion	Failure of left ventricular output to ↑ during exercise.
Paroxysmal nocturnal dyspnea, pulmonary edema	Failure of left heart output to keep up with right heart output → acute rise in pulmonary venous and capillary pressure → transudation of fluid.
Orthopnea (shortness of breath when supine)	Pooling of blood in lungs in supine position adds volume to congested pulmonary vascular system; ↑ venous return not put out by left ventricle.
Cardiac dilation	Greater ventricular end-diastolic volume.

Flowchart:
Decreased myocardial contractility → Decreased cardiac output → ↓ Effective arterial blood volume → ↑ Sympathetic nervous outflow and ↑ Renin release → Angiotensin II → Maintains blood pressure → ↑ Aldosterone secretion → ↑ Tubular reabsorption of Na$^+$ and H$_2$O → ↓ Urinary excretion of Na$^+$ and H$_2$O → ↑ Total body Na$^+$ and H$_2$O → Edema. Also ↑ Venous pressure, Renal vasoconstriction → ↓ GFR.

UCV *Path1.10*

Embolus types

Fat, Air, Thrombus, Bacteria, Amniotic fluid, Tumor. Fat emboli are associated with long bone fractures and liposuction. Amniotic fluid emboli can lead to DIC, especially postpartum. Pulmonary embolus—chest pain, tachypnea, dyspnea.

An embolus moves like a **FAT BAT.** Approximately 95% of pulmonary emboli arise from deep leg veins.

Deep venous thrombosis

Predisposed by Virchow's triad:
1. Stasis
2. Hypercoagulability   factor 5 leiden mutation.
3. Endothelial damage

① Stasis
② Hypercoagulability
③ Endothelial damage

Cardiac tamponade

Compression of heart by fluid (i.e., blood) in pericardium, leading to ↓ CO.
Equilibration of pressures in all 4 chambers.
Pulsus paradoxus; ECG shows electrical alternans (beat-to-beat alterations of QRS complex height).

Bacterial endocarditis

New murmur, anemia, fever, Osler nodes (tender raised lesions on finger or toe pads), Roth's spots (round white spots on retina surrounded by hemorrhage), Janeway lesions (small erythematous lesions on palm or sole), splinter hemorrhages on nail bed. Multiple blood cultures necessary for diagnosis (continuous bacteremia).

1. Acute—*Staphylococcus aureus* (high virulence). Large vegetations on previously normal valves. Rapid onset.
2. Subacute—viridans streptococcus (low virulence). Smaller vegetations on congenitally abnormal or diseased valves. Sequela of dental procedures. More insidious onset.

Endocarditis may also be nonbacterial 2° to metastasis or renal failure (marantic/thrombotic endocarditis).

UCV *Micro1.5*   *Path3.5*

Mitral valve is most frequently involved. Tricuspid valve endocarditis is associated with IV drug abuse.

Complications: chordae rupture, glomerulonephritis, suppurative pericarditis, emboli.

JR = NO FAME:
Janeway lesions
Roth's spots
Nail-bed hemorrhage
Osler nodes
Fever
Anemia
Murmur
Emboli

Rheumatic fever/ rheumatic heart disease

Rheumatic fever is a consequence of pharyngeal infection with group A, β-hemolytic streptococci. Late sequelae include rheumatic heart disease, which affects heart valves— mitral > aortic >> tricuspid (high-pressure valves affected most). Associated with Aschoff bodies, migratory polyarthritis, erythema marginatum, elevated ASO titers.

Due to cross-reactivity, not direct effect of bacteria.

UCV *Micro1.52*

FEVERSS:
Fever
Erythema marginatum
Valvular damage
ESR ↑
Red-hot joints (polyarthritis)
Subcutaneous nodules
St. Vitus' dance (chorea)

Pericarditis

Serous
Fibrinous
Hemorrhagic

Caused by SLE, RA, infection, uremia.
Uremia, MI, rheumatic fever.
TB, malignancy (e.g., melanoma).

Findings: pericardial pain, friction rub, ECG changes (diffuse ST elevations in all leads), pulsus paradoxus, distant heart sounds.

Can resolve without scarring or lead to chronic adhesive or chronic constrictive pericarditis.

UCV *Micro1.3, Path1.11*

Syphilitic heart disease

3° syphilis disrupts the vasa vasorum of the aorta with consequent dilation of the aorta and valve ring. Often affects the aortic root and ascending aorta. Associated with a tree-bark appearance of the aorta.

UCV *Path2.45*

Can result in aneurysm of the ascending aorta or aortic arch and aortic valve incompetence. *Aortic Regurgitation*

Vasa Vasorum

Buerger's disease

Known as smoker's disease and thromboangiitis obliterans; idiopathic, segmental, thrombosing vasculitis of intermediate and small peripheral arteries and veins.

Findings
Intermittent claudication, superficial nodular phlebitis, cold sensitivity (Raynaud's phenomenon), severe pain in affected part; may lead to gangrene.

Treatment
Quit smoking.

UCV *Path1.26*

Takayasu's arteritis

Known as "pulseless disease"—thickening of aortic arch and/or proximal great vessels. Associated with an elevated ESR. Primarily affects young Asian females. **F**ever, **A**rthritis, **N**ight sweats, **MY**algia, **SKIN** nodules, **O**cular disturbances, **W**eak pulses in upper extremities.

Affects medium and large arteries.

FAN MY SKIN On Wednesday.

Temporal arteritis (giant cell arteritis)

Most common vasculitis that affects medium and small arteries, usually branches of carotid artery. Findings include unilateral headache, jaw claudication, impaired vision (occlusion of ophthalmic artery, which can lead to blindness). Half of patients have systemic involvement and syndrome of polymyalgia rheumatica (proximal muscle pain, periarticular pain). Associated with elevated ESR. Responds well to steroids.

TEMporal = signs near **TEM**ples. ESR is markedly elevated. Affects elderly females.

UCV *Path3.34*

Polyarteritis nodosa

Characterized by necrotizing immune complex inflammation of small or medium-sized muscular arteries, typically involving renal and visceral vessels.

Symptoms
Fever, weight loss, malaise, abdominal pain, headache, myalgia, hypertension.

Findings
Cotton-wool spots, microaneurysms, pericarditis, myocarditis, palpable purpura. Increased ESR. Associated with hepatitis B infection in 30% of patients. **P-AN**CA (perinuclear pattern of antineutrophil cytoplasmic antibodies) is often present in the serum and correlates with disease activity, primarily in small vessel disease.

Treatment
Corticosteroids, azathioprine, and/or cyclophosphamide.

PAN = P-ANCA.
Lesions are of different ages.
Churg-Strauss—variant associated with eosinophilia and asthma.

UCV *Path3.86*

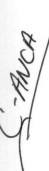

C-ANCA

Wegener's granulomatosis

Characterized by focal necrotizing vasculitis and necrotizing granulomas in the lung and upper airway and by necrotizing glomerulonephritis.

Symptoms
Perforation of nasal septum, chronic sinusitis, otitis media, mastoiditis, cough, dyspnea, hemoptysis.

Findings
C-ANCA is a strong marker of disease; CXR may reveal large nodular densities; hematuria and red cell casts.

Treatment
Cyclophosphamide, corticosteroids, and/or methotrexate.

UCV *Path3.96*

Kawasaki disease

Acute, self-limiting disease of infants/kids. Acute necrotizing vasculitis of small/medium-sized vessels. Fever, congested conjunctiva, changes in lips/oral mucosa, lymphadenitis. May develop coronary aneurysms.

Glomerular pathology

NephrItic syndrome—<u>hematuria</u>, <u>hypertension</u>, <u>oliguria</u>, <u>azotemia</u>.

1. **Acute poststreptococcal glomerulonephritis**—LM: glomeruli enlarged and hypercellular, neutrophils, "lumpy-bumpy." EM: subepithelial humps. IF: granular pattern.

2. **Rapidly progressive (crescentic) glomerulonephritis**—LM and IF: crescent-moon shape.

3. **Goodpasture's syndrome (type II hypersensitivity)**—IF: linear pattern, anti-GBM antibodies.

4. **Membranoproliferative glomerulonephritis**—EM: subendothelial humps, "tram track."

5. **IgA nephropathy (Berger's disease)**—IF and EM: mesangial deposits of IgA.

NephrOtic syndrome—massive proteinuria, hypoalbuminemia, generalized edema, hyperlipidemia.

1. **Membranous glomerulonephritis**—LM: diffuse capillary and basement membrane thickening. IF: granular pattern. EM: "spike and dome."

2. **Minimal change disease (lipoid nephrosis)**—LM: normal glomeruli. EM: foot process effacement.

3. **Focal segmental glomerular sclerosis**—LM: segmental sclerosis and hyalinosis.

4. **Diabetic nephropathy**—LM: Kimmelstiel-Wilson lesions, BM thickening.

5. **SLE** (5 patterns of renal involvement)—LM: wire-loop appearance with extensive granular subendothelial BM deposits in membranous glomerulonephritis pattern.

(LM = light microscopy; EM = electron microscopy; IF = immunofluorescence)

I = inflammation.

Most frequently seen in children. Peripheral, periorbital edema. Resolves spontaneously.

Rapid course to renal failure from one of many causes.

Hemoptysis, hematuria.

Slowly progresses to renal failure.

Mild disease. Often postinfectious.

O = prOteinuria.

A common cause of adult nephrotic syndrome.

Most common cause of childhood nephrotic syndrome. Responds well to steroids.

More severe disease in HIV patients.

[Handwritten margin notes:]
Lumpy Bumpy.
cresent moon shaped.
linear pattern (Anti GBM)
Tram Track
IgA mesangial deposits.

SPIKE + DOME
FOOT Process Effacement
SLE → wire loop

Nodular glomerulosclerosis

EP = epithelium with foot processes
US = urinary space
GBM = glomerular basement membrane
EN = fenestrated endothelium
MC = mesangial cells
EM = extracellular matrix

1 = subepithelium deposits (membranous nephropathy)
2 = large irregular subepithelium deposits or "humps" (acute glomerulonephritis)
3 = subendothelial deposits in lupus glomerulonephritis
4 = mesangial deposits (IgA nephropathy)
5 = antibody binding to GBM—smooth linear pattern on immunofluorescence (Goodpasture's)
6 = effacement of epithelial foot processes (common in all forms of glomerular injury with proteinuria)

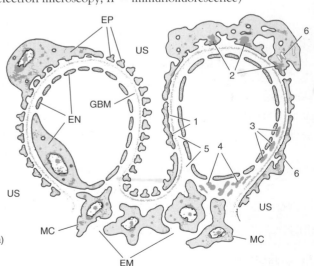

(Adapted, with permission, from Luke RG et al. "Nephrology and hypertension." In *Medical Knowledge Self-Assessment Program IX.* Philadelphia: American College of Physicians, 1992.)

Kidney stones

Can lead to severe complications such as hydronephrosis and pyelonephritis. 4 major types:

1. Calcium—constitute the majority of kidney stones (80–85%). Calcium oxalate or calcium phosphate or both. Stones are radiopaque. Disorders or conditions that cause hypercalcemia (e.g., cancer, increased PTH, increased vitamin D, milk-alkali syndrome) can all lead to hypercalciuria and stones. Tend to recur.
2. Ammonium magnesium phosphate (struvite)—2nd most common kidney stone. Radiopaque and urease-positive bugs such as *Proteus vulgaris* or *Staphylococcus*. Can form large struvite calculi that can be a nidus for UTIs.
3. Uric acid—strong association with hyperuricemia (e.g., gout). Often seen as a result of diseases with increased cell proliferation and turnover, such as leukemia and myeloproliferative disorders. Radiolucent.
4. Cystine—most often 2° to cystinuria. Radiolucent.

Renal cell carcinoma

Most common renal malignancy. Most common in men ages 50–70. ↑ incidence in smokers. Associated with von Hippel–Lindau and gene deletion in chromosome 3. Originates in renal tubule cells → polygonal clear cells. Manifests clinically with hematuria, palpable mass, 2° polycythemia, flank pain, and fever. Invades IVC and spreads hematogenously. Associated with paraneoplastic syndromes (ectopic EPO, ACTH, PTHrP, and prolactin).

Wilms' tumor

Most common renal malignancy of early childhood (ages 2–4). Presents with huge, palpable flank mass, hemihypertrophy. Deletion of tumor suppression gene WT-1 on chromosome 11. Can be part of **WAGR** complex: **W**ilms' tumor, **A**niridia, **G**enitourinary malformation, and mental-motor **R**etardation.

Transitional cell carcinoma

Most common tumor of urinary tract system (can occur in renal calyces, renal pelvis, ureters, and bladder). Often recurs after removal. Presents with hematuria and may spread to adjacent tissue. Associated with problems in your **Pee SAC**: **P**henacetin, **S**moking, **A**niline dyes, and **C**yclophosphamide.

Acid-base physiology

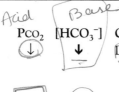

	pH	P_{CO_2}	$[HCO_3^-]$	Cause	Compensatory response
Metabolic acidosis	↓	↓	↓	Diabetic ketoacidosis, diarrhea, lactic acidosis, salicylate OD, acetazolamide OD	Hyperventilation
Respiratory acidosis	↓	↑	↑	COPD, airway obstruction	Renal $[HCO_3^-]$ reabsorption
Respiratory alkalosis	↑	↓	↓	High altitude, hyperventilation	Renal $[HCO_3^-]$ secretion
Metabolic alkalosis	↑	↑	↑	Vomiting	Hypoventilation

Henderson-Hasselbalch equation: $pH = pKa + \log \dfrac{[HCO_3^-]}{0.03\, P_{CO_2}}$

Key: ↑ ↓ = primary disturbance; ↓ ↑ = compensatory response.

Acidosis/alkalosis

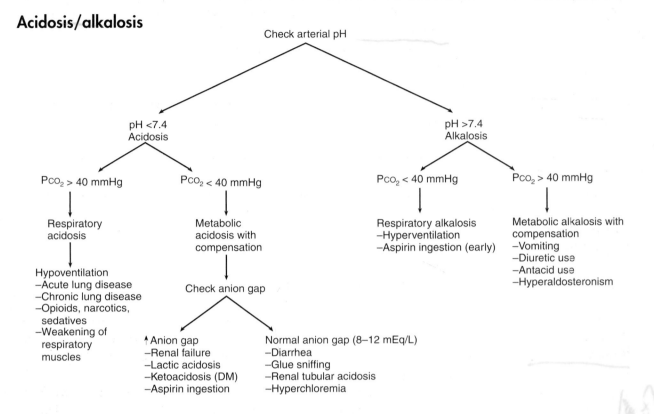

Check arterial pH

pH <7.4
Acidosis

pH >7.4
Alkalosis

P_{CO_2} > 40 mmHg

P_{CO_2} < 40 mmHg

P_{CO_2} < 40 mmHg

P_{CO_2} > 40 mmHg

Respiratory
acidosis

Metabolic
acidosis with
compensation

Respiratory alkalosis
–Hyperventilation
–Aspirin ingestion (early)

Metabolic alkalosis with
compensation
–Vomiting
–Diuretic use
–Antacid use
–Hyperaldosteronism

Hypoventilation
–Acute lung disease
–Chronic lung disease
–Opioids, narcotics,
 sedatives
–Weakening of
 respiratory
 muscles

Check anion gap

↑Anion gap
–Renal failure
–Lactic acidosis
–Ketoacidosis (DM)
–Aspirin ingestion

Normal anion gap (8–12 mEq/L)
–Diarrhea
–Glue sniffing
–Renal tubular acidosis
–Hyperchloremia

UCV *Bio.8, 22, 23, 83*

Anion gap acidosis	Gap is $Na^+ - (Cl^- + HCO_3^-) = 8\text{–}12$ mEq/L.
	  If elevated, may be due to:
	    Methanol
	    Uremia (chronic renal failure)
	    Diabetic ketoacidosis
	    Paraldehyde or **P**henformin
	    Iron tablets or **I**NH
	    Lactic acidosis (CN^-, CO, shock)
	    Ethanol or **E**thylene glycol
	    Salicylates
		MUD PILES.

Acid-base compensations	The following formulas give appropriate compensations for a single disorder. If the formula does not match the actual values, suspect a mixed disorder.
Metabolic acidosis	Winter's formula: $P_{CO_2} = 1.5 \, (HCO_3^-) + 8 \pm 2$.
Metabolic alkalosis	P_{CO_2} ↑ 0.7 mmHg for every ↑ 1 mEq/L HCO_3^-.
Respiratory acidosis	Acute— ↑ 1 mEq/L HCO_3^- for every ↑ 10 mmHg P_{CO_2}. Chronic— ↑ 3.5 mEq/L HCO_3^- for every ↑ 10 mmHg P_{CO_2}.
Respiratory alkalosis	Acute— ↓ 2 mEq/L HCO_3^- for every ↓ 10 mmHg P_{CO_2}. Chronic— ↓ 5 mEq/L HCO_3^- for every ↓ 10 mmHg P_{CO_2}.

HIGH-YIELD FACTS

Pathology

Pyelonephritis

Acute
Affects cortex with relative sparing of glomeruli/vessels. White cell casts in urine are pathognomonic.

Chronic
Coarse, asymmetric corticomedullary scarring. Tubules can contain eosinophilic casts (thyroidization of kidney).

Diffuse cortical necrosis

Acute generalized infarction of cortices of both kidneys. Likely due to a combination of vasospasm and DIC. Associated with obstetric catastrophes (e.g., abruptio placentae) and septic shock.

Acute tubular necrosis

Most common cause of ARF. Reversible, but fatal if left untreated. Associated with renal ischemia (e.g., shock), crush injury (myoglobulinuria), toxins. Death most often occurs during initial oliguric phase. Recovery in 2–3 weeks.

Renal papillary necrosis

Associated with:
1. Diabetes mellitus
2. Acute pyelonephritis
3. Chronic phenacetin use

Acute renal failure

Abrupt decline in renal function with ↑ creatinine and ↑ BUN over a period of several days.
1. Prerenal azotemia—decreased RBF (e.g., hypotension) → ↓ GFR. Na+/H_2O retained by kidney.
2. Intrinsic renal—generally due to ATN or ischemia/toxins. Patchy necrosis leads to debris obstructing tubule and fluid backflow across necrotic tubule → ↓ GFR. Urine has epithelial/granular casts.
3. Postrenal—outflow obstruction (stones, BPH, neoplasia). Develops only with bilateral obstruction.

Variable	Prerenal	Renal	Postrenal
Urine osmolality	> 500	< 350	< 350
Urine Na	< 10	> 20	> 40
Fe_{Na}	< 1%	> 2%	> 4%
BUN/Cr ratio	> 20	< 15	> 15

Renal failure

Failure to make urine and excrete nitrogenous wastes.
Consequences:

1. Anemia (failure of erythropoietin production)
2. Renal osteodystrophy (failure of active vitamin D production)
3. Hyperkalemia, which can lead to cardiac arrhythmias
4. Metabolic acidosis due to ↓ acid secretion and ↓ generation of HCO_3^-
5. Uremia (↑ BUN, creatinine)
6. Sodium and H_2O excess → CHF and pulmonary edema
7. Chronic pyelonephritis
8. Hypertension

2 forms of renal failure—acute renal failure (often due to hypoxia) and chronic renal failure (e.g., due to HTN and diabetes).

Electrolytes

Electrolyte	Functions	Causes and Signs of Deficiency	Causes and Signs of Toxicity
Ca^{2+} Bio.12, 15	Muscle contraction Neurotransmitter release Bones, teeth	Kids—rickets Adults—osteomalacia Contributes to osteoporosis Tetany	Delirium
PO_4^{3-}	ATP Nucleic acids Phosphorylation Bones, teeth	Kids—rickets Adults—osteomalacia	Low serum Ca^{2+} Can cause bone loss Renal stones
Na^+ Bio.18	Extracellular fluid Maintains plasma volume Nerve/muscle function	2° to injury or illness	Delirium
K^+ Bio.16	Intracellular fluid Nerve/muscle function	2° to injury, illness, or diuretics Causes weakness, paralysis, confusion	ECG changes Arrhythmia
Cl^-	Fluid/electrolyte balance Gastric acid HCO_3^-/Cl^- shift in RBC	2° to emesis, diuretics, renal disease	None that are clinically significant
Mg^{2+} Bio.17	Bones, teeth Enzyme cofactor	2° to malabsorption Diarrhea, alcoholism	↓ reflexes ↓ respiration

UCV

Alcoholism

Physiologic tolerance and dependence with symptoms of withdrawal (tremor, tachycardia, hypertension, malaise, nausea, delirium tremens) when intake is interrupted.

Continued drinking despite medical and social contraindications and life disruptions.

Treatment: disulfiram to condition the patient negatively against alcohol use. Supportive treatment of other systemic manifestations. Alcoholics Anonymous and other peer support groups are most successful in sustaining abstinence.

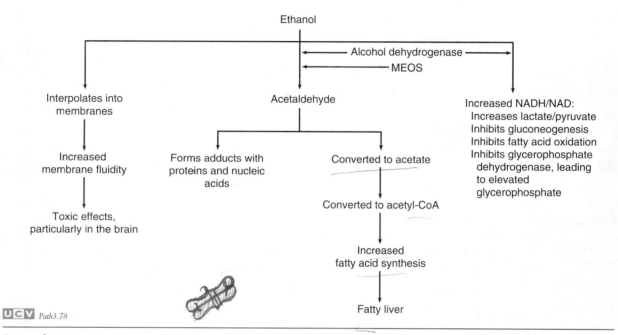

UCV Path3.78

Complications of alcoholism

Alcoholic hepatitis and cirrhosis, pancreatitis, dilated cardiomyopathy, peripheral neuropathy, cerebellar degeneration, Wernicke-Korsakoff syndrome, testicular atrophy and hyperestrinism, and Mallory-Weiss syndrome.

Alcoholic cirrhosis

Long-term alcohol use leads to micronodular cirrhosis with accompanying symptoms of jaundice, hypoalbuminemia, coagulation factor deficiencies, and portal hypertension, leading to peripheral edema and ascites, encephalopathy, and neurologic manifestations (e.g., asterixis, flapping tremor of the hands). Path1.92

Wernicke-Korsakoff syndrome

Caused by vitamin B_1 (thiamine) deficiency in alcoholics. Classically may present with triad of psychosis, ophthalmoplegia, and ataxia (Wernicke's encephalopathy). May progress to memory loss, confabulation, confusion (Korsakoff's syndrome; irreversible). Associated with periventricular hemorrhage/necrosis, especially in mammillary bodies. Treatment: IV vitamin B_1 (thiamine). Bio.86

Mallory-Weiss syndrome

Longitudinal lacerations at the gastroesophageal junction caused by excessive vomiting with failure of LES relaxation that could lead to fatal hematemesis.

UCV

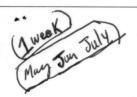

HIGH-YIELD FACTS

Pathology

HIGH-YIELD FACTS

Pathology

Argyll Robertson pupil	Argyll Robertson pupil constricts with accommodation but is not reactive to light. Pathognomonic for 3° syphilis.	Argyll Robertson Pupil— **ARP: A**ccommodation **R**esponse **P**resent.
Amyloidosis	1° (light chain deposition) seen with multiple myeloma (most common cause) or Waldenström's macroglobulinemia; 2° (amyloid associated) can cause nephrotic syndrome in kidney. Apple-green birefringence on Congo red stain.	Alzheimer's disease associated with β-amyloid deposition in the cerebral cortex; islet cell amyloid deposition characteristic of diabetes mellitus type 2.
UCV *Path2.51*		
Aschoff body	Aschoff bodies (granuloma with giant cells) and Anitschkow's cells (activated histiocytes) are found in rheumatic heart disease.	Think of two **RH**ussians with **RH**eumatic heart disease (Aschoff and Anitschkow).
Auer bodies (rods)	Auer rods are peroxidase-positive cytoplasmic inclusions in granulocytes and myeloblasts. Primarily seen in acute promyelocytic leukemia (M3).	
Casts	Casts in urine: RBC casts—glomerular inflammation, ischemia, or malignant hypertension. WBC casts—inflammation in renal interstitium, tubules, and glomeruli. Hyaline casts often seen in normal urine. Waxy casts seen in chronic renal failure.	Presence of casts indicates that hematuria/pyuria is of renal origin. RBC cells—bladder cancer. WBC cells—acute cystitis.

Red blood cell casts   White blood cell casts   Hyaline casts   Granular casts

Erythrocyte sedimentation rate	Nonspecific test that measures acute-phase reactants. Dramatically ↑ with infection, malignancy, connective tissue disease. Also ↑ with pregnancy, inflammatory disease, anemia, and polycythemia. ↓ with sickle cell anemia and congestive heart failure.	Simple and cheap but nonspecific. Should not be used for asymptomatic screening; can be used to diagnose and monitor temporal arteritis and polymyalgia rheumatica.
Ghon complex	TB granulomas with lobar or perihilar lymph node involvement (Ghon focus and lymph node involvement). Reflects 1° infection or exposure.	

Hyperlipidemia signs

Atheromata	Plaques in blood vessel walls.
Xanthoma	Plaques or nodules composed of lipid-laden histiocytes in the skin, especially the eyelids.
Tendinous xanthoma	Lipid deposit in tendon, especially Achilles.
Corneal arcus	Lipid deposit in cornea, nonspecific (arcus senilis).

Psammoma bodies

Laminated, concentric, calcific spherules seen in:

1. Papillary adenocarcinoma of thyroid ←
2. Serous papillary cystadenocarcinoma of ovary
3. Meningioma ←
4. Malignant mesothelioma

PSaMMoma:
Papillary (thyroid)
Serous (ovary)
Meningioma
Mesothelioma

RBC forms

Biconcave	Normal.
Spherocytes	Hereditary spherocytosis, autoimmune hemolysis.
Elliptocyte	Hereditary elliptocytosis.
Macro-ovalocyte	Megaloblastic anemia, marrow failure.
Helmet cell, schistocyte	DIC, traumatic hemolysis.
Sickle cell	Sickle cell anemia.
Teardrop cell	Myeloid metaplasia with myelofibrosis.
Acanthocyte	Spiny appearance in abetalipoproteinemia.
Target cell	Thalassemia, liver disease, HbC.
Poikilocytes	Nonuniform shapes in TTP/HUS, microvascular damage, DIC.
Burr cell	TTP/HUS.

HLA-B27

Associated with **P**soriasis, **A**nkylosing spondylitis, **I**nflammatory bowel disease, **R**eiter's syndrome. 90-fold greater chance of developing ankylosing spondylitis with HLA-B27.

PAIR.

Reed-Sternberg cells

Distinctive tumor giant cell seen in Hodgkin's disease; large cell that is binucleate or bilobed with the 2 halves as mirror images ("owl's eyes"). Necessary but not sufficient for a diagnosis of Hodgkin's disease.

There are 4 types of Hodgkin's disease; nodular sclerosis variant is the only one seen in women > men (excellent prognosis).

Virchow's (sentinel) node

A firm supraclavicular lymph node, often on left side, easily palpable (can be detected by medical students), also known as "jugular gland." Presumptive evidence of malignant visceral neoplasm (classically stomach).

Islet cell amyloid deposition – characteristic of diabetes mellitus type 2.

β-amyloid deposition found in Alzheimer's disease.

Peripheral blood smears

Normal

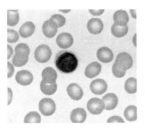

Microcytic hypochromic anemia

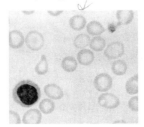

—normally 2° to **iron deficiency**

—low serum ferritin

—elevated serum iron-binding capacity

—lead poisoning

Megaloblastic anemia

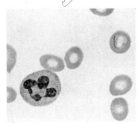

—2° to **folate or B$_{12}$ deficiency**

—hypersegmented (5–7 lobes) PMNs

—large red blood cells (MCV > 100)

—**never** give folate to a patient who is deficient in B$_{12}$

—**pernicious anemia**—autoimmune disease that causes B$_{12}$ deficiency by depleting **intrinsic factor,** which is needed to absorb B$_{12}$ in **terminal ileum**

—anisocytosis, poikilocytosis

Target cells

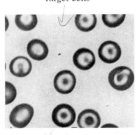

—**HALT:**

    —**H**emoglobin C disease

    —**A**splenia

    —**L**iver disease

    —**T**halassemia

Hemoglobin SS with sickle cells

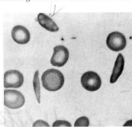

—**HbS**—β-globin GLU → VAL at #6; 8% of U.S. blacks are HbS carriers

—cells will sickle 2° to hypoxia, dehydration, and ↑ blood viscosity

—anemia

—vaso-occlusive crises +/– chest pain

—aplastic crises (B19 virus)

—splenic sequestration crises

—CVA

(Adapted, with permission, from Stobo J et al. *The Principles and Practice of Medicine,* 23rd ed. Stamford, CT: Appleton & Lange, 1996:704.)

Enzyme markers	**Serum enzyme**	**Major diagnostic use**
	Aminotransferases (AST and ALT)	Myocardial infarction (AST only)
		Viral hepatitis (ALT > AST)
		Alcoholic hepatitis (AST > ALT)
	Amylase ✓	Acute pancreatitis, mumps
	Ceruloplasmin (↓)	Wilson's disease
	CPK (creatine phosphokinase)	Muscle disorders (e.g., DMD) and myocardial infarction (CPK-MB)
	GGT (γ-glutamyl transpeptidase)	Various liver diseases
	LDH-1 (lactate dehydrogenase fraction 1)	Myocardial infarction (LDH-1 > LDH-2)
	Lipase	Acute pancreatitis
	Alkaline phosphatase	Bone disease (Paget's disease of bone), obstructive liver disease (hepatocellular carcinoma)

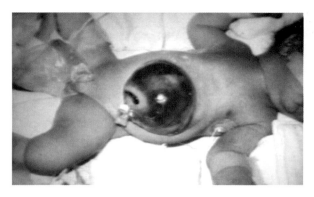

Omphalocele in a newborn. Note that the defect is midline and is covered by peritoneum, as opposed to gastroschisis, which is not covered by peritoneum and is often not midline.*

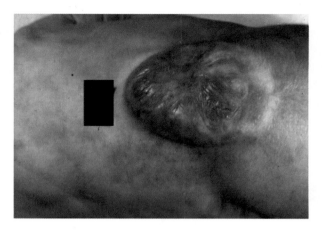

Meningomyelocele. A neural tube defect in which the meninges and spinal cord herniate through the spinal canal; gross image of infant's lower back.*

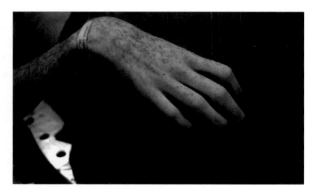

Marfan's syndrome. Patients are tall with very long extremities. The joints are hyperextensible, with slim bone structure and wiry muscles.*

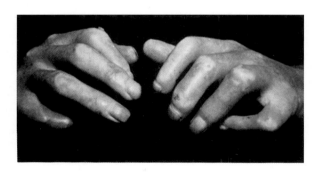

Scleroderma. The progressive "tightening" of the skin has contracted the fingers and eliminated creases over the knuckles. Fibrosis is widespread and may also involve the esophagus (dysphagia), lung (restrictive disease), and small vessels of the kidney (hypertension).

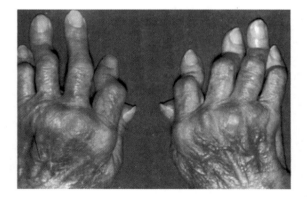

Rheumatoid arthritis. Note the swan-neck deformities of the digits and severe, symmetric involvement of the proximal interphalangeal (PIP) joints.

*(Reproduced courtesy of the Pathology Education Instructional Resource Digital Library at the University of Alabama, Birmingham.)

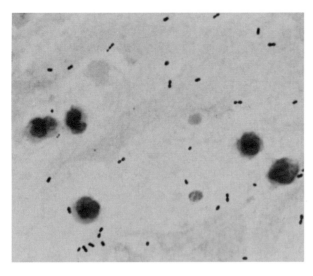

Streptococcus pneumoniae. Sputum sample from a patient with pneumonia shows gram-positive diplococci.

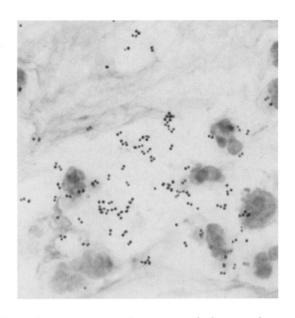

Staphylococcus aureus. Sputum sample from another patient with pneumonia shows gram-positive cocci in clusters.

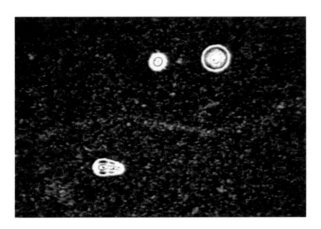

Cryptococcus neoformans. The polysaccharide capsule is visible by India ink preparation in CSF from an AIDS patient with meningoencephalitis.*

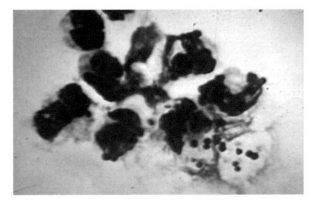

Gram-negative diplococci of ***Neisseria meningitidis*** within neutrophils from CSF.*

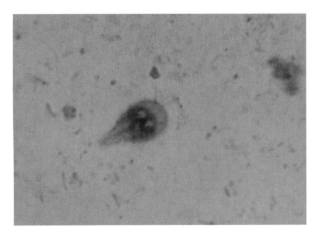

Giardia lamblia, small intestine, microscopic. The trophozoite has a classic pear shape, with double nuclei giving an owl's-eye appearance.

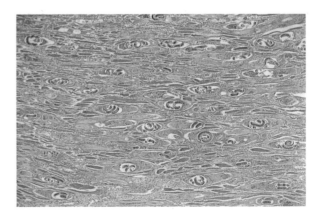

Taenia solium, the pig tapeworm, infesting porcine myocardium. When humans ingest this meat, the larvae attach to the wall of the small intestine and mature to adult worms.

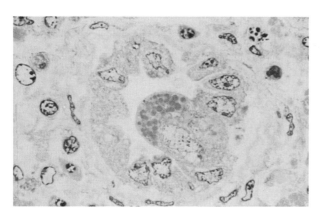

Cytomegalovirus (CMV) giant cell with multiple hyaline inclusions in a renal tubule. Of special concern in HIV patients (CMV retinitis) and organ transplant patients (as here, in a transplanted kidney); however, CMV can infect almost anything. Treatment is ganciclovir or foscarnet.

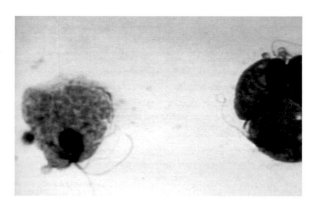

Trichomonas vaginalis demonstrating trophozoites with flagellae.*

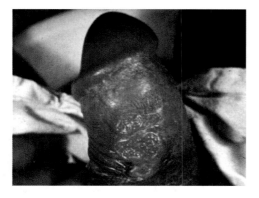

Chancre associated with primary syphilis. These ulcerative lesions are painless.*

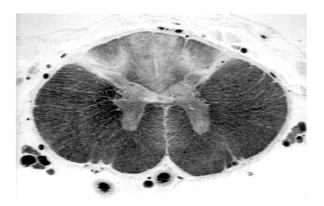

Tabes dorsalis resulting from progressive syphilis infection, thoracic spinal cord. Note degeneration of dorsal columns and dorsal roots.*

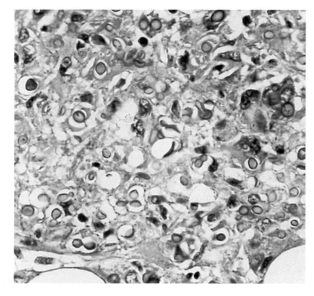

Infectious granuloma in bone marrow, with intracytoplasmic inclusions. Cultures grew *Cryptococcus neoformans*.*

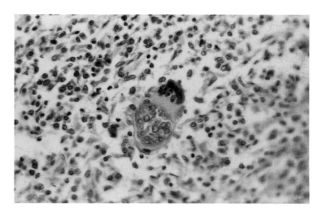

Coccidioidomycosis. Endospores within a spherule in infected lung parenchyma. Initial infection usually resolves spontaneously, but when immunity is compromised, dissemination to almost any organ can occur. Endemic in the southwestern United States.

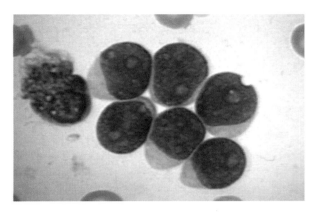

Acute lymphocytic leukemia, peripheral blood smear.*

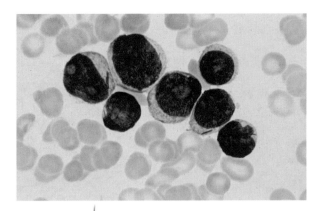

Acute myelocytic leukemia with Auer rods, peripheral blood smear.*

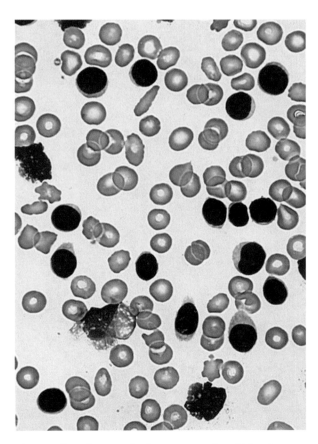

Chronic lymphocytic leukemia, peripheral blood smear. In CLL, the lymphocytes are excessively fragile. These lymphocytes are easily destroyed during slide preparation, forming "smudge cells."*

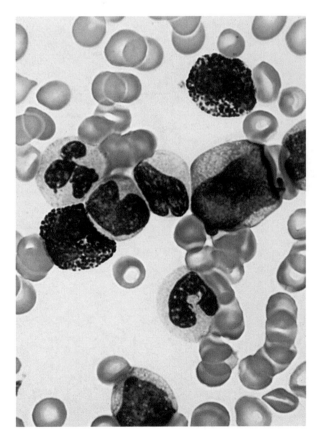

Chronic myeloid leukemia, peripheral blood smear. Promyelocytes and myelocytes are seen adjacent to a vascular structure.*

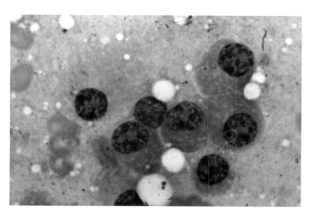

Smears from a patient with **multiple myeloma** displaying an abundance of plasma cells. RBCs will often be seen in rouleaux formation, stacked like poker chips. Multiple myeloma is associated with hypercalcemia, lytic bone lesions, and renal insufficiency due to Bence Jones (light-chain) proteinuria.*

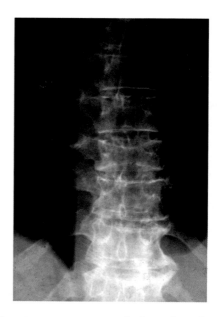

X-ray showing numerous punched-out lytic lesions (lucent areas within the radiograph) typical of **multiple myeloma.** Note the generalized osteopenia and multiple compression fractures.*

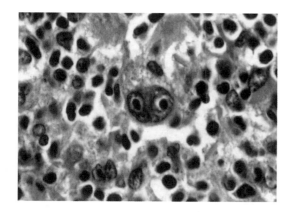

Hodgkin's disease (Reed-Sternberg cells). Binucleate RS cells displaying prominent inclusion-like nucleoli surrounded by lymphocytes and other reacting inflammatory cells. The RS cell is a necessary but insufficient pathologic finding for the diagnosis of Hodgkin's disease.

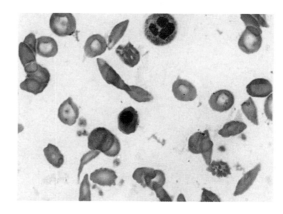

Sickle cell anemia. Note the sickled cells as well as anisocytosis, poikilocytosis, and nucleated RBCs.

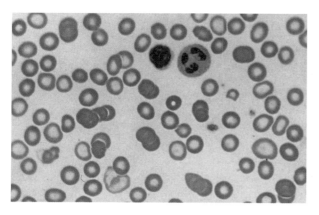

Iron deficiency anemia. Microcytosis and hypochromia.

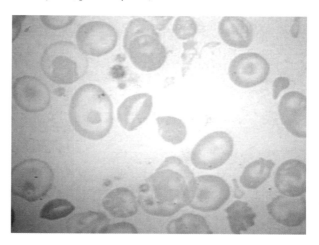

Thalassemia major. A blood dyscrasia caused by a defect in β-chain synthesis in hemoglobin. Note the presence of target cells.*

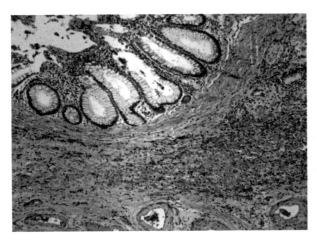

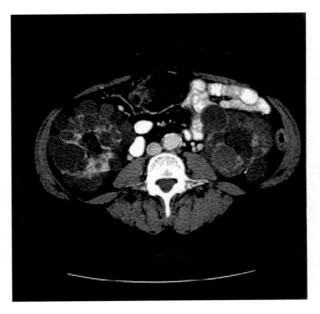

Diverticulitis. Inflammation of diverticula typically causes LLQ pain and can progress to perforation, peritonitis, abscess formation, or bowel stenosis. Note the presence of macrophages. Gut lumen at the top of the photo.*

Polycystic kidney disease. Abdominal CT shows multiple cysts in both kidneys. PKD is an autosomal-dominant disease and is often associated with aneurysm formation in the brain.*

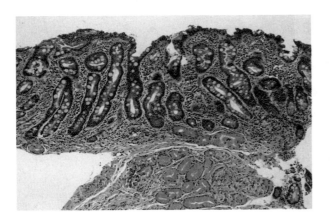

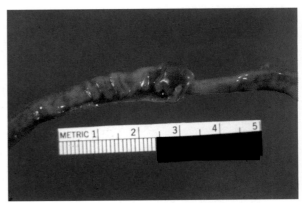

Celiac sprue (gluten-sensitive enteropathy). Histology shows blunting of villi and crypt hyperplasia.

Intussusception of infant gut, gross.*

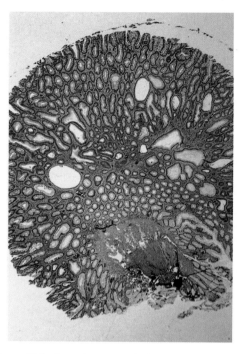

A

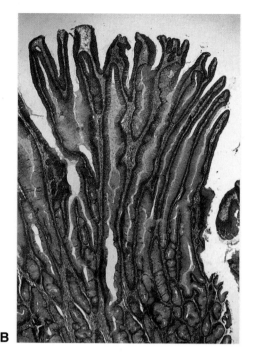

B

Colonic polyps. Tubular adenomas **(A)** are smaller and rounded in morphology and have less malignant potential than do **villous adenomas (B),** which are composed of long, fingerlike projections.

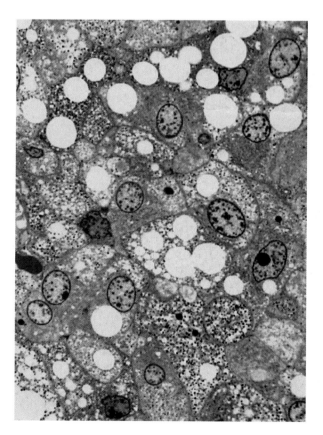

Pheochromocytoma. The tumor cells have numerous vacuolar spaces within the cytoplasm (pseudoacini). Most of the punctate blue-black granules of variable density are dense-core neurosecretory granules.*

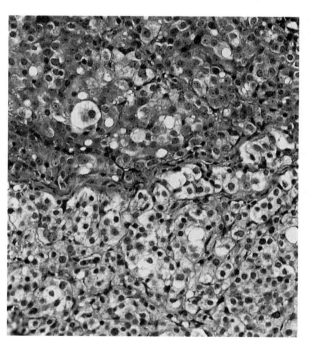

Metastatic prostatic adenocarcinoma in a supraclavicular lymph node. Despite the relatively solid growth, the nuclei do not show great variation in size. Note the typical prominent nucleoli. Some cells have eosinophilic cytoplasm, whereas others have pale cytoplasm.*

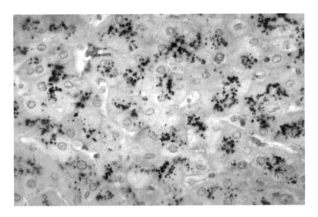

Hemochromatosis with cirrhosis. Prussian blue iron stain shows hemosiderin in the liver parenchyma. Such deposition occurs throughout the body, causing organ damage and the characteristic darkening of the skin.*

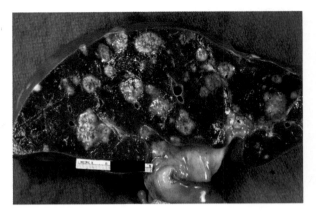

Metastatic carcinoma to the liver. The most common primary sites are the colon, breast, and lung.*

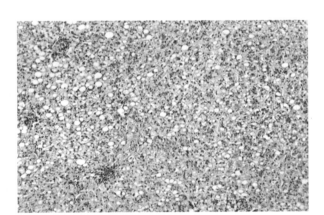

Fatty metamorphosis (macrovesicular steatosis) of the liver, microscopic. Early reversible change associated with alcohol consumption; there are abundant fat-filled vacuoles but no inflammation due to fibrosis of more serious alcoholic liver damage (yet).*

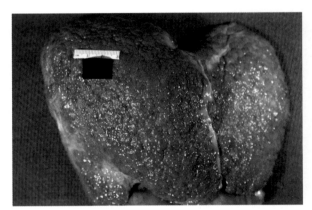

Micronodular cirrhosis of the liver, gross, from an alcoholic patient. The liver is approximately normal in size with a fine, granular appearance. Later stages of disease result in an irregularly shrunken liver with larger nodules.*

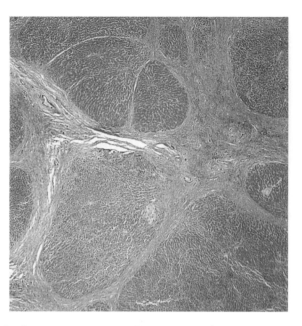

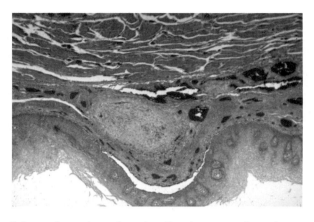

Sclerosed **esophageal varix.** Overlying esophageal mucosa is generally normal.*

Cirrhosis, microscopic. Regenerative lesions are surrounded by fibrotic bands of collagen ("bridging fibrosis"), forming the characteristic nodularity.

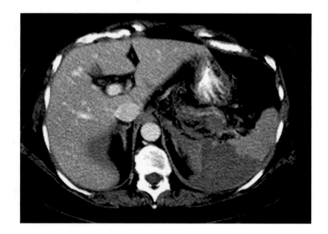

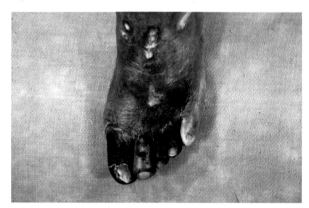

Splenic infarction. The splenic artery lacks collateral supply, making the spleen particularly susceptible to ischemic damage. Coagulative necrosis has occurred in a wedge shape along the pattern of vascular supply.*

Foot gangrene. The first four toes and adjacent skin are dry, shrunken, and blackened with superficial necrosis and peeling of the skin. A well-defined line of demarcation separates the black region from the viable skin.*

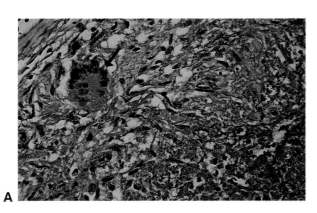 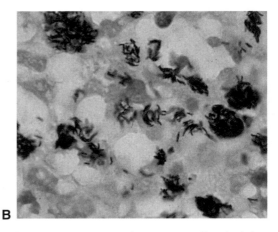

A

B

Microscopically, **tuberculosis (A)** is characterized by caseating granulomas containing Langhans' giant cells, which have a "horseshoe" pattern of nuclei (see arrow). Organisms **(B)** are identified by their red color on acid-fast staining ("red snappers").

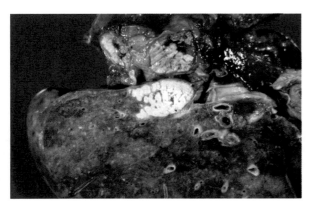 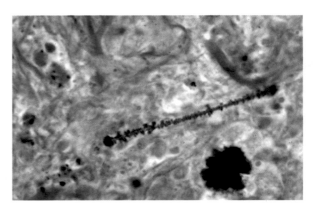

Miliary tuberculosis with large caseous lesions at the left medial upper lobe and miliary lesions in the surrounding hilar node. This life-threatening infection is caused by blood-borne dissemination of *Mycobacterium tuberculosis* to many organs from a quiescent site of infection.*

Asbestosis. Ferruginous bodies (asbestos bodies with Prussian blue iron stain) in lung, microscopic. Inhaled asbestos fibers are ingested by macrophages.*

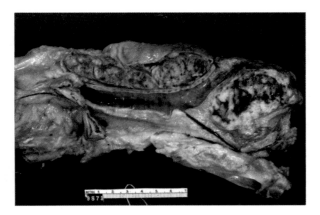 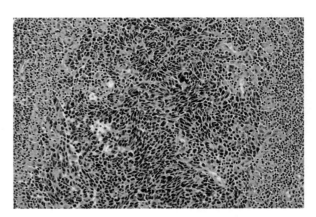

Squamous cell carcinoma of the lung, gross, from a patient with a long smoking history. This tumor arises from the bronchial epithelium and is centrally located.*

Small (oat) cell carcinoma in a pulmonary hilar lymph node. Almost all of these tumors are related to tobacco smoking. They can arise anywhere in the lung, most often near the hilum, and quickly spread along bronchi.*

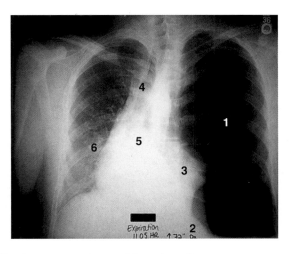

Tension pneumothorax. Note these features:

1—Hyperlucent lung field
2—Hyperexpansion lowers diaphragm
3—Collapsed lung
4—Deviation of trachea
5—Mediastinal shift
6—Compression of opposite lung

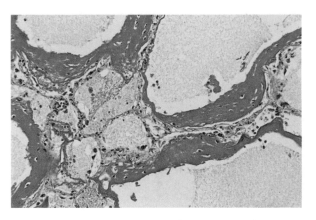

Acute respiratory distress syndrome (ARDS). Persistent inflammation leads to poor pulmonary compliance and edema; note both alveolar fluid and hyaline membranes.

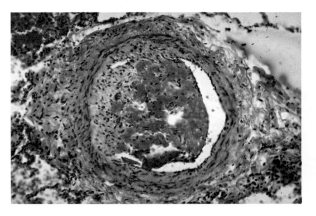

Lung thromboembolus in a small muscular pulmonary artery. The interdigitating areas of pale pink and red within the organizing embolus form the "lines of Zahn" characteristic of a thrombus. These lines represent layers of red cells, platelets, and fibrin that are laid down in the vessel as the thrombus forms.*

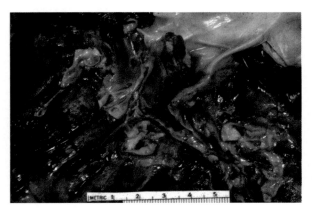

Pulmonary thromboembolus, gross. Most often arises from deep venous thrombosis.*

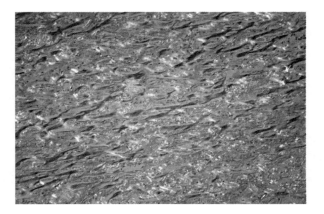

Amyloidosis from tongue tissue with skeletal muscle atrophy. The amyloid deposits stain red with Congo red and exhibit an apple-green birefringence with polarized light (as shown here in a section of cardiac muscle).*

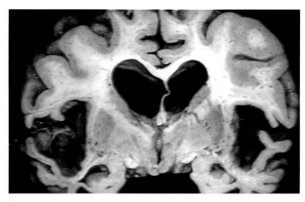

A

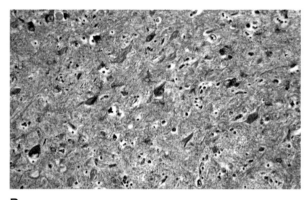

B

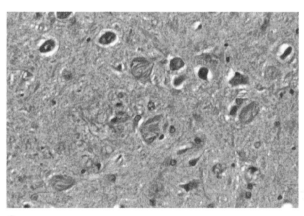

C

Alzheimer's disease. Key histologic features include "senile plaques" (A), a coronal section showing atrophy, especially of the temporal lobes (B); and focal masses of interwoven neuronal processes around an amyloid core. The remnants of neuronal degeneration (C) are also associated with Alzheimer's disease, the most common cause of dementia in older persons.*

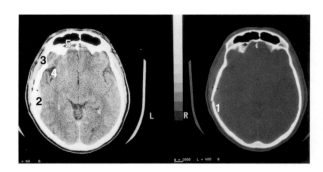

Epidural hematoma from skull fracture. Note lens-shaped (biconcave) dense blood next to fracture. 1—Skull fracture; 2—hematoma in epidural space; 3—temporalis muscle; 4—Sylvian fissure; 5—frontal sinus.

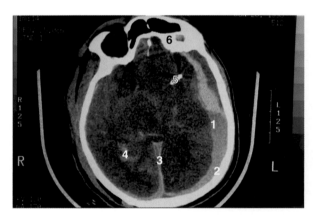

Subdural hemorrhage. Note hyperdense extra-axial blood on the left side. Concomitant subarachnoid hemorrhage. 1—subdural blood, layering; 2—skull; 3—falx; 4—subarachnoid blood; 5—shunt catheter; 6—frontal sinus.

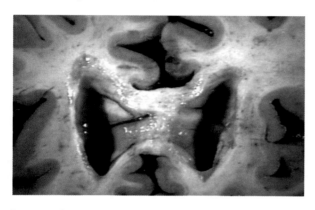

Brain with periventricular white-matter plaques of demyelination due to **multiple sclerosis,** gross. Demyelination occurs in a bilateral asymmetric distribution. Classic
clinical findings are nystagmus, scanning speech, and intention tremor.*

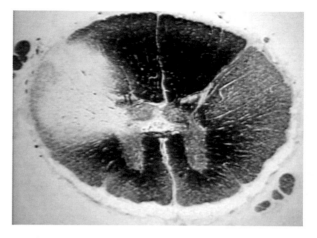

Multiple sclerosis, lumbar spinal cord, mostly random
and asymmetric white-matter lesions.*

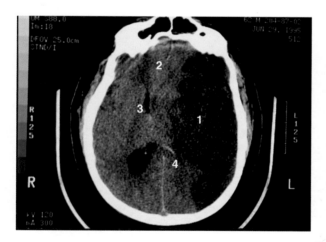

Left MCA stroke. Large left MCA territory stroke with
edema and mass effect but no visible hemorrhage. The
patient experienced deficits in speech and in the right
side of the face and upper extremities. 1—ischemic brain
parenchyma; 2—subtle midline shift to the right; 3—the
right frontal horn of the lateral ventricle; 4—the left lateral ventricles obliterated by edema.

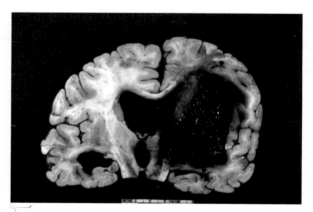

Brain with **hypertensive hemorrhage** in the region of
the basal ganglia, gross.*

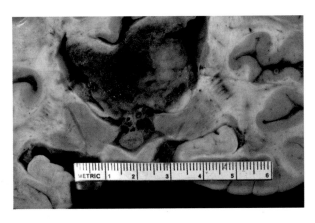

Glioblastoma multiforme extending across the midline of the cerebral cortex, gross.*

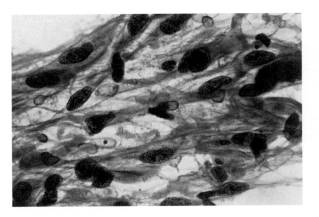

Glioblastoma multiforme. Small cells with elongated nuclei and bipolar processes are characteristic. The chromatin is generally not markedly dense, nor are nucleoli usually prominent.*

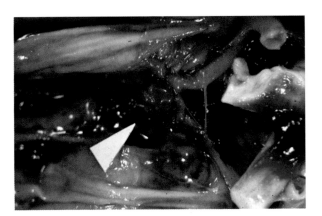

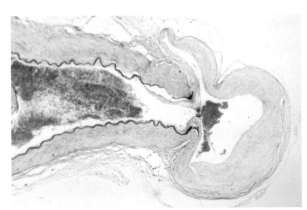

View of a typical **berry aneurysm** located on the anterior cerebral artery. The small, saclike structure can easily rupture during periods of hypertension or stress. The histologic section at the origin of the aneurysm shows lack of internal elastic lamina.*

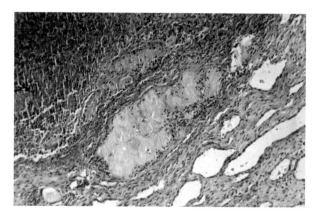

Tophus consisting of a uric acid deposit lesion from the elbow of a patient with gout. Crystals (not visible here) will be needle shaped and negatively birefringent.*

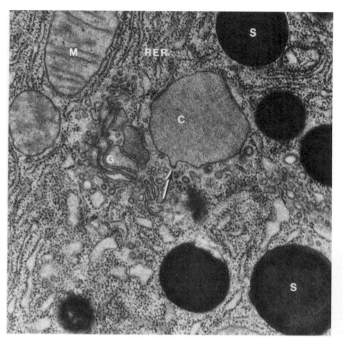

Electron micrograph of a **pancreatic acinar cell.** A condensing vacuole (C) is receiving secretory product (arrow) from the Golgi complex (G). M—mitochondrion; RER—rough endoplasmic reticulum; S—mature condensed secretory zymogen granules.

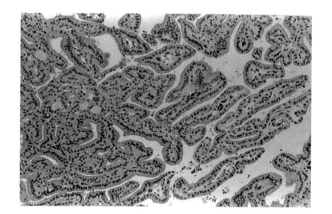

In **Graves' disease,** stimulation of follicular cells by TSH causes the normal uniform architecture to be replaced by hyperplastic papillary, involuted borders, and decreased colloid. Typical medical therapy is propylthiouracil, which inhibits the production of thyroid hormone as well as peripheral conversion of T_4 to T_3.*

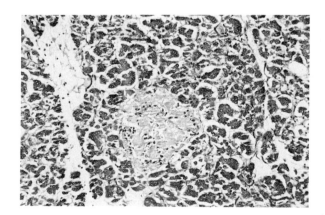

Pancreatic islet cells in **DM type 1.** In patients with diabetes mellitus type 1, autoantibodies against β cells cause a chronic inflammation until, over time, islet cells are entirely replaced by amyloid.

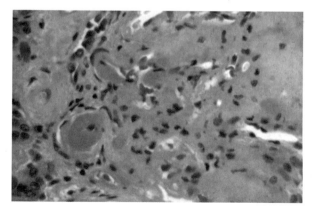

Arteriolar sclerosis showing masses of hyaline material in glomerular afferent and efferent arterioles and in the glomerulus. From a type 1 diabetic patient.*

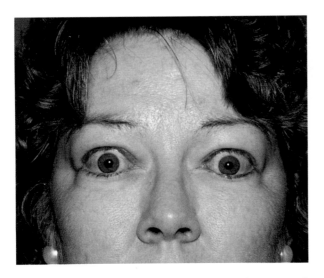

Exophthalmos in a patient with **Graves' disease,** with proptosis and periorbital edema.

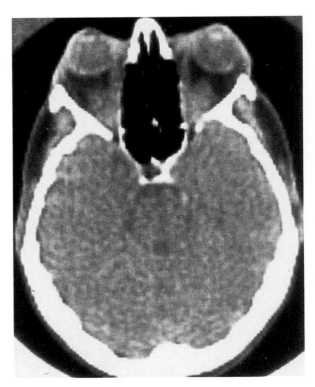

Graves' disease. CT shows extraocular muscle enlargement at the orbital apex.*

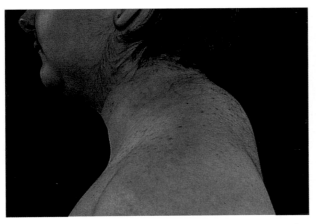

A

Cushing's disease. The clinical picture includes **(A)** moon facies and buffalo hump and **(B)** truncal obesity and abdominal striae.

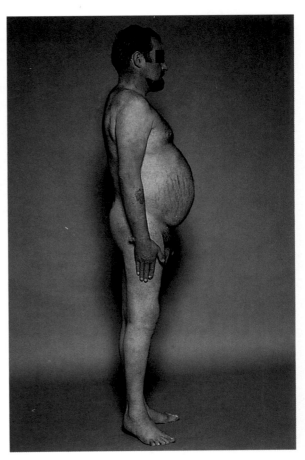

B

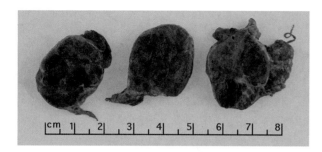

Adrenocortical adenoma, gross. Cause of hypercortisolism (Cushing's syndrome) or hyperaldosteronism (Conn's syndrome)*

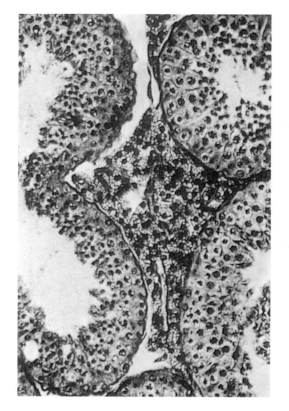

In the **seminiferous tubules,** Sertoli cells play a supportive and protective role in spermatogenesis. Note cells in various stages of differentiation, with spermatogonia near the basal lamina and more mature forms near the lumen.

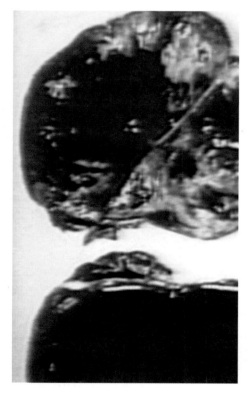

Serosal surface of the uterus with "chocolate cysts" resulting from **endometriosis,** gross. "Powder burn" lesions (not shown here) are another characteristic finding. Patients experience pain with menstruation.*

Hydatidiform mole. The characteristic gross appearance is a "bunch of grapes." Hydatidiform moles are the most common precursors of choriocarcinoma. Complete moles usually display a 46,XX diploid pattern with all the chromosomes derived from the sperm. In partial moles, the karyotype is triploid or tetraploid, and fetal parts may be present.

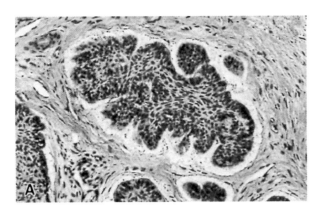
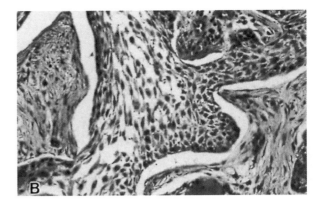

Basal cell carcinoma. Cytologic details show that islands of tumor within a mucinous dermis **(A)** are composed of small, round-to-fusiform cells with inconspicuous cytoplasm and densely hyperchromatic nuclei. Also evident is an early **(A)** and well-developed **(B)** separation artifact.*

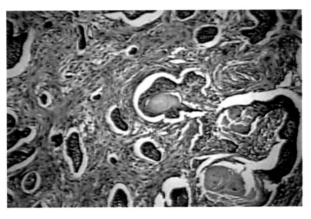
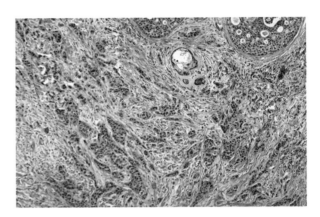

Squamous cell carcinoma. Malignant skin tumor involving epidermal skin layer. Note the presence of keratin pearls.*

Papillary intraductal adenocarcinoma of the breast. Invasive tumor with marked desmoplastic reaction. Intraductal lesions are also seen.*

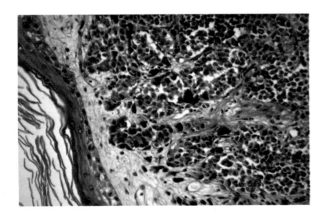
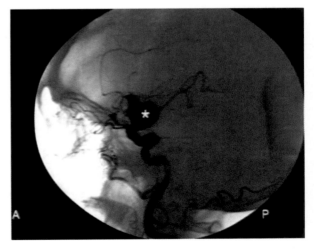

Malignant melanoma, showing lesion just beneath the epidermis with pigmented and nonpigmented cells. The tumor cells are usually polyhedral but may be spindle shaped, dendritic, or ballooned or may resemble oat cells. Many but by no means all melanomas make melanin. Big nucleoli are common.*

Carotid angiogram showing aneurysm. Note the path of the internal carotid artery through the neck and its major branches (ophthalmic artery, anterior cerebral artery, middle cerebral artery). The aneurysm is inferior to the terminal branches in this angiogram.*

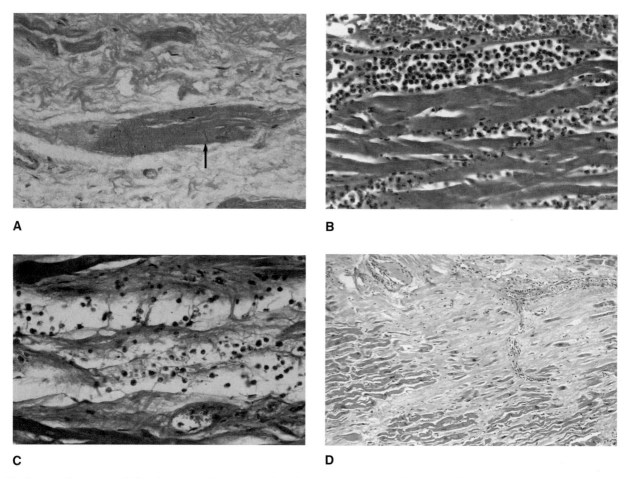

A

B

C

D

Evolution of a **myocardial infarction** Contraction band necrosis (arrow) is the first visible change, occurring in one to two hours **(A).** In the first three days, neutrophilic infiltration and coagulation necrosis occur **(B).** By three to seven days, neutrophils have been replaced by macrophages, and clearing of myocyte debris has begun **(C).** Within weeks, granulation and scarring occur **(D).**

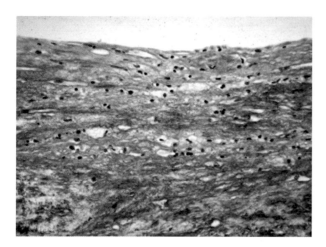

Atherosclerosis. Aorta with fibrous intimal thickening and foam cells dispersed throughout smooth muscle cells, micro.*

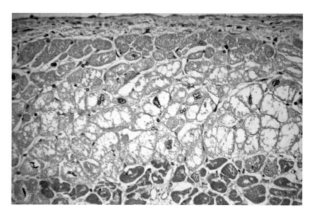

Microscopic example of myocytolysis and coagulation necrosis beneath the endocardium, commonly seen in **chronic ischemia.***

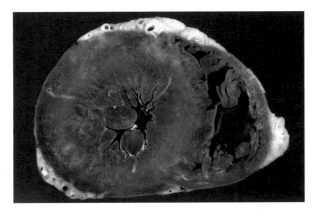

Heart with marked concentric **left ventricular hypertrophy** from hypertension, gross.*

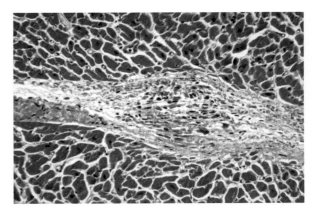

The **Aschoff body,** an area of fibrinoid necrosis surrounded by mononuclear and multinucleated giant cells, is pathognomonic for **rheumatic heart disease.** The mitral valve is most commonly affected.*

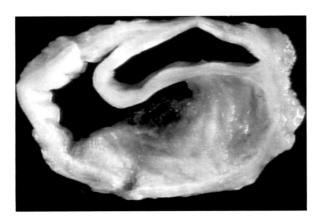

Aortic dissection with a blood clot compressing the aortic lumen. A tear in the intima allowed blood to surge through the muscular layer to the adventitia (may lead to sudden death from hemothorax). Risk factors are hypertension, Marfan's syndrome, pregnancy, Ehlers-Danlos syndrome, and trauma.*

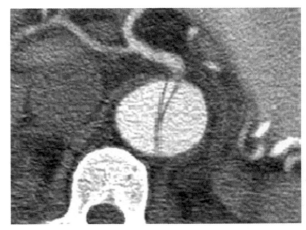

Abdominal aortic dissection demonstrating a double-barrel lumen at the level of the superior mesenteric artery (anterior).*

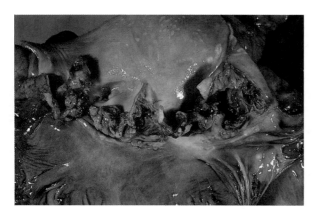

Acute bacterial endocarditis. Virulent organisms (e.g., *Staphylococcus aureus*) infect previously normal valves, causing marked damage (here, in the aortic valve) and potentially giving rise to septic emboli.

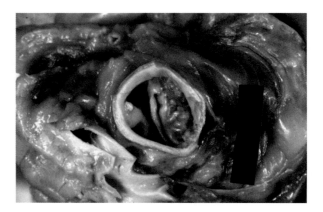

Calcified **bicuspid aortic valve** showing false raphe. The abnormal architecture of the valve makes its leaflets susceptible to otherwise ordinary hemodynamic stresses, which ultimately leads to valvular thickening, calcification, increased rigidity, and stenosis.*

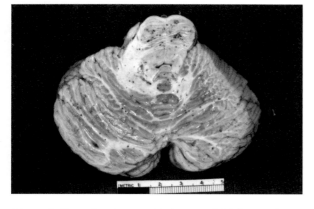

Air embolism showing multiple petechial hemorrhages in the pons and cerebellum.*

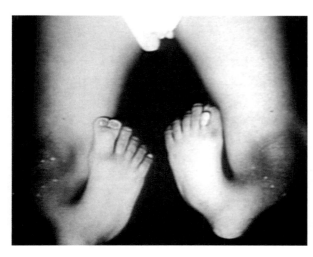

Osteogenesis imperfecta. Abnormal collagen synthesis results from a variety of gene mutations and causes brittle bones and connective tissue malformations.*

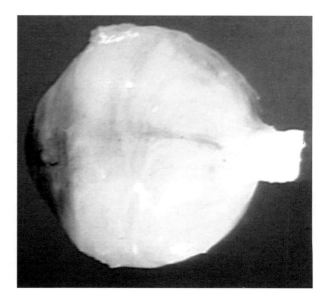

Osteogenesis imperfecta. Blue sclera caused by translucency of connective tissue over the choroid. The optic nerve is on the right side of the image.*

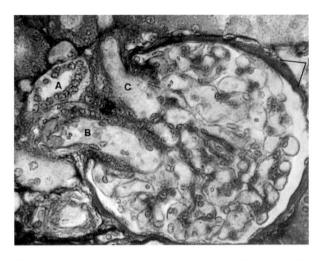

Normal glomerulus, microscopic, with **(A)** macula densa and **(B)** afferent and **(C)** efferent arterioles.

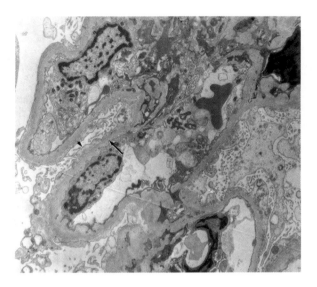

Minimal change disease (lipoid nephrosis) shows normal glomeruli on light microscopy but effacement of foot processes on EM (arrowhead). The full arrow points to a normal foot process.

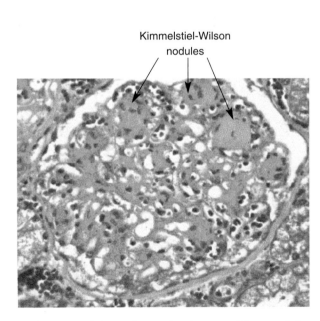

Kimmelstiel-Wilson nodules

Diabetic nodular glomerulosclerosis. The nodular Kimmelstiel-Wilson lesions at the periphery of the glomerulus are pathognomonic for diabetic GS.

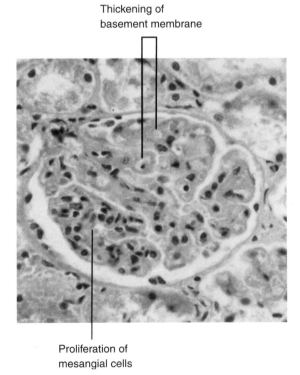

Thickening of basement membrane

Proliferation of mesangial cells

Systemic lupus erythematosus, kidney pathology. In the membranous glomerulonephritic pattern, "wire-loop" thickening occurs as a result of subendothelial immune complex deposition.

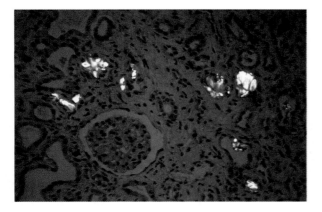

Calcium oxalate crystals in the kidney, viewed with partially crossed polarizers. Tubular failure in oxalate nephropathy can result from vitamin C or antifreeze abuse.*

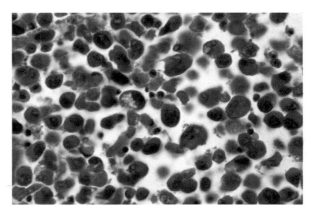

Renal cell carcinoma, microscopic, taken from the urinary tract, showing eosinophilic cell lesions. Glycogen and lipid-filled clear cells derived from tubular epithelium are common but not shown here.*

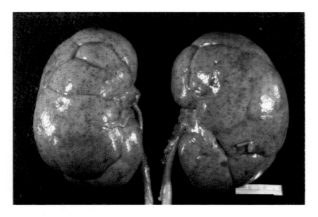

Enlarged, very pale kidneys with "flea bite" or ectasia from a patient with nephrotic syndrome or subacute glomerulonephritis as a result of **lupus erythematosus.***

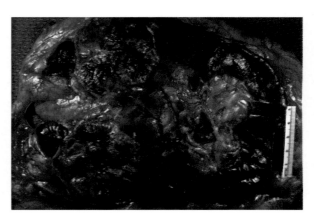

Renal cell carcinoma, gross. Notably, tumor may extend into the renal vein and IVC and spread hematogenously.*

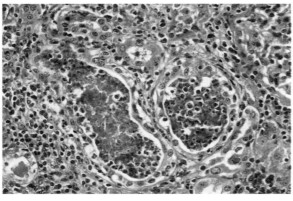

A

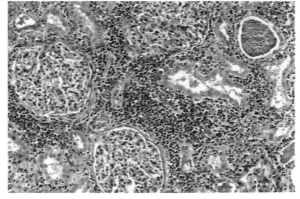

B

Acute pyelonephritis (A) is characterized by neutrophilic infiltration and abscess formation within the renal interstitium. Abscesses may rupture, introducing collections of white cells to the tubular lumen. In contrast, **chronic pyelonephritis (B)** has a lymphocytic invasion with fibrosis.

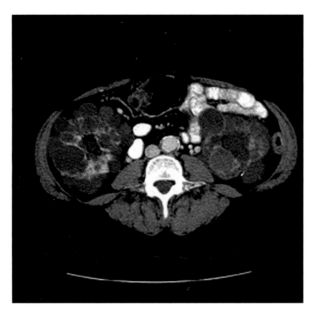

CT showing **autosomal-dominant polycystic kidney disease.** Disease occurs bilaterally and presents with flank pain and hematuria.*

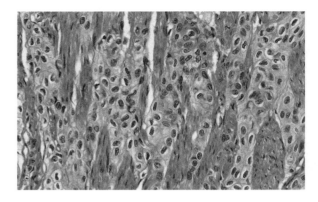

Transitional cell carcinoma of the urinary bladder, microscopic. Malignant urothelial cells have invaded the muscular layer of the bladder wall.

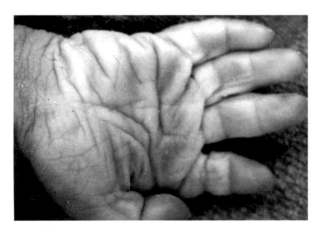

Simian crease. A characteristic feature of Down syndrome (trisomy 21). The palm has a single transverse crease instead of the normal two creases.*

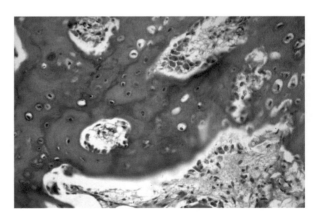

Bone fracture. New bone formation with osteoblasts.*

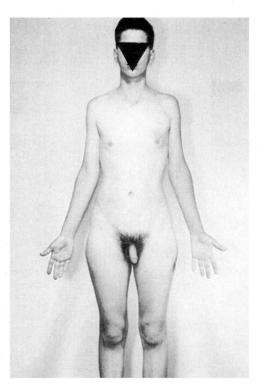

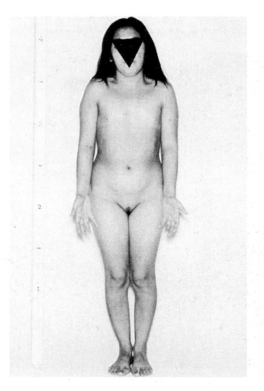

Klinefelter's syndrome (XXY). Phenotype includes a female fat distribution with male external genitalia.

Turner's syndrome (XO). Phenotype includes short stature, webbing of the neck, and poorly developed secondary sex characteristics.

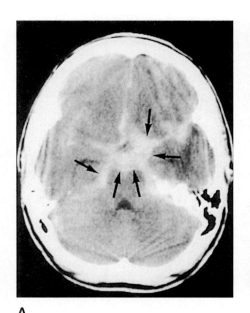

A

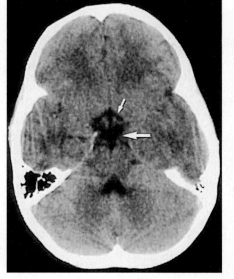

B

Subarachnoid hemorrhage. CT scan with contrast reveals blood in the subarachnoid space at the base of the brain.

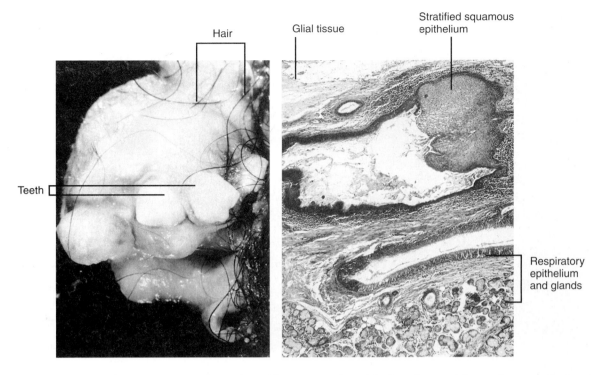

A benign **teratoma** of the ovary containing teeth and hair, an incidental finding during abdominal surgery. In females, teratomas are generally benign, whereas in males they account for about 30% of testicular tumors.

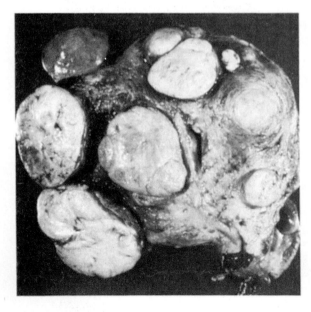

Multiple **leiomyomas** (fibroids) of the uterus. Common benign uterine tumor. Fibroids beneath the endometrium may present with vaginal bleeding; they also develop subserosally or within the myometrium.

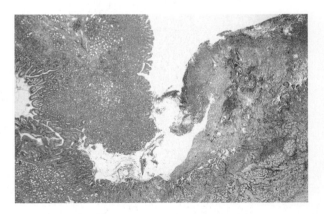

Duodenal ulcer. The epithelium is ulcerated, and the lamina propria is infiltrated with inflammatory cells. Necrotic debris is present in the ulcer crater.

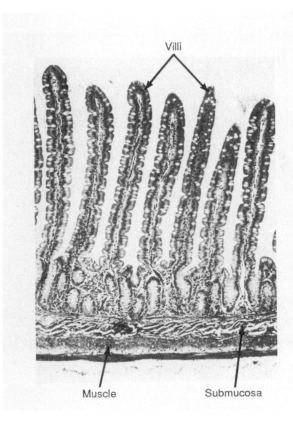

Photomicrograph of the **small intestine.**

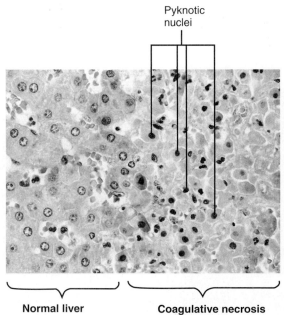

Normal liver cells	Coagulative necrosis of liver cells
Arranged in cords	Disorganized
Normal nuclei	Pyknotic or absent nuclei
Granular cytoplasm	Homogeneous cytoplasm

Coagulative necrosis of hepatocytes.

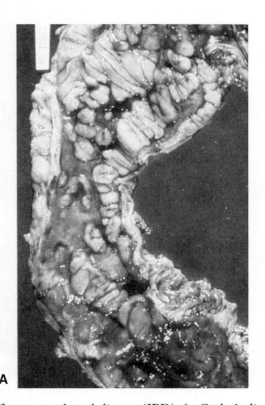

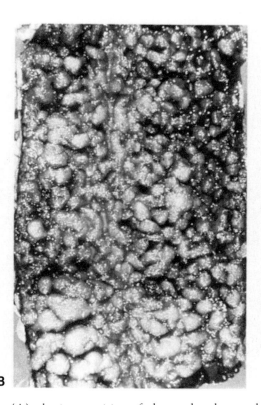

Inflammatory bowel disease (IBD). In **Crohn's disease (A),** the juxtaposition of ulcerated and normal mucosa gives a "cobblestone" appearance. In acute **ulcerative colitis (B),** the intestinal mucosa is inflamed and edematous and has a pseudopolypoid appearance. Chronically, ulcerative colitis has a more atrophic appearance.

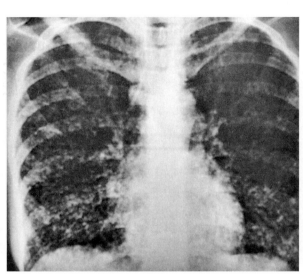

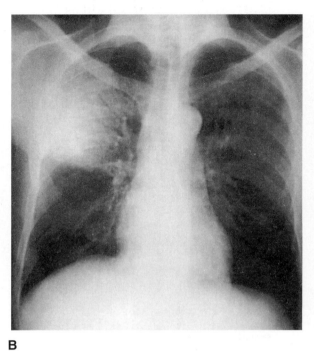

A

B

Compare the diffuse, patchy bilateral infiltrates of "atypical" **interstitial pneumonia (A)** with the localized, dense lesion of **lobar pneumonia (B)**.

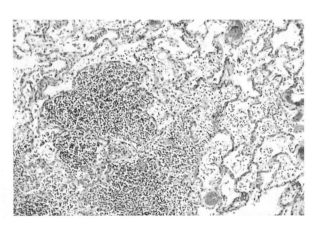

Bronchopneumonia with neutrophils in alveolar spaces, microscopic.

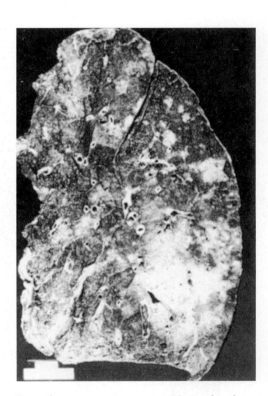

Bronchopneumonia, gross. Note the large area of consolidation at the base plus multiple small areas of consolidation (pale) involving bronchioles and surrounding alveolar sacs throughout the lung.

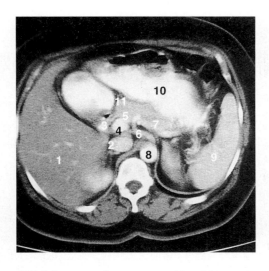

CT abdomen with contrast—normal anatomy.

1—Liver
2—Inferior vena cava
3—Portal vein
4—Hepatic artery
5—Gastroduodenal artery
6—Celiac trunk
7—Splenic vein
8—Aorta
9—Spleen
10—Stomach
11—Pancreas

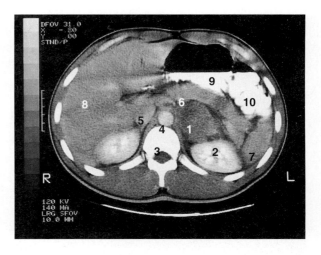

Left adrenal mass.

1—Large left adrenal mass
2—Kidney
3—Vertebral body
4—Aorta
5—IVC
6—Pancreas
7—Spleen
8—Liver
9—Stomach with air and contrast
10—Colon–splenic flexure

Anterior shoulder dislocation. Note the humeral head inferior and medial to the glenoid fossa and fracture fragments from the greater tuberosity.

1—Acromion
2—Coracoid
3—Glenoid fossa
4—Fracture fragments
5—Humeral head
6—Clavicle

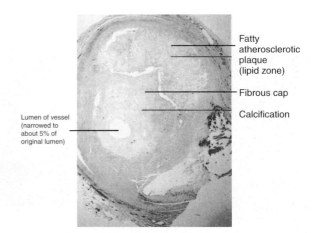

Fatty atherosclerotic plaque (lipid zone)

Fibrous cap

Calcification

Lumen of vessel (narrowed to about 5% of original lumen)

Atherosclerosis in a coronary vessel. Calcified plaques have narrowed the lumen of the artery, increasing the risk for occlusion—i.e., myocardial infarction.

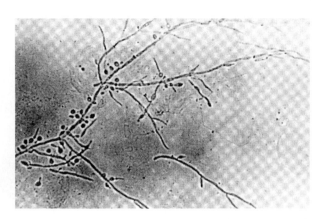

Candidal vaginitis. Branched and budding *Candida albicans* is visible on KOH preparation of whitish vaginal discharge.

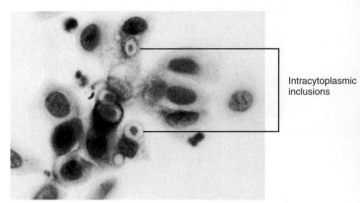

Intracytoplasmic inclusions

Trophozoites of **Trichomonas vaginalis** by Giemsa stain.

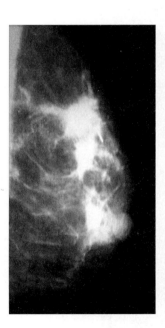

Breast mammogram diagnosis of breast cancer. The upper half of the breast shows a dense, irregularly shaped mass with long, branching tentacles extending toward the nipple. Numerous tiny calcium deposits looking like grains of sand (microcalcifications) are seen both in the mass and in the surrounding tissue.*

Pharmacology

"Take me, I am the drug; take me, I am hallucinogenic."
—Salvador Dali

"I was under medication when I made the decision not to burn the tapes."
—Richard Nixon

Preparation for questions on pharmacology is straightforward. Memorizing all the key drugs and their characteristics (e.g., mechanisms, clinical use, and important side effects) is high yield. Focus on understanding the prototype drugs in each class. Avoid memorizing obscure derivatives. Learn the "classic" and distinguishing toxicities of the major drugs. Do not bother with drug dosages or trade names. Reviewing associated biochemistry, physiology, and microbiology can be useful while studying pharmacology. There is a strong emphasis on autonomic nervous system, central nervous system, antimicrobial, and cardiovascular agents as well as on NSAIDs. Much of the material is clinically relevant. Newer drugs on the market are also fair game.

High-Yield Clinical Vignettes
High-Yield Topics
Pharmacokinetics
Antimicrobial
Central Nervous System
Cardiovascular
Cancer Drugs
Toxicology
Miscellaneous

These abstracted case vignettes are designed to demonstrate the thought processes necessary to answer multistep clinical reasoning questions.

Vignette	Question	Answer
28-year-old chemist presents with MPTP exposure.	What neurotransmitter is depleted?	Dopamine. *Pharm.69*
Woman taking tetracycline exhibits photosensitivity.	What are the clinical manifestations?	Rash on sun-exposed regions of the body. *Pharm.55*
Young girl with congenital valve disease is given penicillin prophylactically. She develops bacterial endocarditis.	What do you give now?	β-lactamase-resistant penicillin. *Pharm.52*
Nondiabetic patient presents with hypoglycemia but low levels of C peptide.	What is the diagnosis?	Surreptitious insulin injection. *Pharm.17*
African-American man who goes to Africa develops anemia after taking prophylactic medicine.	What is the enzyme deficiency?	Glucose-6-phosphate dehydrogenase.
27-year-old female with a history of psychiatric illness now has urinary retention due to a neuroleptic.	What do you treat it with?	Bethanechol.
Farmer presents with dyspnea, salivation, miosis, diarrhea, cramping, and blurry vision.	What caused this, and what is the mechanism of action?	Insecticide poisoning; inhibition of acetylcholinesterase.
55-year-old man undergoing treatment for BPH has decreased levels of testosterone and DHT as well as gynecomastia and edema.	What is the drug?	Estrogen (DES).
Patient with recent kidney transplant is on cyclosporine for immunosuppression. Requires antifungal agent for candidiasis.	What antifungal drug would result in cyclosporine toxicity?	Ketoconazole. *Pharm.51*
Man on several medications, including antidepressants and antihypertensives, has mydriasis and becomes constipated.	What is the cause of his symptoms?	Tricyclic antidepressant. *Pharm.89*
Patient presents with renal insufficiency.	What alterations in doses of digoxin and digitoxin, respectively?	Decreased, same.

Vignette	Question	Answer
55-year-old postmenopausal woman is on tamoxifen therapy.	What is she at increased risk of acquiring?	Endometrial carcinoma.
Woman on MAO inhibitor has hypertensive crisis after a meal.	What did she ingest?	Tyramine (wine or cheese). *Pharm.83*
After taking clindamycin, patient develops toxic megacolon and diarrhea.	What is the mechanism of diarrhea?	*C. difficile* overgrowth.
Man starts a medication for hyperlipidemia. He then develops a rash, pruritus, and GI upset.	What drug was it?	Niacin. *Pharm.7*
Patient is on carbamazepine.	What routine workup should always be done?	LFTs. *Pharm.64*
23-year-old female who is on rifampin for TB prophylaxis and on birth control (estrogen) gets pregnant.	Why?	Rifampin augments estrogen metabolism in the liver. *Pharm.53*
Older female goes into the OR for emergency surgery; after administration of succinylcholine, she requires respiratory support for over 4 hours. Later it is determined that she is receiving medication for glaucoma.	What is she on?	Acetylcholinesterase inhibitor.
Patient develops cough and must discontinue captopril.	What is a good replacement drug, and why doesn't it have the same side effects?	Losartan, an AT II receptor antagonist, does not increase bradykinin as captopril does.

Mechanism, clinical use, and toxicity of:

1. Motion sickness drugs (e.g., scopolamine).
2. Antipsychotics (neuroleptics), low and high potency.
3. Opiates (e.g., analgesic, antidiarrheal, antitussive), receptor types, agonists, mixed agonist-antagonists.
4. Myasthenia gravis drugs.
5. Hormonal treatments of cancer (e.g., leuprolide, flutamide, aminoglutethimide).
6. New oral hypoglycemic agents (acarbose, metformin, rosiglitazone).
7. Stool softeners (e.g., psyllium, methylcellulose).
8. Angiotensin II receptor blockers (e.g., losartan).
9. Dermatologic agents (e.g., corticosteroids, retinoids, antifungal agents).
10. Other new pharmacologic agents (erythropoietin, RU-486).

Know about:

1. Complications of empiric antibiotic use (e.g., resistance, fungal infection, pseudomembranous colitis).
2. Secondary effects of common drugs (e.g., heparin and osteoporosis, thiazides and hyperlipidemia).
3. Fundamental pharmacodynamics (e.g., partial agonists, physiologic antagonists, efficacy).
4. Drug efficacy and potency as demonstrated on dose-response curves.
5. Pharmacogenetics: drugs whose metabolism is affected by inheritance (e.g., isoniazid).
6. Anesthesia: physical properties of gaseous agents (MAC, blood-gas partition coefficient, rate of induction), different IV agents, toxicities (e.g., malignant hyperthermia).
7. Treatment of anemia (e.g., erythropoietin, B_{12}, folate, testosterone, iron supplements).
8. Prevention/treatment of cerebrovascular disease (e.g., aspirin, thrombolytics).
9. Treatment of rheumatoid arthritis.
10. Vaccines: indications, potential side effects.
11. Chemotherapeutic agents: risk of possible secondary cancer.

Pharmacokinetics

Volume of distribution (V_d)	Relates the amount of drug in the body to the plasma concentration. V_d of plasma protein–bound drugs can be altered by liver and kidney disease.

$$V_d = \frac{\text{amount of drug in the body}}{\text{plasma drug concentration}}$$

Clearance (CL)	Relates the rate of elimination to the plasma concentration.

$$CL = \frac{\text{rate of elimination of drug}}{\text{plasma drug concentration}}$$

Half-life ($t_{1/2}$)	The time required to change the amount of drug in the body by ½ during elimination (or during a constant infusion). A drug infused at a constant rate reaches about 94% of steady state after four $t_{1/2}$.

$$t_{1/2} = \frac{0.7 \times V_d}{CL}$$

# of half-lives	1	2	3	3.3
Concentration	50%	75%	87.5%	90%

Dosage calculations

Loading dose = $C_p \times V_d / F$.

Maintenance dose = $C_p \times CL / F$

where C_p = target plasma concentration
and F = bioavailability.

In patients with impaired renal or hepatic function, the loading dose remains unchanged, although the maintenance dose is decreased.

Elimination of drugs

Zero-order elimination	Rate of elimination is constant regardless of C (i.e., constant **amount** of drug eliminated per unit time). C_p decreases linearly with time. Examples of drugs—ethanol, phenytoin, and aspirin (at high or toxic concentrations).
First-order elimination	Rate of elimination is proportional to the drug concentration (i.e., constant **fraction** of drug eliminated per unit time). C_p decreases exponentially with time.

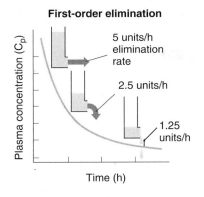
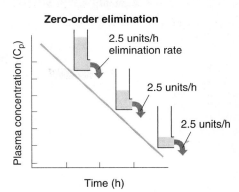

In drugs with first-order kinetics (see left panel above), rate of elimination is proportional to plasma concentration (C_p); in the case of zero-order elimination (right panel), the rate is constant and independent of concentration.

(Adapted, with permission, from Katzung BG, Trevor AJ. *Examination & Board Review: Pharmacology*, 5th ed. Stamford, CT: Appleton & Lange, 1998:5.)

HIGH-YIELD FACTS

Pharmacology

Phase I vs. phase II metabolism

Phase I (reduction, oxidation, hydrolysis) yields slightly polar, water-soluble metabolites (often still active).

~Add groups.~ ← Phase II (acetylation, glucuronidation, sulfation) yields very polar, inactive metabolites (renally excreted).

Phase I—cyt. P450.
Phase II—conjugation.
Geriatric patients lose phase I first.

Drug development

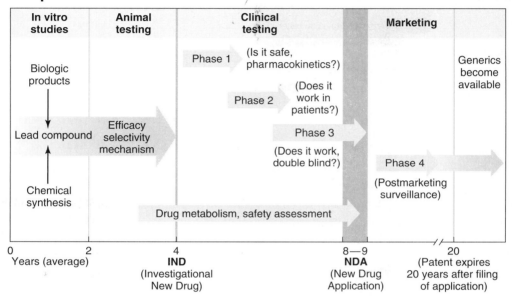

(Adapted, with permission, from Katzung BG, Trevor AJ. *Examination & Board Review: Pharmacology,* 5th ed. Stamford, CT: Appleton & Lange, 1998:365.)

Pharmacodynamics

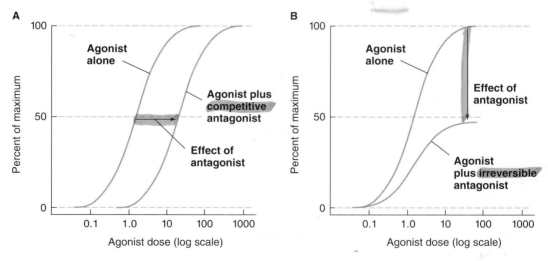

(Adapted, with permission, from Katzung BG and Trevor AJ. *Examination & Board Review: Pharmacology,* 5th ed. Stamford, CT: Appleton & Lange, 1998:13–14.)

Shown above are agonist dose-response curves in the presence of competitive and irreversible antagonists. Note the use of a logarithmic scale for drug concentration. **A.** A competitive antagonist has an effect illustrated by the shift of the agonist curve to the right. **B.** A noncompetitive antagonist shifts the agonist curve downward.

Pharmacodynamics
(continued)

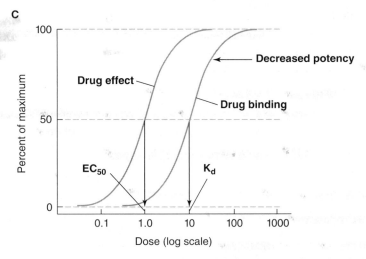

(Adapted, with permission, from Katzung BG. *Basic and Clinical Pharmacology,* 7th ed. Stamford, CT: Appleton & Lange, 1997:13.)

C. In a system with spare receptors, the EC_{50} is lower than the K_d, indicating that to achieve 50% of maximum effect, fewer than 50% of the receptors must be activated.

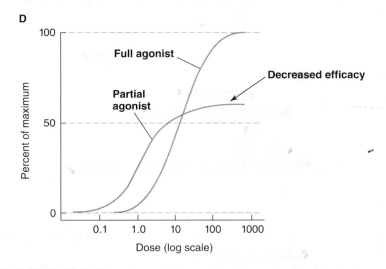

(Adapted, with permission, from Katzung BG. *Basic and Clinical Pharmacology,* 7th ed. Stamford, CT: Appleton & Lange, 1997: 13.)

D. Comparison of dose-response curves for a full agonist and a partial agonist. The partial agonist acts on the same receptor system as the full agonist but cannot produce as large an effect (it has lower maximal efficacy) no matter how much the dose is increased. A partial agonist may be more potent (as in the figure), less potent, or equally potent; potency is an independent factor.

Antimicrobial therapy

Mechanism of action	Drugs
Block cell wall synthesis by inhibition of peptidoglycan cross-linking	Penicillin, ampicillin, ticarcillin, piperacillin, imipenem, aztreonam, cephalosporins
Block peptidoglycan synthesis	Bacitracin, vancomycin
Block protein synthesis at 50S ribosomal subunit	Chloramphenicol, erythromycin/macrolides, lincomycin, clindamycin, streptogramins (quinupristin, dalfopristin)
Block protein synthesis at 30S ribosomal subunit	Aminoglycosides, tetracyclines
Block nucleotide synthesis	Sulfonamides, trimethoprim
Block DNA topoisomerases	Quinolones
Block mRNA synthesis	Rifampin
Bactericidal antibiotics	Penicillin, cephalosporins, vancomycin, aminoglycosides, fluoroquinolones, metronidazole
Disrupt bacterial/fungal cell membranes	Polymyxins
Disrupt fungal cell membranes	Amphotericin B, nystatin, fluconazole/azoles
Unknown	Pentamidine

FAN

Penicillin

Penicillin G (IV form), penicillin V (oral).

Mechanism	1. Binds penicillin-binding proteins
	2. Blocks transpeptidase cross-linking of cell wall
	3. Activates autolytic enzymes
Clinical use	Bactericidal for gram-positive cocci, gram-positive rods, gram-negative cocci, and spirochetes. Not penicillinase resistant.
Toxicity	Hypersensitivity reactions, hemolytic anemia.

UCV *Pharm.52*

Methicillin, nafcillin, dicloxacillin

Mechanism	Same as penicillin. Narrow spectrum; penicillinase resistant because of bulkier R group.
Clinical use	*Staphylococcus aureus.*
Toxicity	Hypersensitivity reactions; methicillin—interstitial nephritis.

Ampicillin, amoxicillin

Mechanism	Same as penicillin. Wider spectrum; penicillinase sensitive. Also combine with clavulanic acid (penicillinase inhibitor) to enhance spectrum. AmOxicillin has greater Oral bioavailability than ampicillin.
Clinical use	Extended-spectrum penicillin—certain gram-positive bacteria and gram-negative rods (*H*aemophilus influenzae, *E*scherichia coli, *L*isteria monocytogenes, *P*roteus mirabilis, *S*almonella, enterococci).
Toxicity	Hypersensitivity reactions; ampicillin rash; pseudomembranous colitis.

Coverage: ampicillin/ amoxicillin **HELPS** kill enterococci.

Carbenicillin, piperacillin, ticarcillin

Mechanism	Same as penicillin. Extended spectrum.
Clinical use	*Pseudomonas* species and gram-negative rods; susceptible to penicillinase; use with clavulanic acid.
Toxicity	Hypersensitivity reactions.

Cephalosporins

Mechanism — β-lactam drugs that inhibit cell wall synthesis but are less susceptible to penicillinases. Bactericidal.

Clinical use —

1st generation—gram-positive cocci, *Proteus mirabilis*, *E. coli*, *Klebsiella pneumoniae*.

1st generation—**PEcK.**

2nd generation—gram-positive cocci, *Haemophilus influenzae*, *Enterobacter aerogenes*, *Neisseria* species, *Proteus mirabilis*, *E. coli*, *Klebsiella pneumoniae*, *Serratia marcescens*.

2nd generation—**HEN PEcKS.**

3rd generation—serious gram-negative infections resistant to other β-lactams; meningitis (most penetrate the blood-brain barrier). Examples: ceftazidime for *Pseudomonas*; ceftriaxone for gonorrhea.

4th generation—increased activity against *Pseudomonas* and gram-positive organisms.

Toxicity — Hypersensitivity reactions, increased nephrotoxicity of aminoglycosides, disulfiram-like reaction with ethanol (in cephalosporins with a methylthiotetrazole group, e.g., cefamandole).

Aztreonam

Mechanism	A monobactam resistant to β-lactamases. Inhibits cell wall synthesis (binds to PBP3). Synergistic with aminoglycosides. No cross-allergenicity with penicillins.
Clinical use	Gram-negative rods—*Klebsiella* species, *Pseudomonas* species, *Serratia* species. No activity against gram-positives or anaerobes. For penicillin-allergic patients and those with renal insufficiency who can't tolerate aminoglycosides.
Toxicity	Usually nontoxic; occasional GI upset.

Imipenem/cilastatin

Mechanism	Imipenem is a broad-spectrum, β-lactamase-resistant carbapenem. Always administered with cilastatin (inhibitor of renal dihydropeptidase 1) to ↓ inactivation in renal tubules.
Clinical use	Gram-positive cocci, gram-negative rods, and anaerobes. Drug of choice for *Enterobacter*.
Toxicity	GI distress, skin rash, and CNS toxicity (seizures) at high plasma levels.

With imipenem, "the kill is **LASTIN'** with ci**LASTATIN**."

Vancomycin

Mechanism	Inhibits cell wall mucopeptide formation by binding D-ala D-ala portion of cell wall precursors. Bactericidal. Resistance occurs with amino acid change of D-ala D-ala to D-ala D-lac.
Clinical use	Used for serious, gram-positive multidrug-resistant organisms, including *Staphylococcus aureus* and *Clostridium difficile* (pseudomembranous colitis).
Toxicity	**N**ephrotoxicity, **O**totoxicity, **T**hrombophlebitis, diffuse flushing—"red man syndrome" (can largely prevent by pretreatment with antihistamines and slow infusion rate). Well tolerated in general: Does **NOT** have many problems.

Protein synthesis inhibitors

30S inhibitors:

A = Aminoglycosides (streptomycin, gentamicin, tobramycin, amikacin) [bactericidal]

⊖ AA binding T = Tetracyclines [bacteriostatic]

50S inhibitors:

Pep X C = Chloramphenicol [bacteriostatic]

Translocase {
E = Erythromycin [bacteriostatic]
L = Lincomycin [bacteriostatic]
L = cLindamycin [bacteriostatic]
}

"Buy **AT 30**, **CELL** at **50**."

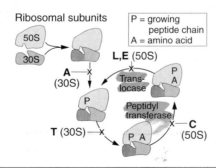

Ribosomal subunits

P = growing peptide chain
A = amino acid

Aminoglycosides

Gentamicin, neomycin, amikacin, tobramycin, streptomycin.

Mechanism Bactericidal; inhibit formation of initiation complex and cause misreading of mRNA. Require O_2 for uptake; therefore ineffective against anaerobes.

Clinical use Severe gram-negative rod infections. Synergistic with β-lactam antibiotics. Neomycin for bowel surgery.

Toxicity Nephrotoxicity (especially when used with cephalosporins), Ototoxicity (especially when used with loop diuretics).

AmiNOglycosides. Teratogen.

→ loop diuretics

cephalosporins

Tetracyclines

Tetracycline, doxycycline, demeclocycline, minocycline.

Mechanism Bacteriostatic; bind to 30S and prevent attachment of aminoacyl-tRNA; limited CNS penetration. Doxycycline is fecally eliminated and can be used in patients with renal failure. Must NOT take with milk, antacids, or iron-containing preparations because divalent cations inhibit its absorption in the gut.

Clinical use Vibrio cholerae, Acne, Chlamydia, Ureaplasma Urealyticum, Mycoplasma pneumoniae, Borrelia burgdorferi (Lyme disease), Rickettsia, tularemia.

VACUUM your BedRoom.

Toxicity GI distress, discolor teeth and inhibit bone growth in children, Fanconi's syndrome, photosensitivity. → sunlight

Macrolides ACE

Erythromycin, azithromycin, clarithromycin.

→ think "MACRO" → cant translocate (more)

Mechanism Inhibit protein synthesis by blocking translocation; bind to the 23S rRNA of the 50S ribosomal subunit. Bacteriostatic.

Clinical use Upper respiratory tract infections, pneumonias, sexually transmitted diseases—gram-positive cocci (streptococcal infections in patients allergic to penicillin), Mycoplasma, Legionella, Chlamydia, Neisseria.

Toxicity GI discomfort (most common cause of noncompliance), acute cholestatic hepatitis, eosinophilia, skin rashes.

Chloramphenicol

Mechanism Inhibits 50S peptidyl transferase. Bacteriostatic.

Clinical use Meningitis (Haemophilus influenzae, Neisseria meningitidis, Streptococcus pneumoniae). Conservative use owing to toxicities.

Toxicity Anemia (dose dependent), aplastic anemia (dose independent), gray baby syndrome (in premature infants because they lack liver UDP-glucuronyl transferase).

Clindamycin

Mechanism Blocks peptide bond formation at 50S ribosomal subunit. Bacteriostatic.

Treats anaerobes above the diaphragm.

Clinical use Treat anaerobic infections (e.g., Bacteroides fragilis, Clostridium perfringens).

Toxicity Pseudomembranous colitis (C. difficile overgrowth), fever, diarrhea.

Sulfonamides

Sulfamethoxazole (SMX), sulfisoxazole, triple sulfas, sulfadiazine.

Mechanism	PABA antimetabolites inhibit dihydropteroate synthase. Bacteriostatic.
Clinical use	Gram-positive, gram-negative, *Nocardia, Chlamydia.* Triple sulfas or SMX for simple UTI.
Toxicity	Hypersensitivity reactions, hemolysis if G6PD deficient, nephrotoxicity (tubulointerstitial nephritis), kernicterus in infants, displace other drugs from albumin (e.g., warfarin).

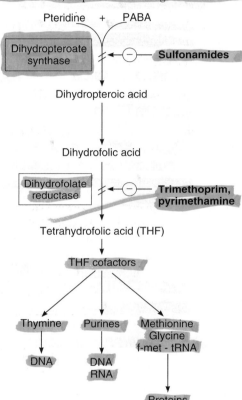

(Adapted, with permission, from Katzung BG. *Basic and Clinical Pharmacology,* 7th ed. Stamford, CT: Appleton & Lange, 1997:762.)

Trimethoprim

Mechanism	Inhibits bacterial dihydrofolate reductase. Bacteriostatic.	**T**rimethoprim = **TMP:** "**T**reats **M**arrow **P**oorly."
Clinical use	Used in combination with sulfonamides (trimethoprim-sulfamethoxazole), causing sequential block of folate synthesis. Combination used for recurrent UTI, *Shigella, Salmonella, Pneumocystis carinii* pneumonia.	
Toxicity	Megaloblastic anemia, leukopenia, granulocytopenia. (May alleviate with supplemental folinic acid.)	

Fluoroquinolones

Ciprofloxacin, norfloxacin, ofloxacin, sparfloxacin, mortifloxacin, gatifloxacin, enoxacin (fluoroquinolones), nalidixic acid (a quinolone).

Mechanism	Inhibit DNA gyrase (topoisomerase II). Bactericidal.	Fluoroquino**LONES** hurt
Clinical use	Gram-negative rods of urinary and GI tracts (including *Pseudomonas*), *Neisseria*, some gram-positive organisms.	attachments to your **BONES.**
Toxicity	GI upset, superinfections, skin rashes, headache, dizziness. Contraindicated in pregnant women and in children because animal studies show damage to cartilage. Tendonitis and tendon rupture in adults.	

Metronidazole

Mechanism	Forms toxic metabolites in the bacterial cell. Bactericidal.
Clinical use	Antiprotozoal. *Giardia*, *Entamoeba*, *Trichomonas*, *Gardnerella vaginalis*, anaerobes (*Bacteroides*, *Clostridium*). Used with bismuth and amoxicillin or tetracycline for "triple therapy" against *H. pylori*.
Toxicity	Disulfiram-like reaction with alcohol, headache.

GET on the **Metro!** Anaerobic infection below the diaphragm.

Polymyxins

Polymyxin B, polymyxin E.

Mechanism	Bind to cell membranes of bacteria and disrupt their osmotic properties. Polymyxins are cationic, basic proteins that act like detergents.
Clinical use	Resistant gram-negative infections.
Toxicity	Neurotoxicity, acute renal tubular necrosis.

Isoniazid (INH)

Mechanism	Decreases synthesis of mycolic acids.
Clinical use	*Mycobacterium tuberculosis*. The only agent used as solo prophylaxis against TB.
Toxicity	Hemolysis if G6PD deficient, neurotoxicity, hepatotoxicity, SLE-like syndrome. Pyridoxine (vitamin B$_6$) can prevent neurotoxicity.

INH Injures Neurons and Hepatocytes.
Different INH half-lives in fast vs. slow acetylators.

UCV *Pharm.29*

Rifampin

Mechanism	Inhibits DNA-dependent RNA polymerase.
Clinical use	*Mycobacterium tuberculosis*; delays resistance to dapsone when used for leprosy. Always used in combination with other drugs except in the treatment of meningococcal carrier state, and chemoprophylaxis in contacts of children with *H. influenzae* type B.
Toxicity	Minor hepatotoxicity and drug interactions (increased P450).

Rifampin's **4 R's:**
RNA polymerase inhibitor
Revs up microsomal P450
Red/orange body fluids
Rapid resistance if used alone

UCV *Pharm.53*

Anti-TB drugs

Rifampin, Ethambutol, Streptomycin, Pyrazinamide, Isoniazid (INH).
Cycloserine (2nd-line therapy)

RESPIre.
INH is used alone for TB prophylaxis.
All are hepatotoxic.

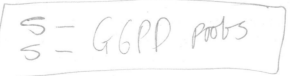

Resistance mechanisms for various antibiotics

Drug	Most common mechanism
Penicillins/ cephalosporins	β-lactamase cleavage of β-lactam ring
Aminoglycosides	Modification via acetylation, adenylation, or phosphorylation
Vancomycin	Terminal D-ala of cell wall component replaced with D-lac; ↓ affinity.
Chloramphenicol	Modification via acetylation
Macrolides	Methylation of rRNA near erythromycin's ribosome-binding site
Tetracycline	↓ uptake or ↑ transport out of cell
Sulfonamides	Altered enzyme (bacterial dihydropteroate synthetase), ↓ uptake, or ↑ PABA synthesis

Nonsurgical antimicrobial prophylaxis

Meningococcal infection	Rifampin (drug of choice), minocycline.
Gonorrhea	Ceftriaxone.
Syphilis	Benzathine penicillin G.
History of recurrent UTIs	Trimethoprim-sulfamethoxazole (TMP-SMX).
PCP	TMP-SMX (drug of choice), aerosolized pentamidine.

[handwritten annotation:] Disulfiram rxn [Cefamandole, Metronidazole]

Amphotericin B

Mechanism	Binds ergosterol (unique to fungi); forms membrane pores that allow leakage of electrolytes and disrupt homeostasis.	Amphotericin "tears" holes in the fungal membrane by forming pores.
Clinical use	Used for wide spectrum of systemic mycoses. *Cryptococcus, Blastomyces, Coccidioides, Aspergillus, Histoplasma, Candida, Mucor* (systemic mycoses). Intrathecally for fungal meningitis; does not cross blood-brain barrier.	
Toxicity	Fever/chills ("shake and bake"), hypotension, nephrotoxicity, arrhythmias ("amphoterrible").	

UCV *Pharm.45*

Nystatin

Mechanism	Binds to ergosterol, disrupting fungal membranes.
Clinical use	"Swish and swallow" for oral candidiasis (thrush).

Fluconazole, ketoconazole, clotrimazole, miconazole, itraconazole

Mechanism	Inhibit fungal steroid (ergosterol) synthesis.
Clinical use	Systemic mycoses. Fluconazole for cryptococcal meningitis in AIDS patients and candidal infections of all types. Ketoconazole for *Blastomyces, Coccidioides, Histoplasma, Candida albicans*; hypercortisolism.
Toxicity	Hormone synthesis inhibition (gynecomastia), liver dysfunction (inhibits cyt. P450), fever, chills.

UCV *Pharm.51*

Griseofulvin

Mechanism	Interferes with microtubule function; disrupts mitosis. Deposits in keratin-containing tissues (e.g., nails).
Clinical use	Oral treatment of superficial infections; inhibits growth of dermatophytes (tinea, ringworm).
Toxicity	Teratogenic, carcinogenic, confusion, headaches, ↑ warfarin metabolism.

Antiviral chemotherapy

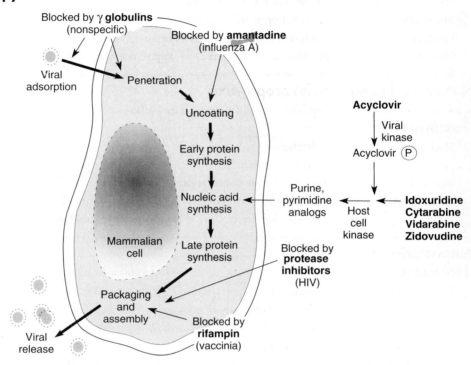

(Adapted, with permission, from Katzung BG, Trevor AJ. *Examination & Board Review: Pharmacology,* 5th ed. Stamford, CT: Appleton & Lange, 1998:359.)

Amantadine

Mechanism	Blocks viral penetration/uncoating; may buffer pH of endosome. Also causes the release of dopamine from intact nerve terminals.	Amantadine blocks influenza **A** and rubell**A** and causes problems with the cerebell**A**.
Clinical use	Prophylaxis for influenza A; Parkinson's disease.	
Toxicity	Ataxia, dizziness, slurred speech.	Rimantidine is a derivative with fewer CNS side effects.

UCV *Pharm.62*

Zanamivir

Mechanism	Inhibits influenza neuraminidase.
Clinical use	Both influenza A and B.

Ribavirin

Mechanism	Inhibits synthesis of guanine nucleotides by competitively inhibiting IMP dehydrogenase.
Clinical use	RSV.
Toxicity	Hemolytic anemia. Severe teratogen.

renal

Acyclovir   HEV

Mechanism	Preferentially inhibits viral DNA polymerase when phosphorylated by viral thymidine kinase.
Clinical use	HSV, VZV, EBV. Mucocutaneous and genital herpes lesions. Prophylaxis in immunocompromised patients.
Toxicity	Delirium, tremor, nephrotoxicity.

renal

Ganciclovir

	DHPG (dihydroxy-2-propoxymethyl guanine)
Mechanism	Phosphorylation by viral kinase; preferentially inhibits CMV DNA polymerase.
Clinical use	CMV, especially in immunocompromised patients.
Toxicity	Leukopenia, neutropenia, thrombocytopenia, renal toxicity. More toxic to host enzymes than acyclovir.

renal

Foscarnet

Mechanism	Viral DNA polymerase inhibitor that binds to the pyrophosphate binding site of the enzyme. Does not require activation by viral kinase.	FOScarnet = pyroFOSphate analog.
Clinical use	CMV retinitis in immunocompromised patients when ganciclovir fails.	
Toxicity	Nephrotoxicity.	

HIV therapy

Protease inhibitors	Saquinavir, ritonavir, indinavir, nelfinavir, amprenavir.
Mechanism	Inhibit assembly of new virus by blocking protease enzyme.
Toxicity	GI intolerance (nausea, diarrhea), hyperglycemia, lipid abnormalities, thrombocytopenia (indinavir).
Reverse transcriptase inhibitors	
Nucleosides	Zidovudine (AZT), didanosine (ddI), zalcitabine (ddC), stavudine (d4T), lamivudine (3TC), abacavir.
Non-nucleosides	Nevirapine, delavirdine, efavirenz.
Mechanism	Preferentially inhibit reverse transcriptase of HIV; prevent incorporation of viral genome into host DNA.
Toxicity	Bone marrow suppression (neutropenia, anemia), peripheral neuropathy, lactic acidosis (nucleosides), rash (non-nucleosides), megaloblastic anemia (AZT).
Clinical use	"Triple therapy" generally entails use of 2 nucleoside reverse transcriptase inhibitors with a protease inhibitor, although other combinations, such as the substitution of a non-nucleoside for a protease inhibitor, are used. Initiated when patients have low CD4 counts (< 500 cells/mm^3) or high viral load. AZT is used during pregnancy to reduce risk of fetal transmission.

Interferons

Mechanism	Glycoproteins from human leukocytes that block various stages of viral RNA and DNA synthesis.
Clinical use	Chronic hepatitis B and C, Kaposi's sarcoma.
Toxicity	Neutropenia.

Antiparasitic drugs

Ivermectin	Onchocerciasis (r**IVER** blindness treated with r**IVER**mectin).
Mebendazole/ thiabendazole	✓ Nematode/roundworm (e.g., pinworm, whipworm) infections. *round the bend.*
Pyrantel pamoate	Giant roundworm (*Ascaris*), hookworm (*Necator/Ancylostoma*), pinworm (*Enterobius*).
Praziquantel	✓ Trematode/fluke (e.g., schistosomes, *Paragonimus, Clonorchis*) and cysticercosis.
Niclosamide	✓ Cestode/tapeworm (e.g., *Diphyllobothrium latum, Taenia* species) infections except cysticercosis.
Pentavalent antimony	Leishmaniasis.
Chloroquine, quinine, mefloquine	Malaria.
Primaquine **VO**	Latent hypnozoite (liver) forms of malaria (*Plasmodium vivax, P. ovale*).
Metronidazole ✓	Giardiasis, amebic dysentery (*Entamoeba histolytica*), bacterial vaginitis (*Gardnerella vaginalis*), *Trichomonas*.
Pentamidine ✓	*Pneumocystis carinii* pneumonia prophylaxis.
Nifurtimox	Chagas' disease, American trypanosomiasis (*Trypanosoma cruzi*).
Suramin	African trypanosomiasis (sleeping sickness).

PHARMACOLOGY—CENTRAL NERVOUS SYSTEM

Central and peripheral nervous system

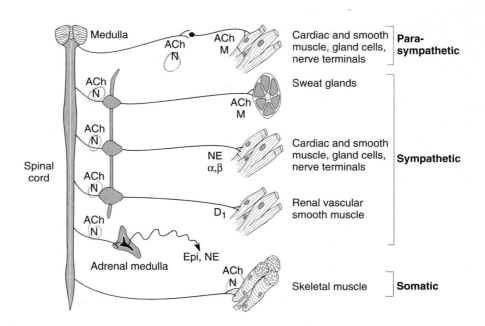

(Adapted, with permission, from Katzung BG. *Basic and Clinical Pharmacology,* 7th ed. Stamford, CT: Appleton & Lange, 1997:74.)

Autonomic drugs

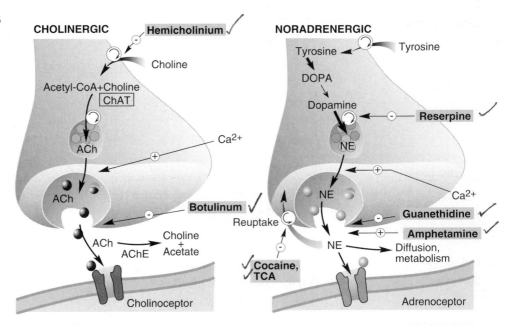

(Adapted, with permission, from Katzung BG, Trevor AJ. *Examination & Board Review: Pharmacology,* 5th ed. Stamford, CT: Appleton & Lange, 1998:42.)

Circles with rotating arrows represent transporters; ChAT, choline acetyltransferase; ACh, acetylcholine; AChE, acetylcholinesterase; NE, norepinephrine.

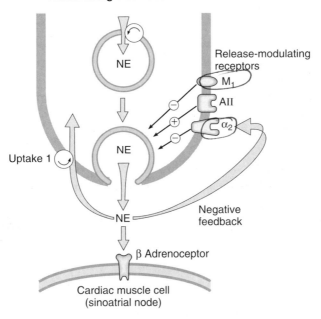

(Adapted, with permission, from Katzung BG, Trevor AJ. *Examination & Board Review: Pharmacology,* 5th ed. Stamford, CT: Appleton & Lange, 1998:42.)

Release of norepinephrine from a sympathetic nerve ending is modulated by norepinephrine itself, acting on presynaptic α_2 autoreceptors, and by acetylcholine, angiotensin II, and other substances.

Cholinomimetics

Drug

Direct agonists	Clinical applications	Action
Bethanechol	Postoperative and neurogenic ileus and urinary retention	Activates bowel and bladder smooth muscle
Carbachol, pilocarpine	Glaucoma	Activates ciliary muscle of eye (open angle), pupillary sphincter (narrow angle)

Indirect agonists (anticholinesterases)

Neostigmine	Postoperative and neurogenic ileus and urinary retention, myasthenia gravis, reversal of NMJ blockade (postoperative)	↑ endogenous ACh
Pyridostigmine	Myasthenia gravis	↑ endogenous ACh; ↑ strength
Edrophonium	Diagnosis of myasthenia gravis (extremely short acting)	↑ endogenous ACh
Physostigmine	Glaucoma (crosses blood-brain barrier → CNS) and atropine overdose	↑ endogenous ACh
Echothiophate	Glaucoma	↑ endogenous ACh

Cholinesterase inhibitor poisoning

Symptoms include **D**iarrhea, **U**rination, **M**iosis, **B**ronchospasm, **B**radycardia, **E**xcitation of skeletal muscle and CNS, **L**acrimation, **S**weating, **S**alivation (also abdominal cramping).

Cholinesterase regenerator (antidote)—pralidoxime regenerates active cholinesterase, chemical antagonist, used to treat organophosphate exposure.

DUMBBELSS.

Parathion and other organophosphates.

Cholinoreceptor blockers

Muscarinic antagonists	Atropine is used to dilate pupil, ↓ acid secretion in acid-peptic disease, ↓ urgency in mild cystitis, ↓ GI motility, reduce airway secretions, and treat organophosphate poisoning. Causes ↑ body temperature, rapid pulse, dry mouth, dry/flushed skin, disorientation, mydriasis with cycloplegia, and constipation.	Blocks **SLUD**: Salivation Lacrimation Urination Defecation Atropine parasympathetic block side effects: Blind as a bat Red as a beet Mad as a hatter Hot as a hare Dry as a bone
Nicotinic antagonists	Hexamethonium—ganglionic blocker.	

Antimuscarinic drugs

Organ system	Drugs	Application
CNS	Benztropine	Parkinson's disease
	Scopolamine	Motion sickness
HAT Eye	Atropine, homatropine, tropicamide	Produce mydriasis and cycloplegia
Respiratory	Ipratropium	Asthma, COPD

Neuromuscular blocking drugs

Used for muscle paralysis in surgery or mechanical ventilation.

Depolarizing

Succinylcholine.

Reversal of blockade:

- Phase I (prolonged depolarization)—no antidote. Block potentiated by cholinesterase inhibitors.
- Phase II (repolarized but blocked)—antidote consists of cholinesterase inhibitors (e.g., neostigmine).

Nondepolarizing

Tubocurarine, atracurium, mivacurium, pancuronium, vecuronium, rapacuronium.

Reversal of blockade—neostigmine, edrophonium, and other cholinesterase inhibitors.

Dantrolene

Used in the treatment of malignant hyperthermia, which is caused by the concomitant use of halothane and succinylcholine. Also used to treat neuroleptic malignant syndrome (a toxicity of antipsychotic drugs).

Mechanism: prevents the release of Ca^{2+} from the sarcoplasmic reticulum of skeletal muscle.

Sympathomimetics

Drug	Mechanism/selectivity	Applications
Catecholamines		
Epinephrine	Direct general agonist (α_1, α_2, β_1, β_2)	Anaphylaxis, glaucoma (open angle), asthma, hypotension
Norepinephrine	α_1, α_2, β_1	Hypotension (but ↓ renal perfusion)
Isoproterenol	$\beta_1 = \beta_2$	AV block (rare)
Dopamine	$D_1 = D_2 > \beta > \alpha$	Shock (↑ renal perfusion), heart failure
Dobutamine	$\beta_1 > \beta_2$	Shock, heart failure
Other		
Amphetamine Pharm.72, 73	Indirect general agonist, releases stored catecholamines	Narcolepsy, obesity, attention deficit disorder
Ephedrine	Indirect general agonist, releases stored catecholamines	Nasal decongestion, urinary incontinence, hypotension
Phenylephrine	$\alpha_1 > \alpha_2$	Pupil dilator, vasoconstriction, nasal decongestion
Albuterol, terbutaline	$\beta_2 > \beta_1$	Asthma
Cocaine Pharm.79	Indirect general agonist, uptake inhibitor	Causes vasoconstriction and local anesthesia
Clonidine, α-methyldopa	Centrally acting alpha agonist, ↓ central adrenergic outflow	Hypertension, especially with renal disease (no ↓ in blood flow to kidney)

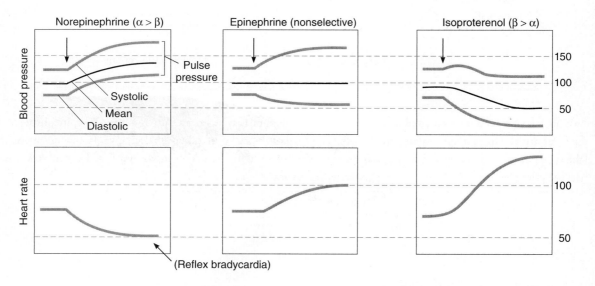

(Adapted, with permission, from Katzung BG, Trevor AJ. *Examination & Board Review: Pharmacology*, 5th ed. Stamford, CT: Appleton & Lange, 1998:72.)

Alpha blockers

Drugs	Application	Toxicity
Nonselective		
Phenoxybenzamine (irreversible) and phentolamine (reversible)	Pheochromocytoma	Orthostatic hypotension, reflex tachycardia
α_1 **selective**		
Prazosin, terazosin, doxazosin	Hypertension, urinary retention in BPH	1st-dose orthostatic hypotension, dizziness, headache
α_2 **selective**		
Yohimbine	Impotence (effectiveness is controversial)	

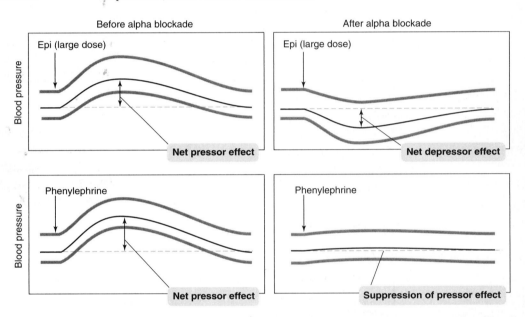

(Adapted, with permission, from Katzung BG, Trevor AJ. *Examination & Board Review: Pharmacology,* 5th ed. Stamford, CT: Appleton & Lange, 1998:80.)

Shown above are the effects of an alpha blocker (e.g., phentolamine) on blood pressure responses to epinephrine and phenylephrine. The epinephrine response exhibits reversal of the mean blood pressure change, from a net increase (the α response) to a net decrease (the β_2 response). The response to phenylephrine is suppressed but not reversed because phenylephrine is a "pure" alpha agonist without beta action.

*Propranol, metoprolol
labetalol are
Lipophilic*

Beta blockers

Propranolol, metoprolol, atenolol, nadolol, timolol, pindolol, esmolol, labetalol.

Application	Effect
Hypertension	↓ cardiac output, ↓ renin secretion.
Angina pectoris	↓ heart rate and contractility, resulting in ↓ oxygen consumption.
MI	Beta blockers ↓ mortality.
SVT (propranolol, esmolol)	↓ AV conduction velocity.
CHF	Slows progression of chronic failure
Glaucoma (timolol)	↓ secretion of aqueous humor

Toxicity Impotence, exacerbation of asthma, cardiovascular adverse effects (bradycardia, AV block, CHF), CNS adverse effects (sedation, sleep alterations); use with caution in diabetics. → mask signs of hypoglycemia.

Selectivity Nonselective ($\beta_1 = \beta_2$)—propranolol, timolol, pindolol, nadolol, and labetalol (also blocks α_1 receptors).

β_1 selective ($\beta_1 > \beta_2$)—Acebutolol, Betaxolol, Esmolol (short acting), Atenolol, Metoprolol.   **A BEAM** of β_1 blockers.

UCV *Pharm.2*

Glaucoma drugs

Drug	Mechanism	Side effects
Alpha agonists		
Epinephrine	↑ outflow of aqueous humor	Mydriasis, stinging; do not use in closed-angle glaucoma
Brimonidine	↓ aqueous humor synthesis	No pupillary or vision changes
Beta blockers		
Timolol, betaxolol, carteolol	↓ aqueous humor secretion	No pupillary or vision changes
Cholinomimetics		
Pilocarpine, carbachol, physostigmine, echothiophate	Ciliary muscle contraction, opening of trabecular meshwork; ↑ outflow of aqueous humor	Miosis, cyclospasm
Diuretics		
Acetazolamide, dorzolamide, brinzolamide	↓ aqueous humor secretion due to decreased HCO_3^- (via inhibition of carbonic anhydrase)	No pupillary or vision changes
Prostaglandin		
Latanoprost	Increased outflow of aqueous humor	Darkens color of iris (browning)

Barbiturates

Phenobarbital, pentobarbital, thiopental, secobarbital.

Mechanism	Facilitate $GABA_A$ action by ↑ **duration** of Cl^- channel opening, thus ↓ neuron firing.	Barbi**DURAT**e (increased **DURAT**ion).
Clinical use	Sedative for anxiety, seizures, insomnia, induction of anesthesia (thiopental).	Contraindicated in porphyria.
Toxicity	Dependence, additive CNS depression effects with alcohol, respiratory or cardiovascular depression (can lead to death), drug interactions owing to induction of liver microsomal enzymes (cyt. P450).	

UCV *Pharm.74*

Benzodiazepines

Diazepam, lorazepam, triazolam, temazepam, oxazepam, midazolam, chlordiazepoxide.

Mechanism	Facilitate $GABA_A$ action by ↑ **frequency** of Cl⁻ channel opening. Most have long half-lives and active metabolites.	FREnzodiazepines (increased FREquency). Short acting = **TOM** Thumb = **T**riazolam, **O**xazepam, **M**idazolam.
Clinical use	Anxiety, spasticity, status epilepticus (diazepam), detoxification (especially alcohol withdrawal–delirium tremens).	
Toxicity	Dependence, additive CNS depression effects with alcohol. Less risk of respiratory depression and coma than with barbiturates. Treat overdose with flumazenil (competitive antagonist at GABA receptor).	

Antipsychotics (neuroleptics)

Thioridazine, haloperidol, fluphenazine, chlorpromazine. CHFT

Mechanism	Most antipsychotics block dopamine D_2 receptors (excess dopamine effects connected with schizophrenia).	Evolution of EPS side effects: 4 h acute dystonia 4 d akinesia
Clinical use	Schizophrenia, psychosis.	4 wk akathisia
Toxicity	Extrapyramidal system side effects, sedation, endocrine side effects, and side effects arising from blocking muscarinic, α, and histamine receptors.	4 mo tardive dyskinesia (often irreversible)
	Neuroleptic malignant syndrome—rigidity, autonomic instability, hyperpyrexia (treat with dantrolene and dopamine agonists). *Pharm.84, 88*	
	Tardive dyskinesia—stereotypic oral-facial movements probably due to dopamine receptor sensitization; results of long-term antipsychotic use. *Pharm.87*	

UCV

Atypical antipsychotics
ROCk

Clozapine, olanzapine, risperidone.

Mechanism	Block $5HT_2$ and dopamine receptors.
Clinical use	Treatment of schizophrenia; useful for positive and negative symptoms. **Olanzapine** is also used for OCD, anxiety disorder, and depression.
Toxicity	Fewer extrapyramidal and anticholinergic side effects than other antipsychotics. **Clozapine** may cause agranulocytosis (requires weekly WBC monitoring).

Lithium

Mechanism	Not established; possibly related to inhibition of phosphoinositol cascade.
Clinical use	Mood stabilizer for bipolar affective disorder; blocks relapse and acute manic events.
Toxicity	Tremor, hypothyroidism, polyuria (ADH antagonist causing nephrogenic DI), teratogenesis. Narrow therapeutic window requiring close monitoring of serum levels.

UCV *Pharm.81*

Tricyclic antidepressants

Imipramine, amitriptyline, desipramine, nortriptyline, clomipramine, doxepin.

Mechanism	Block reuptake of norepinephrine and serotonin.
Clinical use	Endogenous depression, bedwetting (imipramine), obsessive-compulsive disorder (clomipramine).
Side effects	Sedation, alpha-blocking effects, atropine-like (anticholinergic) side effects (tachycardia, urinary retention). 3° TCAs (amitriptyline) have more anticholinergic effects than do 2° TCAs (nortriptyline). Desipramine is the least sedating.
Toxicity	**Tri-Cs**: Convulsions, Coma, Cardiotoxicity (arrhythmias); also respiratory depression, hyperpyrexia. Confusion and hallucinations in elderly due to anticholinergic side effects.

UCV Pharm.89

SSRIs

Fluoxetine, sertraline, paroxetine, citalopram.

Mechanism	Serotonin-specific reuptake inhibitors.	It normally takes 2–3 weeks for antidepressants to have an effect.
Clinical use	Endogenous depression.	
Toxicity	Fewer than TCAs. CNS stimulation—anxiety, insomnia, tremor, anorexia, nausea, and vomiting. "Serotonin syndrome" with MAOIs—hyperthermia, muscle rigidity, CV collapse.	

Heterocyclics

2nd- and 3rd-generation antidepressants with varied and mixed mechanisms of action. Used in major depressive disorders.

Trazodone	Primarily inhibit serotonin reuptake. Toxicity: sedation, nausea, priapism, postural hypotension.
Buproprion	Also used for smoking cessation. Mechanism not well known. Toxicity: stimulant effects (tachycardia, agitation), dry mouth, aggravation of psychosis.
Venlafaxine	Also used in generalized anxiety disorder. Inhibits serotonin and dopamine reuptake. Toxicity: stimulant effects (anxiety, agitation, headache, insomnia).
Mirtazapine	α_2 antagonist (increases release of norepinephrine and serotonin) and potent $5HT_2$ receptor antagonist. Toxicity: sedation, increased serum cholesterol, increased appetite.

Monoamine oxidase (MAO) inhibitors

Phenelzine, tranylcypromine.

Mechanism	Nonselective MAO inhibition.
Clinical use	Atypical depressions (i.e., with psychotic or phobic features), anxiety, hypochondriasis.
Toxicity	Hypertensive crisis with tyramine ingestion (in many foods) and meperidine; CNS stimulation. Contraindication with SSRIs or beta agonists.

UCV Pharm.83

Selegiline (deprenyl)

Mechanism	Selectively inhibits MAO-B, thereby increasing the availability of dopamine.
Clinical use	Adjunctive agent to L-dopa in treatment of Parkinson's disease.
Toxicity	May enhance adverse effects of L-dopa.

L-dopa (levodopa)/carbidopa

Mechanism	↑ level of dopamine in brain. Parkinsonism thought to be due to loss of dopaminergic neurons and excess cholinergic function. Unlike dopamine, L-dopa can cross blood-brain barrier and is converted by dopa decarboxylase in the CNS to dopamine.
Clinical use	Parkinsonism.
Toxicity	Arrhythmias from peripheral conversion to dopamine. Carbidopa, a peripheral decarboxylase inhibitor, is given with L-dopa in order to ↑ the bioavailability of L-dopa in the brain and to limit peripheral side effects. Dyskinesias also occur.

UCV *Pharm.67*

Parkinson's disease drugs

Dopamine agonists	L-dopa/carbidopa, bromocriptine (an ergot alkaloid and partial dopamine agonist), amantadine (enhances dopamine release).	**BALSA:** Bromocriptine Amantadine
MAO inhibitors	Selegiline (selective MAO type B inhibitor).	Levodopa
Antimuscarinics	Benztropine (improves tremor and rigidity but has little effect on bradykinesia).	Selegiline Antimuscarinics

Opioid analgesics

Morphine, fentanyl, codeine, heroin, methadone, meperidine, dextromethorphan.

Mechanism	Act as agonists at opioid receptors (mu = morphine, delta = enkephalin, kappa = dynorphin) to modulate synaptic transmission.
Clinical use	Pain, cough suppression (dextromethorphan), diarrhea (loperamide and diphenoxylate), acute pulmonary edema, maintenance programs for addicts (methadone).
Toxicity	Addiction, **respiratory depression,** constipation, miosis (**pinpoint pupils**), additive **CNS depression** with other drugs. Tolerance does not develop to miosis and constipation. Toxicity treated with naloxone or naltrexone (opioid receptor antagonist).

UCV *Pharm.80, 86*

Sumatriptan

Mechanism	5-HT_{1D} agonist. Half-life < 2 hours.
Clinical use	Acute migraine, cluster headache attacks.
Toxicity	Chest discomfort, mild tingling (contraindicated in patients with CAD or Prinzmetal's angina).

Ondansetron

Mechanism	5-HT_3 antagonist. Powerful central-acting antiemetic.
Clinical use	Control vomiting postoperatively and in patients undergoing cancer chemotherapy.
Toxicity	Headache, diarrhea.

You will not vomit with **ONDANS**etron, so you can go **ON DANC**ing.

Epilepsy drugs

	PARTIAL		GENERALIZED			
	Simple	Complex	Tonic-Clonic	Absence	Status	Notes
Phenytoin	✓	✓	✓		✓	Also a Class IB antiarrhythmic
Carbamazepine	✓	✓	✓			Monitor LFTs weekly
Lamotrigine	✓	✓	✓			
Gabapentin	✓	✓	✓			Adjunct in refractory seizures, renal excretion
Topiramate	✓	✓				Adjunct use
Phenobarbital			✓			Safer in pregnant women Crigler-Najjar II
Valproate			✓	✓		
Ethosuximide				✓		
Benzodiazepines (diazepam or lorazepam)					✓	

Epilepsy drug toxicities

Benzodiazepines	Sedation, tolerance, dependence.
Carbamazepine	Diplopia, ataxia, induction of cyt. P450, blood dyscrasias (agranulocytosis, aplastic anemia), liver toxicity (always check LFTs).
Ethosuximide	Gastrointestinal distress, lethargy, headache, urticaria, Stevens-Johnson syndrome.
Phenobarbital	Sedation, induction of cyt. P450, tolerance, dependence.
Phenytoin	Nystagmus, diplopia, ataxia, sedation, gingival hyperplasia, hirsutism, anemias, birth defects (teratogenic).
Valproic acid	Gastrointestinal distress, rare but fatal hepatotoxicity (measure LFTs), neural tube defects in fetus (spina bifida).
Lamotrigine	Life-threatening rash, Stevens-Johnson syndrome.
Gabapentin	Sedation, movement disorders.
Topiramate	Sedation, mental dulling, kidney stones, weight loss.

UCV Pharm. 63, 64, 70, 74

Phenytoin

Mechanism	Use-dependent blockade of Na^+ channels.
Clinical use	Grand mal seizures.
Toxicity	Nystagmus, ataxia, diplopia, lethargy. Chronic use produces gingival hyperplasia in children, peripheral neuropathy, hirsutism, megaloblastic anemia ($\downarrow$ vitamin B_{12}), and malignant hyperthermia (rare); teratogenic (fetal hydantoin syndrome).

UCV Pharm. 70

Pharmacology

Anesthetics— general principles

Drugs with ↓ solubility in blood = rapid induction and recovery times.

Drugs with ↑ solubility in lipids = ↑ potency = $\dfrac{1}{\text{MAC}}$.

Examples: N_2O has low blood and lipid solubility, and thus fast induction and low potency. Halothane, in contrast, has ↑ lipid and blood solubility, and thus high potency and slow induction.

Inhaled anesthetics

Halothane, enflurane, isoflurane, sevoflurane, methoxyflurane, nitrous oxide.

Mechanism | The lower the solubility in blood, the quicker the anesthetic induction and the quicker the recovery.

Effects | Myocardial depression, respiratory depression, nausea/emesis, ↑ cerebral blood flow.

Toxicity | Hepatotoxicity (halothane), nephrotoxicity (methoxyflurane), proconvulsant (enflurane), malignant hyperthermia (rare).

UCV *Pharm.28, 68*

Intravenous anesthetics

Barbiturates | Thiopental—high lipid solubility, rapid entry into brain. Used for induction of anesthesia and short surgical procedures. Effect terminated by redistribution from brain. ↓ cerebral blood flow.

Benzodiazepines | Midazolam most common drug used for endoscopy; used adjunctively with gaseous anesthetics and narcotics. May cause severe postoperative respiratory depression and amnesia.

Arylcyclohexylamines | Ketamine (PCP analog) acts as dissociative anesthetic. Cardiovascular stimulant. Causes disorientation, hallucination, and bad dreams. Increases cerebral blood flow. *Pharm.66*

Narcotic analgesics | Morphine, fentanyl used with other CNS depressants during general anesthesia.

Other | Propofol used for rapid anesthesia induction and short procedures. Less postoperative nausea than thiopental.

Local anesthetics

Esters—procaine, cocaine, tetracaine; amides—lIdocaine, bupIvacaine (amIdes have 2 I's in name).

Mechanism | Block Na^+ channels by binding to specific receptors on inner portion of channel. 3° amine local anesthetics penetrate membrane in uncharged form, then bind in charged form.

Principle | 1. In infected (acidic) tissue, anesthetics are charged and cannot penetrate membrane effectively. Therefore more anesthetic is needed in these cases.
2. Order of nerve blockade—small-diameter fibers > large diameter. Myelinated fibers > unmyelinated fibers. Overall, size factor predominates over myelination such that small unmyelinated pain fibers > small myelinated autonomic fibers > large myelinated autonomic fibers. Order of loss—pain (lose first) > temperature > touch > pressure (lose last).
3. Given with vasoconstrictors (usually epinephrine) to enhance local action.

Clinical use | Minor surgical procedures, spinal anesthesia. If allergic to esters, give amides.

Toxicity | CNS excitation, severe cardiovascular toxicity (bupivacaine), hypertension and arrhythmias (cocaine).

Antihypertensive drugs

Drug	Adverse effects
Diuretics	
Hydrochlorothiazide	Hypokalemia, slight hyperlipidemia, hyperuricemia, lassitude, hypercalcemia, hyperglycemia
Loop diuretics	Potassium wasting, metabolic alkalosis, hypotension, ototoxicity
Sympathoplegics	
Clonidine	Dry mouth, sedation, severe rebound hypertension
Methyldopa	Sedation, positive Coombs' test *Pharm.7*
Ganglionic blockers	Severe orthostatic hypotension, blurred vision, constipation, sexual dysfunction
Reserpine	Sedation, depression, nasal stuffiness, diarrhea
Guanethidine	Orthostatic and exercise hypotension, sexual dysfunction, diarrhea
Prazosin	1st-dose orthostatic hypotension, dizziness, headache
Beta blockers	Impotence, asthma, CV effects (bradycardia, CHF, AV block), CNS effects (sedation, sleep alterations)
Vasodilators	
Hydralazine[a]	Nausea, headache, lupus-like syndrome, reflex tachycardia, angina, salt retention
Minoxidil[a]	Hypertrichosis, pericardial effusion, reflex tachycardia, angina, salt retention
Nifedipine, verapamil	Dizziness, flushing, constipation (verapamil), nausea
Nitroprusside	Cyanide toxicity (releases CN)
ACE inhibitors	
Captopril	Fetal renal toxicity, hyperkalemia, **C**ough, **A**ngioedema, **P**roteinuria, **T**aste changes, hyp**O**tension, **P**regnancy problems (fetal renal damage), **R**ash, **I**ncreased renin, **L**ower AII
AII receptor inhibitors	
Losartan	Fetal renal toxicity, hyperkalemia

[a]Use with beta blockers to prevent reflex tachycardia; diuretic to block salt retention.

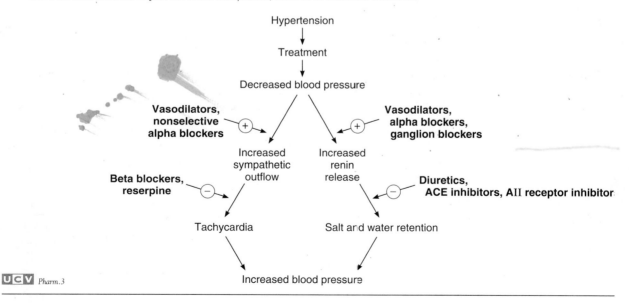

Hydralazine

Mechanism	$\uparrow$ cGMP $\rightarrow$ smooth muscle relaxation. Vasodilates arterioles > veins; afterload reduction.
Clinical use	Severe hypertension, CHF.
Toxicity	Compensatory tachycardia, fluid retention. Lupus-like syndrome.

Calcium channel blockers

Nifedipine, verapamil, diltiazem.

Mechanism	Block voltage-dependent L-type calcium channels of cardiac and smooth muscle and thereby reduce muscle contractility.
	Vascular smooth muscle—nifedipine > diltiazem > verapamil.
	Heart—verapamil > diltiazem > nifedipine.
Clinical use	Hypertension, angina, arrhythmias.
Toxicity	Cardiac depression, peripheral edema, flushing, dizziness, and constipation.

UCV *Pharm.11*

ACE inhibitors

Captopril, enalapril, lisinopril.

Mechanism	Inhibit angiotensin-converting enzyme, reducing levels of angiotensin II and preventing inactivation of bradykinin, a potent vasodilator. Renin release is $\uparrow$ due to loss of feedback inhibition.	**Losartan** is an angiotensin II receptor antagonist. It is **not** an ACE inhibitor and does not cause cough.
Clinical use	Hypertension, congestive heart failure, diabetic renal disease.	
Toxicity	**C**ough, **A**ngioedema, **P**roteinuria, **T**aste changes, hyp**O**tension, **P**regnancy problems (fetal renal damage), **R**ash, **I**ncreased renin, **L**ower AII, hyperkalemia.	**CAPTOPRIL.**

Acetazolamide

Mechanism	Carbonic anhydrase inhibitor. Causes self-limited $NaHCO_3$ diuresis and reduction in total-body HCO_3^- stores. Acts at the proximal convoluted tubule.	
Clinical use	Glaucoma, urinary alkalinization, metabolic alkalosis, altitude sickness.	
Toxicity	Hyperchloremic metabolic acidosis, neuropathy, NH_3 toxicity, sulfa allergy.	**ACID**azolamide causes **ACID**osis.

Furosemide

Mechanism	Sulfonamide loop diuretic. Inhibits cotransport system (Na^+, K^+, $2\ Cl^-$) of thick ascending limb of loop of Henle. Abolishes hypertonicity of medulla, preventing concentration of urine. $\uparrow Ca^{2+}$ excretion.	Loops Lose calcium.
Clinical use	Edematous states (CHF, cirrhosis, nephrotic syndrome, pulmonary edema), HTN, hypercalcemia.	
Toxicity	**O**totoxicity, **H**ypokalemia, **D**ehydration, **A**llergy (sulfa), **N**ephritis (interstitial), **G**out.	**OH DANG!**

UCV *Pharm.57*

Ethacrynic acid

Mechanism	Phenoxyacetic acid derivative (NOT a sulfonamide). Essentially same action as furosemide.
Clinical use	Diuresis in patients allergic to sulfa drugs.
Toxicity	Similar to furosemide except no hyperuricemia, no sulfa allergies.

Hydrochlorothiazide

Mechanism	Thiazide diuretic. Inhibits NaCl reabsorption in early distal tubule, reducing diluting capacity of the nephron. Decreases Ca^{2+} excretion.	
Clinical use	Hypertension, congestive heart failure, idiopathic hypercalciuria, nephrogenic diabetes insipidus.	
Toxicity	Hypokalemic metabolic alkalosis, hyponatremia, hyperGlycemia, hyperLipidemia, hyperUricemia, and hyperCalcemia. Sulfa allergy.	HyperGLUC.

K⁺-sparing diuretics

Spironolactone, Triamterene, Amiloride. The K⁺ STAys.

Mechanism	Spironolactone is a competitive aldosterone receptor antagonist in the cortical collecting tubule. Triamterene and amiloride act at the same part of the tubule by blocking Na^+ channels in the CCT.
Clinical use	Hyperaldosteronism, K⁺ depletion, CHF.
Toxicity	Hyperkalemia, endocrine effects (e.g. spironolactone causes gynecomastia, antiandrogen effects).

Mannitol

Mechanism	Osmotic diuretic, ↑ tubular fluid osmolarity, producing ↑ urine flow.
Clinical use	Shock, drug overdose, ↓ intracranial/intraocular pressure.
Toxicity	Pulmonary edema, dehydration. Contraindicated in anuria, CHF.

Diuretics: electrolyte changes

Urine NaCl	↑ (all diuretics—carbonic anhydrase inhibitors, loop diuretics, thiazides, K⁺-sparing diuretics).
Urine K⁺	↑ (all except K⁺-sparing diuretics).
Blood pH	↓ (acidosis)—carbonic anhydrase inhibitors, K⁺-sparing diuretics; ↑ (alkalosis)—loop diuretics, thiazides.
Urine Ca⁺	↑ loop diuretics, ↓ thiazides.

Diuretics: site of action

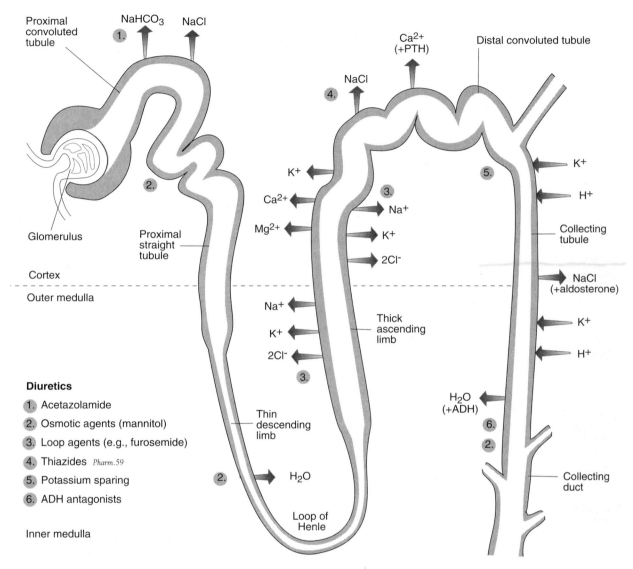

Diuretics

1. Acetazolamide
2. Osmotic agents (mannitol)
3. Loop agents (e.g., furosemide)
4. Thiazides *Pharm.59*
5. Potassium sparing
6. ADH antagonists

(Adapted, with permission, from Katzung BG. *Basic and Clinical Pharmacology*, 7th ed. Stamford, CT: Appleton & Lange, 1997:243.)

Antianginal therapy

Goal—reduction of myocardial O_2 consumption (MVO_2) by decreasing 1 or more of the determinants of MVO_2: end diastolic volume, blood pressure, heart rate, contractility, ejection time.

Component	Nitrates (affect preload)	Beta blockers (affect afterload)	Nitrates + beta blockers
End diastolic volume	↓	↑	No effect or ↓
Blood pressure	↓	↓	↓
Contractility	↑ (reflex response)	↓	Little/no effect
Heart rate	↑ (reflex response)	↓	↓
Ejection time	↓	↑	Little/no effect
MVO_2	↓	↓	↓↓

Calcium channel blockers—**N**ifedipine is similar to **N**itrates in effect; verapamil is similar to beta blockers in effect.

UCV *Pharm.9*

Nitroglycerin, isosorbide dinitrate

Mechanism	Vasodilate by releasing nitric oxide in smooth muscle, causing ↑ in cGMP and smooth muscle relaxation. Dilate veins >> arteries.
Clinical use	Angina, pulmonary edema. Also used as an aphrodisiac and erection enhancer.
Toxicity	Tachycardia, hypotension, headache, "Monday disease" in industrial exposure, development of tolerance for the vasodilating action during the work week and loss of tolerance over the weekend, resulting in tachycardia, dizziness, and headache.

Cardiac glycosides

Digoxin—75% bioavailability, 20–40% protein bound, $T_{1/2}$ = 40 hours, urinary excretion.

Mechanism	Inhibit the Na^+/K^+ ATPase of cell membrane, causing ↑ intracellular Na^+. Na^+-Ca^{2+} antiport does not function as efficiently, causing ↑ intracellular Ca^{2+}; leads to positive inotropy. May cause ↑ PR, ↓ QT, scooping of ST segment, T-wave inversion on ECG.
Clinical use	CHF, atrial fibrillation.
Toxicity	Nausea, vomiting, diarrhea. Blurry yellow vision (think Van Gogh). Arrhythmia. Toxicities of digoxin are ↑ by renal failure (↓ excretion), hypokalemia (potentiates drug's effects), and quinidine (↓ digoxin clearance; displaces digoxin from tissue binding sites).
Antidote	Slowly normalize K^+, lidocaine, cardiac pacer, anti-dig Fab fragments.

Cardiac drugs: sites of action

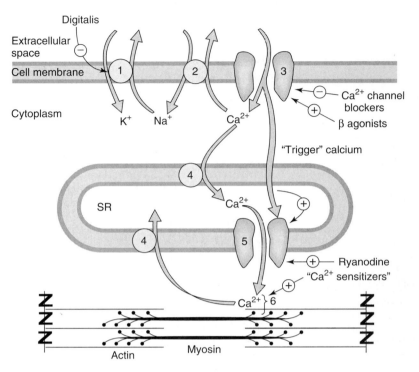

(Adapted, with permission, from Katzung BG. *Basic and Clinical Pharmacology*, 7th ed. Stamford, CT: Appleton & Lange, 1998:198.)

Cardiac sarcomere is shown above with the cellular components involved in excitation-contraction coupling. Factors involved in excitation-contraction coupling are numbered. (1) Na^+/K^+ ATPase; (2) Na^+-Ca^{2+} exchanger; (3) voltage-gated calcium channel; (4) calcium pump in the wall of the sarcoplasmic reticulum (SR); (5) calcium release channel in the SR; (6) site of calcium interaction with troponin-tropomyosin system.

Antiarrhythmics—Na⁺ channel blockers (class I)	Local anesthetics. Slow or block (↓) conduction (especially in depolarized cells). ↓ slope of phase 4 depolarization and ↑ threshold for firing in abnormal pacemaker cells. Are state dependent (selectively depress tissue that is frequently depolarized, e.g., fast tachycardia).	
Class IA	Quinidine, Amiodarone, Procainamide, Disopyramide. ↑ AP duration, ↑ effective refractory period (ERP), ↑ QT interval. Affect both atrial and ventricular arrhythmias. *Pharm.10* Toxicity: quinidine (cinchonism—headache, tinnitus; thrombocytopenia; torsades de pointes due to increased QT interval); procainamide (reversible SLE-like syndrome).	"Queen Amy Proclaims Diso's pyramid."
Class IB	Lidocaine, mexiletine, tocainide. ↓ AP duration. Affect ischemic or depolarized Purkinje and ventricular tissue. Useful in acute ventricular arrhythmias (especially post-MI) and in digitalis-induced arrhythmias. *Pharm.5* Toxicity: Local anesthetic. CNS stimulation/depression, cardiovascular depression.	
Class IC	Flecainide, encainide, propafenone. No effect on AP duration. Useful in V-tachs that progress to VF and in intractable SVT. Usually used only as last resort in refractory tachyarrhythmias because of toxicities. Toxicity: proarrhythmic.	

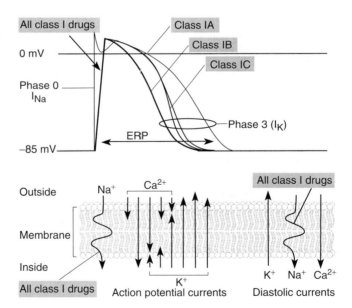

(Adapted, with permission, from Katzung BG, Trevor AJ. *Examination & Board Review: Pharmacology*, 5th ed. Stamford, CT: Appleton & Lange, 1998:118.)

HIGH-YIELD FACTS

Pharmacology

Antiarrhythmics— beta blockers (class II)

Propranolol, esmolol, metoprolol, atenolol, timolol.

Mechanism
$\downarrow$ cAMP, $\downarrow$ Ca^{2+} currents. Suppress abnormal pacemakers by $\downarrow$ slope of phase 4. AV node particularly sensitive—$\uparrow$ PR interval. Esmolol very short acting.

Toxicity
Impotence, exacerbation of asthma, CV effects (bradycardia, AV block, CHF), CNS effects (sedation, sleep alterations). May mask the signs of hypoglycemia.

UCV *Pharm.2*

Antiarrhythmics— K+ channel blockers (class III)

Sotalol, ibutilide, bretylium, amiodarone. *Pharm.1*

Mechanism
$\uparrow$ AP duration, $\uparrow$ ERP. Used when other antiarrhythmics fail. $\uparrow$ QT interval.

Remember to check **PFTs**, **LFTs**, and **TFTs** when using amiodarone.

Toxicity
Sotalol—torsades de pointes, excessive beta block; ibutilide—torsades; bretylium—new arrhythmias, hypotension; amiodarone—**pulmonary fibrosis,** corneal deposits, **hepatotoxicity,** skin deposits resulting in photodermatitis, neurologic effects, constipation, CV effects (bradycardia, heart block, CHF), **hypothyroidism/hyperthyroidism.**

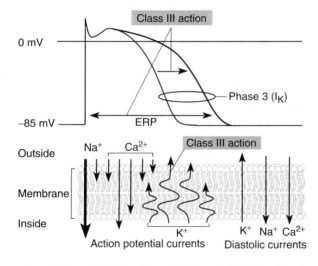

(Adapted, with permission, from Katzung BG, Trevor AJ. *Examination & Board Review: Pharmacology,* 5th ed. Stamford, CT: Appleton & Lange, 1998:120.)

UCV

Antiarrhythmics—Ca²⁺ channel blockers (class IV)

Verapamil, diltiazem.

Mechanism
: Primarily affect AV nodal cells. ↓ conduction velocity, ↑ ERP, ↑ PR interval. Used in prevention of nodal arrhythmias (e.g., SVT).

Toxicity
: Constipation, flushing, edema, CV effects (CHF, AV block, sinus node depression); torsades de pointes (bepridil).

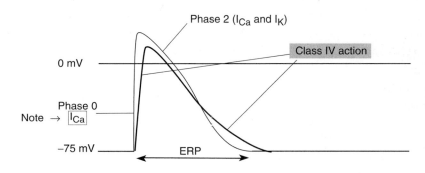

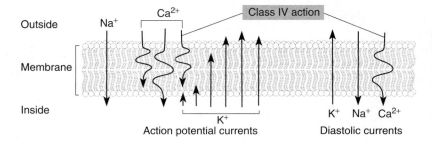

(Adapted, with permission, from Katzung BG, Trevor AJ. *Examination & Board Review: Pharmacology,* 5th ed. Stamford, CT: Appleton & Lange, 1998:121.)

Antiarrhythmics—miscellaneous

Adenosine
: Drug of choice in diagnosing/abolishing AV nodal arrhythmias.

K⁺
: Depresses ectopic pacemakers, especially in digoxin toxicity.

Mg⁺
: Effective in torsades de pointes and digoxin toxicity.

Lipid-lowering agents

Drug	Effect on LDL "bad cholesterol"	Effect on HDL "good cholesterol"	Effect on triglycerides	Side effects/problems
Bile acid resins (cholestyramine, colestipol)	↓↓	No effect	Slightly ↑	Patients hate it—tastes bad and causes GI discomfort
HMG-CoA reductase inhibitors (lovastatin, pravastatin, simvastatin, atorvastatin)	↓↓↓	↑	↓	Expensive, reversible ↑ LFTs, myositis
Niacin	↓↓	↑↑	↓	Red, flushed face, which is ↓ by aspirin or long-term use
Lipoprotein lipase stimulators (gemfibrozil, clofibrate)	↓	↑	↓↓↓	Myositis, ↑ LFTs

Pharm.7

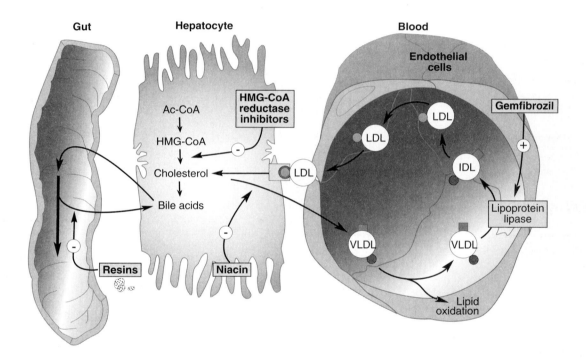

Cancer drugs—site of action

Nucleotide synthesis

1. Methotrexate— ↓ thymidine + purine synthesis
2. 5-FU— ↓ thymidine + purine synthesis
3. 6-MP

DNA

4. Alkylating agents + cisplatin—DNA cross-linkage
5. Dactinomycin + doxorubicin—intercalate DNA strands
6. Bleomycin
7. Etoposide—strand breakage

mRNA

8. Steroids
9. Tamoxifen

Protein

10. Vinca alkaloids—inhibit microtubule formation
11. Paclitaxel

Cell cycle specific— antimetabolites, plant alkaloids, steroid hormones, bleomycin, paclitaxel, etoposide.
Cell cycle nonspecific— alkylating agents, antibiotics.

Methotrexate

Mechanism	S-phase-specific antimetabolite. Folic acid analog that inhibits dihydrofolate reductase, resulting in decreased dTMP and therefore decreased DNA and protein synthesis.
Clinical use	Leukemias, lymphomas, choriocarcinoma, sarcomas. Abortion, ectopic pregnancy, rheumatoid arthritis, psoriasis.
Toxicity	Myelosuppression, which is reversible with leucovorin (folinic acid) "rescue." Macrovesicular fatty change in liver.

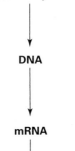 *Pharm.40*

5-fluorouracil (5-FU)

Mechanism	S-phase-specific antimetabolite. Pyrimidine analog bioactivated to 5F-dUMP, which covalently complexes folic acid. This complex inhibits thymidylate synthase, resulting in decreased dTMP and same effects as methotrexate.
Clinical use	Colon cancer and other solid tumors, basal cell carcinoma (topical). Synergy with methotrexate.
Toxicity	Myelosuppression, which is NOT reversible with leucovorin; photosensitivity.

6-mercaptopurine (6-MP)

Mechanism	Blocks purine synthesis.
Clinical use	Leukemias, lymphomas (not CLL or Hodgkin's).
Toxicity	Bone marrow, GI, liver. Metabolized by xanthine oxidase; thus ↑ toxicity with allopurinol.

Busulfan

Mechanism	Alkylates DNA.
Clinical use	CML.
Toxicity	Pulmonary fibrosis, hyperpigmentation.

HIGH-YIELD FACTS

Pharmacology

Cyclophosphamide

Mechanism	Alkylating agent; covalently x-links (interstrand) DNA at guanine N-7. Requires bioactivation by liver.
Clinical use	Non-Hodgkin's lymphoma, breast and ovarian carcinomas. Also an immunosuppressant.
Toxicity	Myelosuppression, hemorrhagic cystitis.

UCV *Pharm.36*

Nitrosoureas

Carmustine, lomustine, semustine, streptozocin.

Mechanism	Alkylate DNA. Require bioactivation. Cross blood-brain barrier → CNS.
Clinical use	Brain tumors (including glioblastoma multiforme).
Toxicity	CNS toxicity (dizziness, ataxia).

Cisplatin

Mechanism	Acts like an alkylating agent. X-links via hydrolysis of Cl^- groups and reaction with platinum.
Clinical use	Testicular, bladder, ovary, and lung carcinomas.
Toxicity	Nephrotoxicity and acoustic nerve damage.

UCV *Pharm.35*

Doxorubicin (Adriamycin)

Mechanism	Noncovalently intercalates in DNA, creating breaks to ↓ replication and transcription and generate free radicals.
Clinical use	Part of the **A**BVD combination regimen for Hodgkin's and for myelomas, sarcomas, and solid tumors (breast, ovary, lung).
Toxicity	Cardiotoxicity; also myelosuppression and marked alopecia. Toxic extravasation.

Bleomycin

Mechanism	Intercalates DNA strands and induces free radical formation, causing strand breaks.
Clinical use	Testicular cancer, lymphomas.
Toxicity	Pulmonary fibrosis, skin changes, minimal myelosuppression.

UCV *Pharm.34*

Etoposide

Mechanism	G_2-phase-specific inhibits topoisomerase II so that double-strand breaks remain in DNA following replication with subsequent DNA degradation.
Clinical use	Oat cell carcinoma of the lung and prostate, testicular carcinoma.
Toxicity	Myelosuppression, GI irritation, alopecia.

Prednisone

Mechanism	May trigger apoptosis. May even work on nondividing cells.
Clinical use	Most commonly used glucocorticoid in cancer chemotherapy. Used in CLL, Hodgkin's lymphomas (part of the MOPP regimen). Also an immunosuppressant used in autoimmune diseases.
Toxicity	Cushing-like symptoms; immunosuppression, cataracts, acne, osteoporosis, hypertension, peptic ulcers, hyperglycemia, psychosis.

Tamoxifen/raloxifene

Mechanism	Estrogen receptor mixed agonist/antagonist that blocks the binding of estrogen to ER+ cells.
Clinical use	Breast cancer.
Toxicity	Tamoxifen may increase the risk of endometrial carcinoma via partial agonist effects; "hot flashes."

Vincristine and vinblastine

Mechanism	M-phase-specific alkaloid that binds to tubulin and blocks polymerization of microtubules so that mitotic spindle can't form.
Clinical use	Part of the MOPP (Oncovin [vincristine]) regimen for lymphoma, Wilms' tumor, choriocarcinoma.
Toxicity	Vincristine—neurotoxicity (areflexia, peripheral neuritis), paralytic ileus. VinBLASTine BLASTs Bone marrow (suppression).

Paclitaxel

Mechanism	M-phase-specific agent obtained from yew tree that binds to tubulin and hyperstabilizes polymerized microtubules so that mitotic spindle can't break down (anaphase cannot occur).
Clinical use	Ovarian and breast carcinomas.
Toxicity	Myelosuppression and hypersensitivity.

HIGH-YIELD FACTS

Pharmacology

HIGH-YIELD FACTS

Pharmacology

Specific antidotes

Toxin	Antidote/treatment
1. Acetaminophen	1. N-acetylcysteine
2. Salicylates	2. Alkalinize urine, dialysis
3. Anticholinesterases, organophosphates	3. Atropine, pralidoxime
4. Antimuscarinic, anticholinergic agents	4. Physostigmine salicylate
5. Beta blockers	5. Glucagon
6. Digitalis	6. Stop dig, normalize K^+, lidocaine, anti-dig Fab fragments, Mg^{2+}
7. Iron	7. Deferoxamine
8. Lead	8. CaEDTA, dimercaprol, succimer, penicillamine
9. Arsenic, mercury, gold	9. Dimercaprol (BAL), succimer
10. Copper, arsenic, gold	10. Penicillamine
11. Cyanide	11. Nitrite, hydroxocobalamin, thiosulfate
12. Methemoglobin	12. Methylene blue
13. Carbon monoxide	13. 100% O_2, hyperbaric O_2
14. Methanol, ethylene glycol (antifreeze)	14. Ethanol, dialysis, fomepizole
15. Opioids	15. Naloxone/naltrexone
16. Benzodiazepines	16. Flumazenil
17. Tricyclic antidepressants	17. $NaHCO_3$ (nonspecific)
18. Heparin	18. Protamine
19. Warfarin	19. Vitamin K, fresh frozen plasma
20. t-PA, streptokinase	20. Aminocaproic acid

UCV *Pharm. 39, 92, 94, 96, 97, 99, 101, 102, 103*

Lead poisoning

Lead **L**ines on gingivae and on epiphyses of long bones on x-ray.
Encephalopathy and **E**rythrocyte basophilic stippling.
Abdominal colic and sideroblastic **A**nemia.
Drops—wrist and foot drop. Dimercaprol and EDTA first line of treatment.

LEAD.
High risk in houses with chipped paint.

UCV *Pharm. 101*

Urine pH and drug elimination

Weak acids (phenobarbital, methotrexate, aspirin) alkalinize urine with bicarbonate to ↑ clearance.
Weak bases (amphetamines) acidify urine to ↑ clearance (give NH_4Cl).

Drug reactions

Drug reaction	Causal agent
1. Pulmonary fibrosis	1. Bleomycin, amiodarone, busulfan *Pharm.34*
2. Hepatitis	2. Isoniazid (INH), halothane
3. Focal to massive hepatic necrosis	3. Halothane, valproic acid, acetaminophen, *Amanita phalloides*
4. Anaphylaxis	4. Penicillin
5. SLE-like syndrome *Pharm.91*	5. **H**ydralazine, **INH**, **P**rocainamide, **P**henytoin (it's not **HIPP** to have lupus)
6. Hemolysis in G6PD-deficient patients	6. Sulfonamides, INH, aspirin, ibuprofen, primaquine, nitrofurantoin, pyrimethamine, chloramphenicol
7. Thrombotic complications	7. Oral contraceptives (e.g., estrogens and progestins)
8. Adrenocortical insufficiency	8. Withdrawal of glucocorticoids (HPA suppression)
9. Photosensitivity reactions	9. **S**ulfonamides, **A**miodarone, **T**etracycline (**SAT** for a photo)
10. Induce (↑) P450 system	10. Barbiturates, phenytoin, carbamazepine, rifampin, griseofulvin, quinidine
11. Inhibit (↓) P450 system	11. Cimetidine, ketoconazole, grapefruit, erythromycin, INH, sulfonamides
12. Tubulointerstitial nephritis *Pharm.60*	12. Sulfonamides, furosemide, methicillin, rifampin, NSAIDs (except aspirin)
13. Hot flashes	13. Tamoxifen
14. Cutaneous flushing	14. Niacin, Ca^{2+} channel blockers, adenosine, vancomycin
15. Cardiac toxicity	15. Doxorubicin (Adriamycin), daunorubicin
16. Agranulocytosis	16. Clozapine, carbamazepine, colchicine
17. Stevens-Johnson syndrome	17. Ethosuximide, sulfonamides, lamotrigine *Pharm.12*
18. Cinchonism	18. Quinidine, quinine
19. Tendonitis, tendon rupture and cartilage damage (kids)	19. Fluoroquinolones *Pharm.49*
20. Disulfiram-like reaction	20. Metronidazole, certain cephalosporins, procarbazine, sulfonylureas
21. Ototoxicity and nephrotoxicity	21. Aminoglycosides, loop diuretics, cisplatin
22. Drug-induced Parkinson's	22. Haloperidol, chlorpromazine, reserpine, MPTP
23. Torsades de pointes	23. Class III (sotalol), class IA (quinidine) antiarrhythmics
24. Aplastic anemia	24. Chloramphenicol, benzene, NSAIDs
25. Neuro/nephrotoxicity	25. Polymyxins
26. Pseudomembranous colitis	26. Clindamycin, ampicillin
27. Gynecomastia	27. **S**pironolactone, **D**igitalis, **C**imetidine, chronic **A**lcohol use, estrogens, **K**etoconazole (**S**ome **D**rugs **C**reate **A**wesome **K**nockers)

HIGH-YIELD FACTS

Pharmacology

Drug reactions (continued)

28. Atropine-like side effects	28. Tricyclics
29. Cough	29. ACE inhibitors (losartan → no cough)
30. Gingival hyperplasia	30. Phenytoin
31. Diabetes insipidus	31. Lithium
32. Tardive dyskinesia	32. Antipsychotics
33. Fanconi's syndrome	33. Tetracycline
34. Gray baby syndrome	34. Chloramphenicol
35. Extrapyramidal side effects	35. Chlorpromazine, thioridazine, haloperidol
36. Osteoporosis	36. Corticosteroids, heparin

Alcohol toxicity

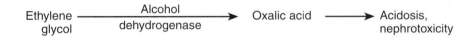

Ethylene glycol ──Alcohol dehydrogenase──▶ Oxalic acid ──▶ Acidosis, nephrotoxicity

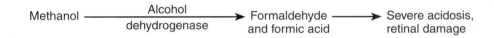

Methanol ──Alcohol dehydrogenase──▶ Formaldehyde and formic acid ──▶ Severe acidosis, retinal damage

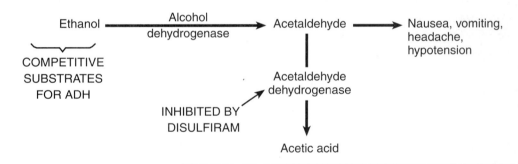

Ethanol ──Alcohol dehydrogenase──▶ Acetaldehyde ──▶ Nausea, vomiting, headache, hypotension

COMPETITIVE SUBSTRATES FOR ADH

Acetaldehyde dehydrogenase

INHIBITED BY DISULFIRAM

Acetic acid

UCV *Pharm.65, 99*

Coma treatment

ER treatment	Airway (protect)	**ABC,** then do the **DON'T**
	Breathing (assist)	(in that order):
	Circulation (assist)	Dextrose
	Dextrose (and thiamine, naloxone IV)	Oxygen
		Naloxone
		Thiamine
Rule out	Infections (lumbar puncture)	**IT'S COMA!**
	Trauma (bleeding, consider CT scan)	
	Seizure	
	Carbon monoxide (give O_2)	
	Overdose (pills)/Opioids (give naloxone)	
	Metabolic (hypothermia/hyperthermia, hypoglycemia/hyperglycemia, thiamine deficiency)	
	Alcohol (check serum osmolality)	

Sildenafil

Mechanism	Inhibits cGMP phosphodiesterase, causing ↑ cGMP, smooth muscle relaxation in the corpus cavernosum, ↑ blood flow, and penile erection.	Sildenafil **fills** the penis.
Clinical use	Treatment of erectile dysfunction.	
Toxicity	Headache, flushing, dyspepsia, blue-green color vision. Risk of life-threatening hypotension in patients taking nitrates.	

Clomiphene

Mechanism	A partial agonist at estrogen receptors in the pituitary gland. Prevents normal feedback inhibition and ↑ release of LH and FSH from the pituitary, which stimulates ovulation.
Clinical use	Treatment of infertility.
Toxicity	Hot flashes, ovarian enlargement, multiple simultaneous pregnancies, visual disturbances.

Mifepristone (RU-486)

Mechanism	Competitive inhibitor of progestins at progesterone receptors.
Clinical use	Abortifacient.
Toxicity	Heavy bleeding, GI effects (nausea, vomiting, anorexia), abdominal pain.

Oral contraception (synthetic progestins, estrogen)

Advantages	Disadvantages
Reliable (<1% failure)	Taken daily
↓ risk of endometrial and ovarian cancer	No protection against STDs
	↑ triglycerides
↓ incidence of ectopic pregnancy	Depression, weight gain, nausea, HTN
↓ pelvic infections	Hypercoagulable state
Regulation of menses	

H₂ blockers

	Cimetidine, ranitidine, famotidine, nizatidine.
Mechanism	Reversible block of histamine H₂ receptors.
Clinical use	Peptic ulcer, gastritis, esophageal reflux, Zollinger-Ellison syndrome.
Toxicity	Cimetidine is a potent inhibitor of P450; it also has an antiandrogenic effect and ↓ renal excretion of creatinine. Other H₂ blockers are relatively free of these effects.

UCV *Pharm.27*

Omeprazole, lansoprazole

Mechanism	Irreversibly inhibits H^+/K^+ ATPase in stomach parietal cells.
Clinical use	Peptic ulcer, gastritis, esophageal reflux, Zollinger-Ellison syndrome.

Sucralfate

Mechanism	Aluminum sucrose sulfate polymerizes in the acid environment of the stomach and selectively binds necrotic peptic ulcer tissue. Acts as a barrier to acid, pepsin, and bile. Sucralfate cannot work in the presence of antacids, H₂ blockers, or proton pump inhibitors (requires acidic environment to polymerize).
Clinical use	Peptic ulcer disease.

HIGH-YIELD FACTS

Pharmacology

Misoprostol

Mechanism	A PGE$_1$ analog. Increases production and secretion of gastric mucous barrier.
Clinical use	Prevention of NSAID-induced peptic ulcers, maintains a PDA. Also used to induce labor.
Toxicity	Diarrhea. Contraindicated in women of childbearing potential (abortifacient).

Antacid overuse

Can affect absorption, bioavailability, or urinary excretion of other drugs by altering gastric and urinary pH or by delaying gastric emptying.

Overuse can also cause the following problems:

1. Aluminum hydroxide—constipation and hypophosphatemia
2. Magnesium hydroxide—diarrhea
3. Calcium carbonate—hypercalcemia, rebound acid ↑

All can cause hypokalemia.

Al**uminimum** amount of feces.

Mg = **M**ust **g**o to the bathroom.

Heparin

Mechanism	Catalyzes the activation of antithrombin III. Short half-life. Check the aPTT.
Clinical use	Immediate anticoagulation for PE, stroke, angina, MI, DVT. Used during pregnancy (does not cross placenta). Follow PTT.
Toxicity	Bleeding, thrombocytopenia, drug-drug interactions. Use **protamine sulfate** for rapid reversal of heparinization (positively charged molecule that acts by binding negatively charged heparin).
Note	Newer **low-molecular-weight heparins** (enoxaparin) have better bioavailability and 2–4 times longer half-life. Can be administered subcutaneously and without laboratory monitoring.

UCV *Pharm.38*

Warfarin (Coumadin)

Mechanism	Interferes with normal synthesis and γ-carboxylation of vitamin K–dependent clotting factors II, VII, IX, and X, protein C and S via vitamin K antagonism. Long half-life.
Clinical use	Chronic anticoagulation. Not used in pregnant women (because warfarin, unlike heparin, can cross the placenta). Follow PT values.
Toxicity	Bleeding, teratogenic, drug-drug interactions.

WEPT—**W**arfarin affects the **E**xtrinsic **p**athway and prolongs the **PT.**

UCV *Pharm.42*

HIGH-YIELD FACTS

Pharmacology

Heparin vs. warfarin

	Heparin	Warfarin
Structure	Large anionic polymer, acidic	Small lipid-soluble molecule
Route of administration	Parenteral (IV, SC)	Oral
Site of action	Blood	Liver
Onset of action	Rapid (seconds)	Slow, limited by half-lives of normal clotting factors
Mechanism of action	Activates antithrombin III	Impairs the synthesis of vitamin K–dependent clotting factors II, VII, IX, and X (vitamin K antagonist)
Duration of action	Acute (hours)	Chronic (weeks or months)
Inhibits coagulation in vitro	Yes	No
Treatment of acute overdose	Protamine sulfate	IV vitamin K and fresh frozen plasma
Monitoring	aPTT (intrinsic pathway)	PT (extrinsic pathway)

Thrombolytics
Streptokinase, urokinase, t-PA (alteplase), APSAC (anistreplase).

Mechanism Directly or indirectly aid conversion of plasminogen to plasmin, which cleaves thrombin and fibrin clots. It is claimed that t-PA specifically converts fibrin-bound plasminogen to plasmin.

Clinical use Early myocardial infarction.

Toxicity Bleeding.

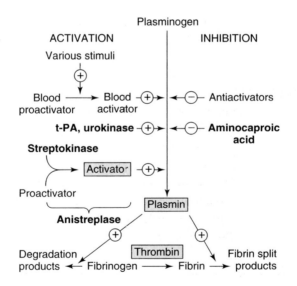

(Adapted, with permission, from Katzung BG. *Basic and Clinical Examination & Board Review: Pharmacology,* 7th ed. Stamford, CT: Appleton & Lange, 1997:550.)

Thrombolytic drugs are shown on the left in bold type. These drugs ↑ the formation of plasmin, the major fibrinolytic enzyme. Aminocaproic acid, a useful inhibitor of fibrinolysis, is shown on the right.

Clopidogrel, ticlopidine

Mechanism	Inhibit platelet aggregation by irreversibly inhibiting the ADP pathway involved in the binding of fibrinogen.
Clinical use	Acute coronary syndrome; coronary stenting. ↓ incidence or recurrence of thrombotic stroke.
Toxicity	Neutropenia (ticlopidine); reserved for those who cannot tolerate aspirin.

Arachidonic acid products

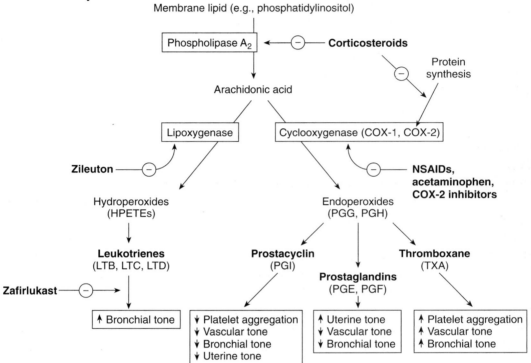

(Adapted, with permission, from Katzung BG and Trevor AJ. *Examination & Board Review: Pharmacology*, 5th ed. Stamford, CT: Appleton & Lange, 1998:150.)

Aspirin

Mechanism	Acetylates and irreversibly inhibits cyclooxygenase (both COX-1 and COX-2) to prevent conversion of arachidonic acid to prostaglandins.
Clinical use	Antipyretic, analgesic, anti-inflammatory, antiplatelet drug.
Toxicity	Gastric ulceration, bleeding, hyperventilation, Reye's syndrome, tinnitus (CN VIII).

UCV *Pharm.32, 110*

Other NSAIDs

	Ibuprofen, naproxen, indomethacin.
Mechanism	Reversibly inhibit cyclooxygenase (both COX-1 and COX-2). Block prostaglandin synthesis.
Clinical use	Antipyretic, analgesic, anti-inflammatory. Indomethacin is used to close a patent ductus arteriosus.
Toxicity	Renal damage, aplastic anemia, GI distress.

COX-2 inhibitors (celecoxib, rofecoxib)

Mechanism	Selectively inhibit cyclooxygenase (COX) isoform 2, which is found in inflammatory cells and mediates inflammation and pain; spares COX-1, which helps maintain the gastric mucosa. Thus, should not have the corrosive effects of other NSAIDs on the gastrointestinal lining.
Clinical use	Rheumatoid and osteoarthritis.
Toxicity	Similar to other NSAIDs; may have less toxicity to GI mucosa (i.e., lower incidence of ulcers, bleeding).

Acetaminophen

Mechanism	Reversibly inhibits cyclooxygenase, mostly in CNS. Inactivated peripherally.
Clinical use	Antipyretic, analgesic, but lacking anti-inflammatory properties.
Toxicity	Overdose produces hepatic necrosis; acetaminophen metabolite depletes glutathione and forms toxic tissue adducts in liver.

UCV Pharm.92

Glucocorticoids

	Hydrocortisone, prednisone, triamcinolone, dexamethasone, beclomethasone.
Mechanism	↓ the production of leukotrienes and prostaglandins by inhibiting phospholipase A_2 and expression of COX-2.
Clinical use	Addison's disease, inflammation, immune suppression, asthma.
Toxicity	Iatrogenic Cushing's syndrome—buffalo hump, moon facies, truncal obesity, muscle wasting, thin skin, easy bruisability, osteoporosis, adrenocortical atrophy, peptic ulcers.

UCV Pharm.15

Asthma drugs

Nonspecific beta agonists	**Isoproterenol**—relaxes bronchial smooth muscle (β_2). Adverse effect is tachycardia (β_1).
β_2 agonists	**Albuterol**—relaxes bronchial smooth muscle (β_2). Use during acute exacerbation.
	Salmeterol—long-acting agent for prophylaxis. Adverse effects are tremor and arrhythmia.
Methylxanthines	**Theophylline**—likely causes bronchodilation by inhibiting phosphodiesterase, thereby ↓ cAMP hydrolysis. The usage is limited because of narrow therapeutic index (cardiotoxicity, neurotoxicity).
Muscarinic antagonists	**Ipratropium**—competitive block of muscarinic receptors, preventing bronchoconstriction.
Cromolyn	Prevents release of mediators from mast cells. Effective only for the prophylaxis of asthma. Not effective during an acute asthmatic attack. Toxicity is rare.
Corticosteroids	**Beclomethasone, prednisone**—inhibits the synthesis of virtually all cytokines. Inactivates NF-κB, the transcription factor that induces the production of TNFα, among other inflammatory agents. 1st-line therapy for chronic asthma.
Antileukotrienes	**Zileuton**—A 5-lipoxygenase pathway inhibitor. Blocks conversion of arachidonic acid to leukotrienes.
	Zafirlukast—blocks leukotriene receptors.

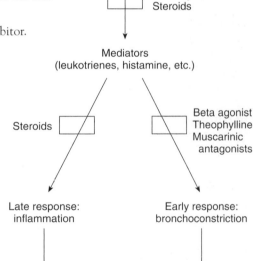

Treatment strategies in asthma

UCV *Pharm.90*   (Adapted, with permission, from Katzung BG, Trevor AJ. *Examination & Board Review: Pharmacology*, 5th ed. Stamford, CT: Appleton & Lange, 1998:159 and 161.)

Gout drugs

Colchicine	Acute gout. Depolymerizes microtubules, impairing leukocyte chemotaxis and degranulation. GI side effects, especially if given orally. (Note: Indomethacin is less toxic, more commonly used.)
Probenecid	Chronic gout. Inhibits reabsorption of uric acid (also inhibits secretion of penicillin).
Allopurinol	Chronic gout. Inhibits xanthine oxidase, ↓ conversion of xanthine to uric acid.

Diabetes drugs

Insulin	Binds insulin receptor, which has tyrosine kinase activity. In liver, ↑ storage of glucose as glycogen. In muscle, stimulates glycogen and protein synthesis, and K^+ uptake. In adipose tissue, facilitates triglyceride storage.
	Clinical use includes life-threatening hyperkalemia and stress-induced hyperglycemia.
	Toxicities are hypoglycemia and (rarely) hypersensitivity reaction.
Sulfonylureas	Tolbutamide, chlorpropamide, glyburide, glipizide.
	Oral hypoglycemic agents used to stimulate release of endogenous insulin in NIDDM (type 2).
	Close K^+ channels in β-cell membrane → cell depolarizes → insulin release triggered owing to ↑ Ca^{2+} influx.
	Inactive in IDDM (type 1) because requires some residual islet function.
	Toxicities includes hypoglycemia (more common with 2nd-generation drugs—glyburide, glipizide) and disulfiram-like effects (not seen with 2nd-generation drugs—glyburide, glipizide).
Metformin	Mechanism unknown; possibly inhibits gluconeogenesis and increases glycolysis; ↓ serum glucose levels.
	Used as an oral hypoglycemic. Can be used in patients without islet function.
	Most grave adverse effect is lactic acidosis.
Glitazones	Pioglitazone, rosiglitazone, troglitazone.
	↑ target cell response to insulin. Used as monotherapy in type 2 diabetes or in combination with above agents.
	Toxicity: weight gain, hepatotoxic (troglitazone).
α-glucosidase inhibitors	Acarbose, miglitol.
	Inhibit intestinal brush border α-glucosidases; delayed hydrolysis of sugars and absorption of glucose lead to ↓ postprandial hyperglycemia.
	Used as monotherapy in type 2 diabetes or in combination with above agents.
	Toxicity: GI disturbances.

UCV *Pharm.17*

Leuprolide

Mechanism	GnRH analog with agonist properties when used in pulsatile fashion; antagonist properties when used in continuous fashion.	When used in continuous fashion, it causes a transient initial burst of LH and FSH.
Clinical use	Infertility (pulsatile), prostate cancer (continuous—use with flutamide), uterine fibroids.	
Toxicity	Antiandrogen, nausea, vomiting.	

Propylthiouracil

Mechanism	Inhibits organification and coupling of thyroid hormone synthesis. Also ↓ peripheral conversion of T_4 to T_3.
Clinical use	Hyperthyroidism.
Toxicity	Skin rash, agranulocytosis (rare), aplastic anemia.

Antiandrogens

Finasteride	A 5α-reductase inhibitor (↓ conversion of testosterone to dihydrotestosterone). Useful in BPH.
Flutamide	A nonsteroidal competitive inhibitor of androgens at the testosterone receptor. Used in prostate carcinoma.
Ketoconazole, spironolactone	Inhibit steroid synthesis; used in the treatment of polycystic ovarian syndrome to prevent hirsutism.

Immunosuppressive agents: sites of action

Agent	Site
Prednisone	2, 5
Cyclosporine	2, 3
Azathioprine	2
Methotrexate	2
Dactinomycin	2, 3
Cyclophosphamide	2
Antilymphocytic globulin and monoclonal anti-T-cell antibodies	1, 2, 3
Rh$_3$(D) immune globulin	1
Tacrolimus	4

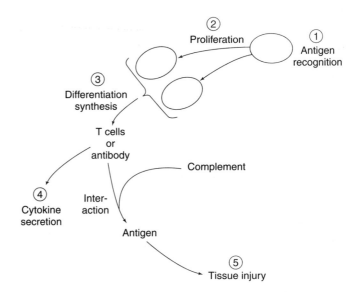

(Adapted, with permission, from Katzung BG. *Basic and Clinical Pharmacology*, 7th ed. Stamford, CT: Appleton & Lange, 1997:924.)

Cyclosporine

Mechanism	Binds to cyclophilins (peptidyl proline *cis-trans* isomerase), blocking the differentiation and activation of T cells mainly by inhibiting the production of IL-2 and its receptor.
Clinical use	Suppresses organ rejection after transplantation; selected autoimmune disorders.
Toxicity	Predisposes patients to viral infections and lymphoma; nephrotoxic (preventable with mannitol diuresis).

UCV *Pharm.43*

Azathioprine

Mechanism	Antimetabolite derivative of 6-mercaptopurine that interferes with the metabolism and synthesis of nucleic acid. Toxic to proliferating lymphocytes after antigenic stimulus.
Clinical use	Kidney transplantation, autoimmune disorders (including glomerulonephritis and hemolytic anemia).

Tacrolimus (FK506)

Mechanism	Similar to cyclosporine; binds to FK-binding protein, inhibiting secretion of IL-2 and other cytokines.
Clinical use	Potent immunosuppressive used in organ transplant recipients.
Toxicity	Significant—nephrotoxicity, peripheral neuropathy, hypertension, pleural effusion, hyperglycemia.

Drug name

Ending	Category	Example
-ane	Inhalational general anesthetic	Halothane
-azepam	Benzodiazepine	Diazepam
-azine	Phenothiazine (neuroleptic, antiemetic)	Chlorpromazine
-azole	Antifungal	Ketoconazole
-barbital	Barbiturate	Phenobarbital
-caine	Local anesthetic	Lidocaine
-cillin	Penicillin	Methicillin
-cycline	Antibiotic, protein synthesis inhibitor	Tetracycline
-ipramine	Tricyclic antidepressant	Imipramine
-navir	Protease inhibitor	Saquinavir
-olol	Beta antagonist	Propranolol
-operidol	Butyrophenone (neuroleptic)	Haloperidol
-oxin	Cardiac glycoside (inotropic agent)	Digoxin
-phylline	Methylxanthine	Theophylline
-pril	ACE inhibitor	Captopril
-terol	β_2 agonist	Albuterol
-tidine	H_2 antagonist	Cimetidine
-triptyline	Tricyclic antidepressant	Amitriptyline
-tropin	Pituitary hormone	Somatotropin
-zosin	α_1 antagonist	Prazosin

NOTES

Physiology

"When I investigate and when I discover that the forces of the heavens and the planets are within ourselves, then truly I seem to be living among the gods."
—Leon Battista Alberti

The portion of the examination dealing with physiology is broad and concept oriented and thus does not lend itself as well to fact-based review. Diagrams are often the best study aids, especially given the increasing number of questions requiring the interpretation of diagrams. Learn to apply basic physiologic relationships in a variety of ways (e.g., Fick equation, clearance equations). You are seldom asked to perform complex calculations. Hormones are the focus of many questions. Learn their sites of production and action as well as their regulatory mechanisms.

A large portion of the physiology tested on the USMLE Step 1 is now clinically relevant and involves understanding physiologic changes associated with pathologic processes (e.g., changes in pulmonary function with chronic obstructive pulmonary disease). Thus, it is worthwhile to review the physiologic changes that are found with common pathologies of the major organ systems (e.g., heart, lungs, kidneys, gastrointestinal tract) and endocrine glands.

High-Yield Topics
Cardiovascular
Renal
Endocrine/Reproductive
Respiratory
Gastrointestinal

Cardiovascular

1. Basic electrocardiographic changes (e.g., Q waves, ST-segment elevation).
2. Effects of electrolyte abnormalities (e.g., potassium or calcium imbalances).
3. Physiologic effects of the Valsalva maneuver.
4. Cardiopulmonary changes with pregnancy.
5. Responses to hemorrhage.
6. Responses to changes in position.

Pulmonary

1. Alveolar – arterial oxygen difference and changes seen in lung disease.
2. Mechanical differences between inspiration and expiration.
3. Characteristic pulmonary function curves for common lung diseases (e.g., bronchitis, emphysema, asthma, interstitial lung disease).
4. Gas diffusion across the alveolocapillary membrane.
5. Responses to high altitude.

Gastrointestinal

1. Sites of absorption of major nutrients (e.g., ileum—vitamin B_{12}).
2. Bile production and enterohepatic circulation.
3. Glucose cotransport into cells of gut.
4. Fat digestion and absorption.
5. Secretion and actions of GI hormones.

Renal/Acid-Base

1. Differences between active transport, facilitated diffusion, and diffusion.
2. Differences between central and nephrogenic diabetes insipidus.
3. Major transporters in each nephron segment.
4. Clearance calculation.
5. Effects of afferent and efferent arteriolar constriction on GFR and RPF.

Endocrine/Reproductive

1. Physiologic features of parathyroid diseases, associated laboratory findings; physiology and pathophysiology of PTHrP.
2. Clinical tests for endocrine abnormalities (e.g., dexamethasone suppression tests, glucose tolerance tests, TSH measurement).
3. Diseases associated with adrenocortical abnormalities (e.g., Cushing's, Addison's, Conn's).
4. Sites of hormone production during pregnancy (e.g., corpus luteum, placenta).
5. Regulation of prolactin secretion.
6. All aspects of diabetes mellitus.

General

1. Role of calmodulin, troponin C, and tropomyosin in muscle contraction.
2. Role of ions (e.g., calcium, sodium, magnesium, potassium) in skeletal muscle, cardiac muscle, and nerve cells (e.g., muscle contraction, membrane and action potentials, neurotransmitter release).
3. The clotting cascade, including those factors which require vitamin K for synthesis (II, VII, IX, X).
4. Regulation of core body temperature.

Myocardial action potential

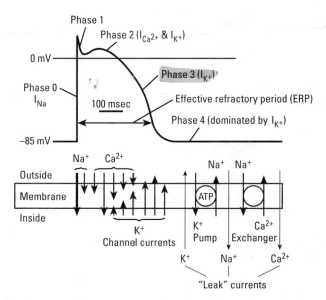

Occurs in atrial and ventricular myocytes and Purkinje fibers.

Phase 0 = rapid upstroke—voltage-gated Na⁺ channels open. ✓

Phase 1 = initial repolarization—inactivation of voltage-gated Na⁺ channels. Voltage-gated K⁺ channels begin to open.

Phase 2 = plateau—Ca^{2+} influx through voltage-gated Ca^{2+} channels balances K⁺ efflux. Ca^{2+} influx triggers another Ca^{2+} release from SR and myocyte contraction.

Phase 3 = rapid repolarization—massive K⁺ efflux due to opening of voltage-gated slow K⁺ channels and closure of voltage-gated Ca^{2+} channels.

Phase 4 = resting potential—high K⁺ permeability through K⁺ channels.

Pacemaker action potential

Occurs in the SA and AV nodes. Key differences from the ventricular action potential include:

Phase 0 = upstroke—opening of voltage-gated Ca^{2+} channels. These cells lack fast voltage-gated Na⁺ channels. Results in a slow conduction velocity that is utilized by the AV node to prolong transmission from the atria to ventricles.

Phase 2 = plateau is absent.

Phase 4 = slow diastolic depolarization—membrane potential spontaneously depolarizes as Na⁺ conductance increases. Accounts for automaticity of SA and AV nodes. The slope of phase 4 in the SA node determines heart rate. Acetylcholine ↓ and catecholamines ↑ the rate of diastolic depolarization, decreasing or increasing heart rate, respectively.

Ach ↓ and Catecholamine ↑ the rate of diastolic depolarization.

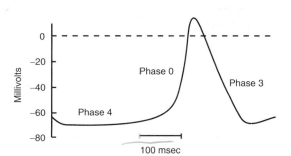

(Adapted, with permission, from Ganong WF et al. *Review of Medical Physiology*, 20th ed. New York: McGraw-Hill, 2001.)

HIGH-YIELD FACTS

Physiology

$$CO = SV \times HR$$

Cardiac output (CO)

Cardiac output = (stroke volume) × (heart rate).

Fick principle

$$CO = \frac{\text{rate of } O_2 \text{ consumption}}{\text{arterial } O_2 \text{ content} - \text{venous } O_2 \text{ content}}$$

$$\begin{pmatrix}\text{Mean arterial} \\ \text{pressure}\end{pmatrix} = \begin{pmatrix}\text{cardiac} \\ \text{output}\end{pmatrix} \times \begin{pmatrix}\text{total peripheral} \\ \text{resistance}\end{pmatrix}$$

Similar to Ohm's law:
Voltage = (current) × (resistance)
MAP = ⅓ systolic + ⅔ diastolic.
Pulse pressure = systolic − diastolic.
Pulse pressure ≈ stroke volume.

$$SV = \frac{CO}{HR} = EDV - ESV$$

$$EF = \frac{SV}{EDV} \times 100\% \text{ (normal} \approx 55\text{–}80\%)$$

UCV *Path1.10*

During exercise, CO ↑ initially as a result of an ↑ in SV. After prolonged exercise, CO ↑ as a result of an ↑ in HR.
If HR is too high, diastolic filling is incomplete and CO ↓ (e.g., ventricular tachycardia).

Cardiac output variables

Stroke volume affected by **C**ontractility, **A**fterload, and **P**reload. Increased SV when ↑ preload, ↓ afterload, or ↑ contractility.
Contractility (and SV) ↑ with:
1. Catecholamines (↑ activity of Ca^{2+} pump in sarcoplasmic reticulum)
2. ↑ intracellular calcium
3. ↓ extracellular sodium
4. Digitalis (↑ intracellular Na^+, resulting in ↑ Ca^{2+})

Contractility (and SV) ↓ with:
1. β_1 blockade ✓
2. Heart failure ✓
3. Acidosis ✓
4. Hypoxia/hypercapnea ✓

SV **CAP.**

Stroke volume ↑ in anxiety, exercise, and pregnancy.
A failing heart has ↓ stroke volume.
Myocardial O_2 demand is ↑ by:
1. ↑ afterload (∝ diastolic BP)
2. ↑ contractility
3. ↑ heart rate
4. ↑ heart size (↑ wall tension)

Preload and afterload

Preload = ventricular end-diastolic volume.
Afterload = diastolic arterial pressure (proportional to peripheral resistance).
Venous dilators (e.g., nitroglycerin) ↓ preload. ✓
Vasodilators (e.g., hydralazine) ↓ afterload. ✓

Preload ↑ with exercise (slightly), ↑ blood volume (overtransfusion), and excitement (sympathetics).
Preload pumps up the heart.

Starling curve Force of contraction is proportional to initial length of cardiac muscle fiber (preload).

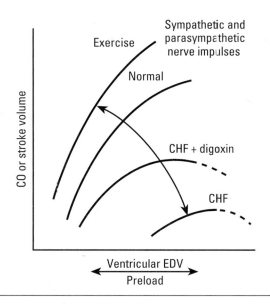

CONTRACTILE STATE OF MYOCARDIUM

⊕

Circulating
  catecholamines
Digitalis
Sympathetic
  stimulation

⊖

Pharmacologic
  depressants
Loss of
  myocardium (MI)

Ejection fraction

$$\text{Ejection fraction} = \frac{\text{end-diastolic volume} - \text{end-systolic volume}}{\text{end-diastolic volume}} = \frac{\text{stroke volume}}{\text{end-diastolic volume}}$$

Ejection fraction is an index of ventricular contractility.
Ejection fraction is normally 60–70%.

Resistance, pressure, flow

$$\text{Resistance} = \frac{\text{driving pressure }(\Delta P)}{\text{flow }(Q)} = \frac{8\eta\ (\text{viscosity}) \times \text{length}}{\pi\ r^4}$$

Viscosity depends mostly on hematocrit.
Viscosity increases in:
1. Polycythemia
2. Hyperproteinemic states (e.g., multiple myeloma)
3. Hereditary spherocytosis

Resistance is directly
  proportional to viscosity
  and inversely proportional
  to the radius to the 4th
  power.

Cardiac cycle

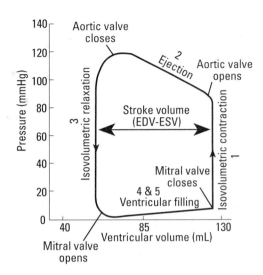

Phases:

1. Isovolumetric contraction—period between mitral valve closure and aortic valve opening; period of highest oxygen consumption
2. Systolic ejection—period between aortic valve opening and closing
3. Isovolumetric relaxation—period between aortic valve closing and mitral valve opening
4. Rapid filling—period just after mitral valve opening
5. Slow filling—period just before mitral valve closure

Sounds:

S1—mitral and tricuspid valve closure.
S2—aortic and pulmonary valve closure.
S3—at end of rapid ventricular filling.
S4—high atrial pressure/stiff ventricle.

S3 is associated with dilated CHF.
S4 ("atrial kick") is associated with a hypertrophic ventricle.

a wave—atrial contraction.
c wave—RV contraction (tricuspid valve bulging into atrium).
v wave— ↑ atrial pressure due to filling against closed tricuspid valve.

Jugular venous distention is seen in right heart failure.

S4 = Hypertrophic ventricle.

S3 = ↑ dilated CHF.

(Adapted, with permission, from Ganong WF. *Review of Medical Physiology,* 19th ed. Stamford, CT: Appleton & Lange, 1999:541.)

Conduction to contraction

A.

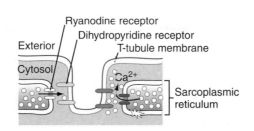

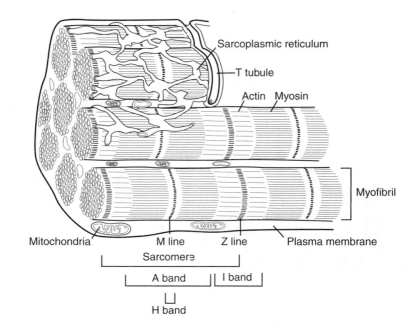

Action potential reaches axon terminal → depolarization opens voltage-gated Ca^{2+} channels and causes neurotransmitter vesicle fusion and exocytosis. Postsynaptic ligand binding leads to depolarization of the postsynaptic (muscle) cell **(A).** Depolarization travels down T tubule. A dihydropyridine receptor (voltage-sensing Ca^{2+} channel protein) lies in the T-tubule membrane next to a ryanodine receptor (voltage-sensing Ca^{2+} channel protein), which lies in the sarcoplasmic reticulum **(B).** Released calcium binds to troponin C, which causes a conformational change and moves tropomyosin out of myosin-binding groove on actin filament. Myosin hydrolyzes its bound ATP and is displaced on the actin filament (power stroke). Contraction results in **HIZ** shrinkage—H, I, and Z bands contract **(B).**

Smooth muscle contraction

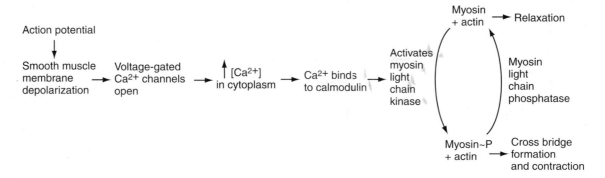

Skeletal muscle contraction

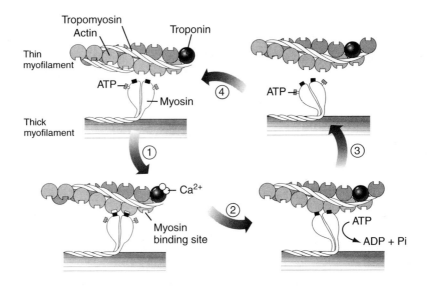

Electrocardiogram

P wave—atrial depolarization.

PR segment—conduction delay through AV node (normally < 200 msec).

QRS complex—ventricular depolarization (normally < 120 msec).

Q-T interval—mechanical contraction of the ventricles.

T wave—ventricular repolarization.

Atrial repolarization is masked by QRS complex.

ST segment—isoelectric, ventricles depolarized.

U wave—caused by hypokalemia.

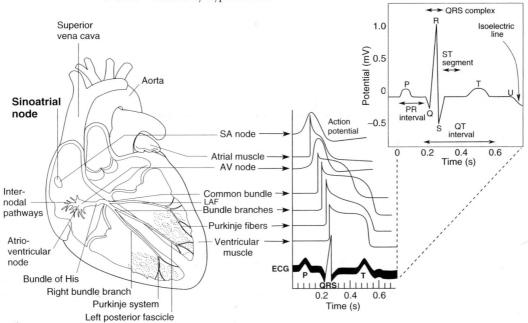

SA node "pacemaker" inherent dominance with slow phase of upstroke
AV node - 100-msec atrial-ventricular delay

(Adapted, with permission, from Ganong WF. *Review of Medical Physiology*, 20th ed. New York: McGraw-Hill, 2001.)

ECG tracings

Atrial fibrillation   A series of chaotic and erratic spikes in between irregularly spaced QRS complexes. Note: These spikes are not true P waves, as they do not depolarize the atria.

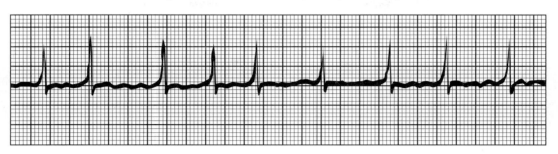

Atrial flutter   A rapid succession of identical, back-to-back atrial depolarization waves. The identical appearance accounts for the "sawtooth" appearance of the flutter waves.

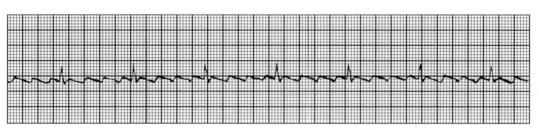

AV block

1st degree   The PR interval is prolonged (> 200 msec). A prolonged PR interval does not usually present symptomatically.

Prolonged PR interval

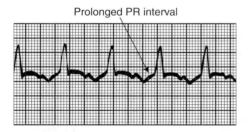

2nd degree
Mobitz type I   Progressive lengthening of the PR interval until a beat is "dropped" (a P wave not
(Wenckebach)   followed by a QRS complex). This condition is usually asymptomatic.

Note progressive increase in PR length before dropped beat

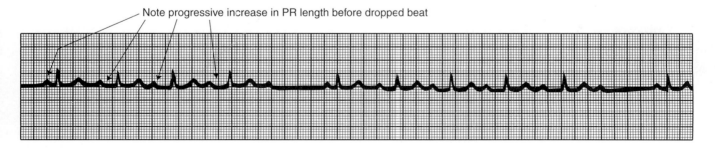

ECG tracings (continued)

Mobitz type II

Dropped beats that are not preceded by a change in the length of the PR interval (as in type I). These abrupt, nonconducted P waves result in a pathologic condition. It is often found as 2:1 block, where there are 2 P waves to 1 QRS response.

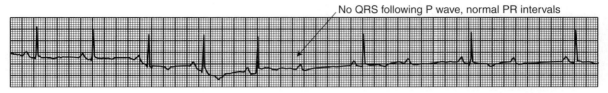

No QRS following P wave, normal PR intervals

3rd degree
(complete)

The atria and ventricles are paced evenly, but independently. Both P waves and QRS complexes are present, although the P waves bear no relation to the QRS complexes. The atrial rate is faster than the ventricular rate.

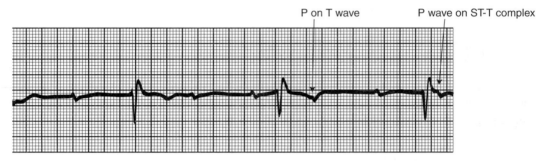

P on T wave   P wave on ST-T complex

Ventricular
fibrillation

A completely erratic rhythm with no identifiable waves. This is a fatal arrhythmia requiring immediate defibrillation.

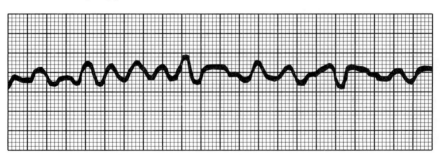

(Adapted, with permission, from Hurst JW. *Introduction to Electrocardiography.* New York: McGraw-Hill, 2001.)

Cardiac myocyte physiology

Cardiac muscle contraction is dependent on extracellular calcium, which enters the cells during plateau of action potential and stimulates calcium release from the cardiac muscle sarcoplasmic reticulum (calcium-induced calcium release).

In contrast to skeletal muscle:
1. Cardiac muscle action potential has a plateau, which is due to Ca^{2+} influx
2. Cardiac nodal cells spontaneously depolarize, resulting in automaticity
3. Cardiac myocytes are electrically coupled to each other by gap junctions

Control of mean arterial pressure

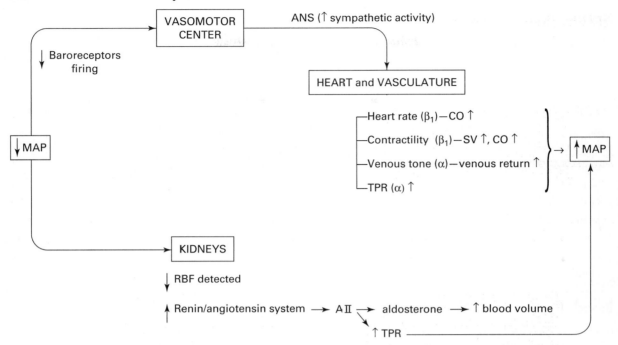

Arterial baroreceptors

Carotid and Aortic bodies receptors (handwritten)

Receptors:
1. Aortic arch transmits via vagus nerve to medulla (responds only to ↑ blood pressure)
2. Carotid sinus transmits via glossopharyngeal nerve to medulla

Hypotension— ↓ arterial pressure → ↓ stretch → ↓ afferent baroreceptor firing → ↑ efferent sympathetic firing and ↓ efferent parasympathetic stimulation → vasoconstriction, ↑ HR, ↑ contractility, ↑ BP. Important in the response to severe hemorrhage.

Carotid massage— ↑ pressure on carotid artery → ↑ stretch → ↓ HR.

Chemoreceptors

Peripheral

Carotid and aortic bodies respond to ↓ P_{O_2} (< 60 mmHg), increased P_{CO_2}, and decreased pH of blood.

Central

Respond to changes in pH and P_{CO_2} of brain interstitial fluid, which in turn are influenced by arterial CO_2. Do not directly respond to P_{O_2}. Responsible for Cushing reaction, response to cerebral ischemia, response to increased intracranial pressure → hypertension (sympathetic response) and bradycardia (parasympathetic response).

Circulation through organs

Liver	Largest share of systemic cardiac output.
Kidney	Highest blood flow per gram of tissue.
Heart	Large arteriovenous O_2 difference. ↑ O_2 demand is met by ↑ coronary blood flow, not by ↑ extraction of O_2.

Normal pressures

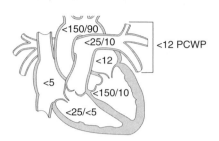

PCWP—pulmonary capillary wedge pressure (in mmHg) is a good approximation of left atrial pressure. Measured with Swan-Ganz catheter.

Autoregulation

Mechanism—blood flow is altered to meet demands of tissue.

Organ	Factors determining autoregulation
Heart	Local metabolites: $-O_2$, adenosine, NO
Brain	Local metabolites: ΔCO_2 (pH)
Kidneys	Myogenic and tubuloglomerular feedback
Lungs	Hypoxia causes vasoconstriction
Skeletal muscle	Local metabolites: lactate, adenosine, K^+

Note: The pulmonary vasculature is unique in that hypoxia causes vasoconstriction (in some organs hypoxia causes vasodilation).

Blood

Normal adult blood composition. Note that serum = plasma – clotting factors (e.g., fibrinogen).

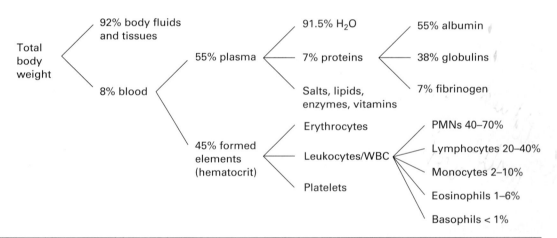

Serum is only plasma without the clotting factors.

Convergence of coagulation, complement, and kinin pathways

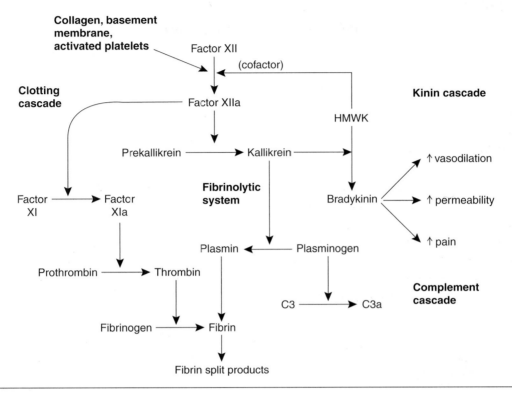

Collagen, basement membrane, activated platelets → Factor XII

(cofactor)

Clotting cascade

Factor XIIa

Kinin cascade

HMWK

Prekallikrein ⟶ Kallikrein

Factor XI → Factor XIa

Fibrinolytic system

Bradykinin → ↑ vasodilation

↑ permeability

↑ pain

Plasmin ← Plasminogen

Prothrombin ⟶ Thrombin

C3 ⟶ C3a

Complement cascade

Fibrinogen ⟶ Fibrin

Fibrin split products

Capillary fluid exchange

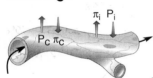

Starling forces determine fluid movement by osmosis through capillary membranes:

1. P_c = capillary pressure—tends to move fluid out of capillary
2. P_i = interstitial fluid pressure—tends to move fluid into capillary
3. π_c = plasma colloid osmotic pressure—tends to move fluid into capillary
4. π_i = interstitial fluid colloid osmotic pressure—tends to move fluid out of capillary

Thus net filtration pressure = $P_{net} = [(P_c - P_i) - (\pi_c - \pi_i)]$.

K_f = filtration constant (capillary permeability).

Net fluid flow = $(P_{net})(K_f)$.

Edema—excess fluid outflow into interstitium that is commonly caused by:

1. ↑ capillary pressure (↑ P_c; heart failure)
2. ↓ plasma proteins (↓ π_c; nephrotic syndrome, liver failure)
3. ↑ capillary permeability (↑ K_f; toxins, infections, burns)
4. ↑ interstitial fluid colloid osmotic pressure (↑ π_i; lymphatic blockage)

Fluid compartments

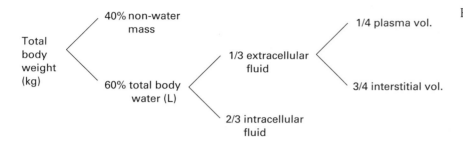

TBW – ECF = ICF.
ECF – PV = interstitial volume.

Renal clearance	$C_x = U_x V / P_x$ = volume of plasma from which the substance is cleared completely per unit time. If $C_x < $ GFR, then there is net tubular reabsorption of X. If $C_x > $ GFR, then there is net tubular secretion of X. If $C_x = $ GFR, then there is no net secretion or reabsorption.	Be familiar with calculations.
Glomerular filtration barrier	Composed of: 1. Fenestrated capillary endothelium (size barrier) 2. Fused basement membrane with heparan sulfate (negative charge barrier) 3. Epithelial layer consisting of podocyte foot processes	The charge barrier is lost in nephrotic syndrome, resulting in albuminuria, hypoproteinemia, generalized edema, and hyperlipidemia.
Glomerular filtration rate	$GFR = U_{inulin} \times V / P_{inulin} = C_{inulin}$ $= K_f [(P_{GC} - P_{BS}) - (\pi_{GC} - \pi_{BS})]$ (GC = glomerular capillary; BS = Bowman's space.) π_{BS} normally equals zero.	Inulin is freely filtered and is neither reabsorbed nor secreted. Clinically, creatinine clearance is a good measure of GFR.
PAH	Secreted in proximal tubule. 2° active transport. Mediated by a carrier system for organic acids; competitively inhibited by probenecid.	
Effective renal plasma flow	$ERPF = U_{PAH} \times V / P_{PAH} = C_{PAH}$ $RBF = RPF / 1 - Hct$	PAH is filtered and secreted.

Filtration fraction

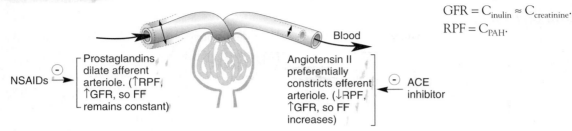

$$FF = GFR/RPF.$$
$$GFR = C_{inulin} \approx C_{creatinine}.$$
$$RPF = C_{PAH}.$$

NSAIDs $\xrightarrow{\ominus}$ Prostaglandins dilate afferent arteriole. ($\uparrow$RPF, $\uparrow$GFR, so FF remains constant)

Angiotensin II preferentially constricts efferent arteriole. ($\downarrow$RPF, $\uparrow$GFR, so FF increases) $\xleftarrow{\ominus}$ ACE inhibitor

Blood

Free water clearance

Given urine flow rate, urine osmolarity, and plasma osmolarity, be able to calculate free water clearance:

$$C_{H_2O} = V - C_{osm}$$
$$V = \text{urine flow rate; } C_{osm} = U_{osm}V/P_{osm}$$

Glucose clearance

Glucose at a normal level is completely reabsorbed in proximal tubule. At plasma glucose of 200 mg/dL, glucosuria begins (threshold). At 350 mg/dL, transport mechanism is saturated (T_m).

Glucosuria is an important clinical clue to diabetes mellitus.

Amino acid clearance

Reabsorption by at least 3 distinct carrier systems, with competitive inhibition within each group. 2° active transport occurs in proximal tubule and is saturable.

HIGH-YIELD FACTS

Physiology

Nephron physiology

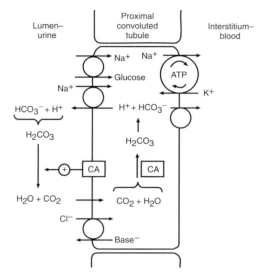

A. Early proximal convoluted tubule—"workhorse of the nephron." Reabsorbs all of the glucose and amino acids and most of the bicarbonate, sodium, and water. Secretes ammonia, which acts as a buffer for secreted H⁺.

B. Thin descending loop of Henle—passively reabsorbs water via medullary hypertonicity (impermeable to sodium).

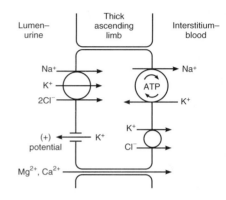

C. Thick ascending loop of Henle—actively reabsorbs Na^+, K^+, and Cl^- and indirectly induces the reabsorption of Mg^{2+} and Ca^{2+}. Impermeable to H_2O.

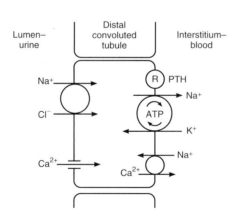

D. Early distal convoluted tubule—actively reabsorbs Na^+, Cl^-. Reabsorption of Ca^{2+} is under the control of PTH.

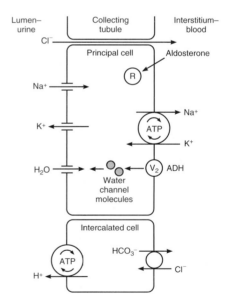

E. Collecting tubules—reabsorb Na^+ in exchange for secreting K^+ or H^+ (regulated by aldosterone). Reabsorption of water is regulated by ADH (vasopressin). Osmolarity of medulla can reach 1200 mOsm.

Relative concentrations along renal tubule

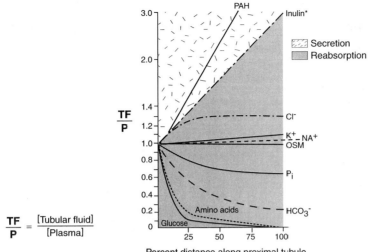

$$\frac{TF}{P} = \frac{[Tubular\ fluid]}{[Plasma]}$$

Percent distance along proximal tubule

* Neither secreted nor reabsorbed; concentration increases as water is reabsorbed.

(Adapted, with permission, from Ganong WF. *Review of Medical Physiology*, 20th ed. New York: McGraw-Hill, 2001.)

Renin-angiotensin system

Mechanism	Renin is released by the kidneys upon sensing ↓ BP and cleaves angiotensinogen to angiotensin I (AI, a decapeptide). AI is then cleaved by angiotensin-converting enzyme (ACE), primarily in the lung capillaries, to angiotensin II (AII, an octapeptide).
Actions of AII	1. Potent vasoconstriction
	2. Release of aldosterone from the adrenal cortex
	3. Release of ADH from posterior pituitary
	4. Stimulates hypothalamus → ↑ thirst
	Overall, AII serves to ↑ intravascular volume and ↑ BP.
	ANP released from atria may act as a "check" on the renin-angiotensin system (e.g., in heart failure).

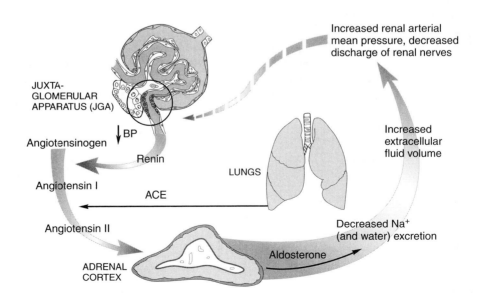

(Adapted, with permission, from Ganong WF. *Review of Medical Physiology*, 20th ed. New York: McGraw-Hill, 2001.)

Kidney endocrine functions

Endocrine functions of the kidney:

1. Endothelial cells of peritubular capillaries secrete erythropoietin in response to hypoxia
2. Conversion of 25-OH vitamin D to 1,25-(OH)$_2$ vitamin D by 1α-hydroxylase, which is activated by PTH
3. JG cells secrete renin in response to $\downarrow$ renal arterial pressure and $\uparrow$ renal nerve discharge (β_1 effect)
4. Secretion of prostaglandins that vasodilate the afferent arterioles to increase GFR

NSAIDs can cause renal failure by inhibiting the renal production of prostaglandins, which normally keep the afferent arterioles vasodilated to maintain GFR.

Hormones acting on kidney

	Stimulus for secretion	Action on kidneys
Vasopressin (ADH)	$\uparrow$ plasma osmolarity $\downarrow\downarrow$ blood volume	$\uparrow$ H$_2$O permeability of principal cells in collecting ducts $\uparrow$ urea absorption in collecting duct $\uparrow$ Na$^+$/K$^+$/2Cl$^-$ transporter in thick ascending limb
Aldosterone	$\downarrow$ blood volume (via AII) $\uparrow$ plasma [K$^+$]	$\uparrow$ Na$^+$ reabsorption, $\uparrow$ K$^+$ secretion, $\uparrow$ H$^+$ secretion in distal tubule
Angiotensin II	$\downarrow$ blood volume (via renin)	Contraction of efferent arteriole $\rightarrow$ $\uparrow$ GFR $\uparrow$ Na$^+$ and HCO$_3^-$ reabsorption in proximal tubule
Atrial natriuretic peptide (ANP)	$\uparrow$ atrial pressure	$\downarrow$ Na$^+$ reabsorption, $\uparrow$ GFR
PTH	$\downarrow$ plasma [Ca^{2+}]	$\uparrow$ Ca^{2+} reabsorption, $\downarrow$ (PO$_4$)$^{3-}$ reabsorption, $\uparrow$ 1,25-(OH)$_2$ vitamin D production

Pituitary gland

Posterior pituitary $\rightarrow$ vasopressin and oxytocin, made in the hypothalamus and shipped to pituitary. Derived from neuroectoderm.

Anterior pituitary $\rightarrow$ FSH, LH, ACTH, GH, TSH, melanotropin (MSH), prolactin. Derived from oral ectoderm.

α subunit—common subunit to TSH, LH, FSH, and hCG.

β subunit—determines hormone specificity.

BFLAT Major:

Basophilic

FSH

LH

ACTH

TSH

MSH

T.S.H. and **TSH** = The Sex Hormones and **TSH.**

PTH

Source	Chief cells of parathyroid.
Function	1. ↑ bone resorption of calcium and phosphate
	2. ↑ kidney reabsorption of calcium in DCT
	3. ↓ kidney reabsorption of phosphate
	4. ↑ 1,25-(OH)$_2$ vitamin D (cholecalciferol) production by stimulating kidney 1α-hydroxylase
Regulation	↓ in free serum Ca^{2+} ↑ PTH secretion.

PTH ↑ serum Ca^{2+}, ↓ serum (PO$_4$)$^{3-}$, ↑ urine (PO$_4$)$^{3-}$.
PTH stimulates both osteoclasts and osteoblasts.

PTH = **P**hosphate **T**rashing **H**ormone.

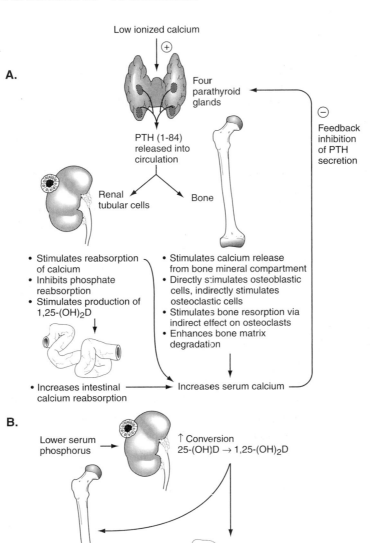

(Adapted, with permission, from Chandrasoma P et al. *Concise Pathology*, 3rd ed. Stamford, CT: Appleton & Lange, 1998:857.)

Shown above are the main actions of PTH and 1,25-(OH)$_2$D in the maintenance of calcium (**A**) and phosphate (**B**) homeostasis.

HIGH-YIELD FACTS

Physiology

Vitamin D

Source	Vitamin D_3 from sun exposure in skin. D_2 from plants. Both converted to 25-OH vitamin D in liver and to 1,25-$(OH)_2$ vitamin D (active form) in kidney.	If you do not get vitamin D, you get rickets (kids) or osteomalacia (adults).
Function	1. ↑ absorption of dietary calcium 2. ↑ absorption of dietary phosphate 3. ↑ bone resorption of Ca^{2+} and $(PO_4)^{3-}$	24,25-$(OH)_2$ vitamin D is an inactive form of vitamin D.
Regulation	↑ PTH causes ↑ 1,25-$(OH)_2$ vitamin D formation. ↓ $[Ca^{2+}]$ ↑ 1,25-$(OH)_2$ vitamin D production. ↓ phosphate causes ↑ 1,25-$(OH)_2$ vitamin D conversion. 1,25-$(OH)_2$ vitamin D feedback inhibits its own production.	

Calcium, phosphate, and alkaline phosphatase levels

	Ca^{2+}	Phosphate	Alkaline phosphatase	
Hyperparathyroidism	↑	↓	↑	Common causes of hypercalcemia—**MISHAP:**
Paget's disease of bone			↑	**M**alignancy
Vitamin D intoxication	↑	↑		**I**ntoxication with vitamin D
Osteoporosis				**S**arcoidosis
Renal insufficiency	↓	↑		**H**yperparathyroidism
				Alkali syndrome
				Paget's disease of bone

Calcitonin

Source	Parafollicular cells (C cells) of thyroid.	Calcitonin opposes actions of PTH and acts faster than PTH. It is probably not important in normal calcium homeostasis.
Function	↓ bone resorption of calcium.	
Regulation	↑ in serum Ca^{2+} ↑ secretion.	

Thyroid hormones (T₃/T₄)

Iodine-containing hormones that control the body's metabolic rate.

Source — Follicles of thyroid.

Function
1. Bone growth (synergism with GH)
2. CNS maturation
3. β-adrenergic effects
4. ↑ basal metabolic rate via ↑ Na^+/K^+ ATPase activity = ↑ O_2 consumption, ↑ body temp
5. Increased glycogenolysis, gluconeogenesis, lipolysis
6. CV— ↑ CO, HR, SV, contractility, RR

Regulation — TRH (hypothalamus) stimulates TSH (pituitary), which stimulates follicular cells. Negative feedback by T_3 to anterior pituitary ↓ sensitivity to TRH. TSI, like TSH, stimulates follicular cells (Graves' disease).

T_3 functions—**4B's**:

Brain maturation
Bone growth
Beta-adrenergic effects
BMR ↑

Steroid/thyroid hormone mechanism

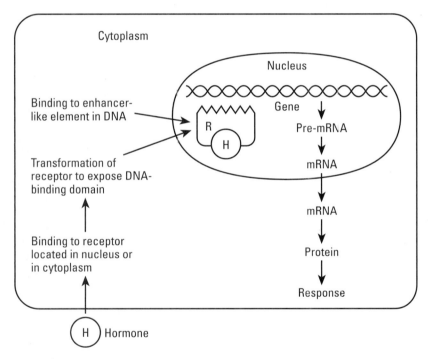

Cytoplasm

Nucleus

Binding to enhancer-like element in DNA

Gene

R

H

Pre-mRNA

Transformation of receptor to expose DNA-binding domain

mRNA

Binding to receptor located in nucleus or in cytoplasm

mRNA

Protein

Response

H Hormone

The need for gene transcription and protein synthesis delays the onset of action of these hormones.

Steroid/thyroid hormones—
PET CAT:

Progesterone
Estrogen
Testosterone
Cortisol
Aldosterone
Thyroxine

(Adapted, with permission, from Ganong WF. *Review of Medical Physiology*, 20th ed. New York: McGraw-Hill, 2001.)

Steroid hormones are lipophilic and insoluble in plasma; therefore, they must circulate bound to specific binding globulins, which ↑ solubility and allows for ↑ delivery of steroid to the target organ.

Adrenal steroids

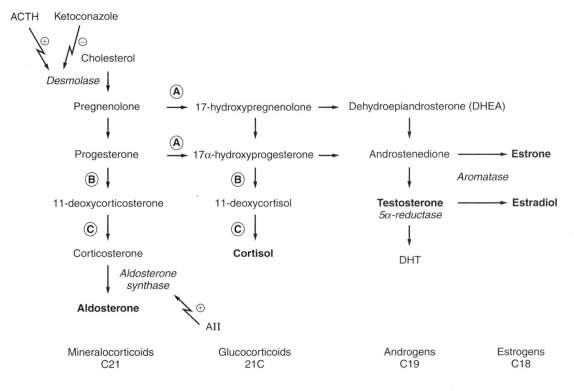

Mineralocorticoids   Glucocorticoids   Androgens   Estrogens
C21   21C   C19   C18

Congenital adrenal hyperplasias

A = 17α-hydroxylase deficiency. ↓ sex hormones, ↓ cortisol, ↑ mineralocorticoids. Cx = **HYPER**tension, hypokalemia; phenotypically female but no maturation.

B = 21β-hydroxylase deficiency. Most common form. ↓ cortisol (increased ACTH), ↓ mineralocorticoids, ↑ sex hormones. Cx = masculinization, female pseudohermaphroditism, **HYPO**tension, hyponatremia, hyperkalemia, ↑ plasma renin activity, and volume depletion. Salt-wasting can lead to hypovolemic shock in the newborn.

C = 11β-hydroxylase deficiency. ↓ cortisol, ↓ aldosterone and corticosterone, ↑ sex hormones. Cx = masculinization, **HYPER**tension (11-deoxycorticosterone acts as a weak mineralocorticoid).

UCV *Bio.1*

Insulin-independent organs	Muscle and adipose tissue depend on insulin for ↑ glucose uptake. Brain and RBCs take up glucose independent of insulin levels.	Brain and RBCs depend on glucose for metabolism under normal circumstances. Brain uses ketone bodies in starvation.

Prolactin regulation

Prolactin increases dopamine synthesis and secretion from the hypothalamus. Dopamine subsequently **inhibits** prolactin secretion. Dopamine agonists (e.g., bromocriptine) therefore **inhibit** prolactin secretion, whereas dopamine antagonists stimulate prolactin secretion. In females, prolactin inhibits GnRH synthesis and release, which inhibits ovulation.

Prolactin regulation

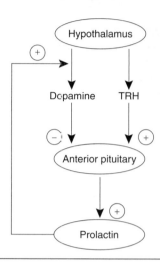

Estrogen

Source	Ovary (estradiol), placenta (estriol), blood (aromatization), testes.	Potency—estradiol > estrone > estriol.
Function	1. Growth of follicle	Estrogen hormone replacement therapy after menopause → ↓ hot flashes and ↓ postmenopausal bone loss.
	2. Endometrial proliferation, myometrial excitability	
	3. Development of genitalia	
	4. Stromal development of breast	
	5. Female fat distribution	Unopposed estrogen therapy— ↑ risk of endometrial cancer; use of progesterone with estrogen ↓ this risk.
	6. Hepatic synthesis of transport proteins	
	7. Feedback inhibition of FSH	
	8. LH surge (estrogen feedback on LH secretion switches to positive from negative just before LH surge)	
	9. ↑ myometrial excitability	

Progesterone

Source	Corpus luteum, placenta, adrenal cortex, testes.	Elevation of progesterone is indicative of ovulation.
Function	1. Stimulation of endometrial glandular secretions and spiral artery development	
	2. Maintenance of pregnancy	
	3. ↓ myometrial excitability	
	4. Production of thick cervical mucus, which inhibits sperm entry into the uterus	
	5. ↑ body temperature	
	6. Inhibition of gonadotropins (LH, FSH)	
	7. Uterine smooth muscle relaxation	

Menstrual cycle

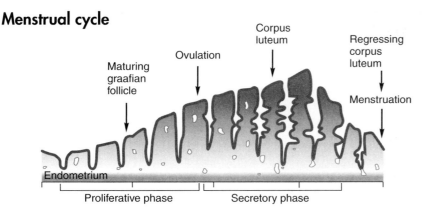

Follicular growth is fastest during 2nd week of proliferative phase.

Blood hormone levels

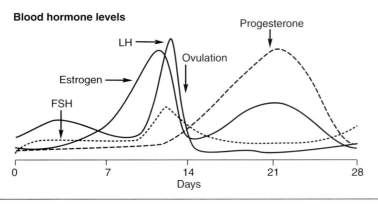

---

hCG

Source — Syncytiotrophoblast of placenta.

Function
1. Maintains the corpus luteum for the 1st trimester by acting like LH. In the 2nd and 3rd trimester, the placenta synthesizes its own estrogen and progesterone and the corpus luteum degenerates.
2. Used to detect pregnancy because it appears in the urine 8 days after successful fertilization (blood and urine tests available).
3. Elevated hCG in women with hydatidiform moles or choriocarcinoma.

Menopause

Cessation of estrogen production with age-linked decline in number of ovarian follicles. Average age of onset is 51 years (earlier in smokers).

Hormonal changes:
↓ estrogen, ↑↑ FSH, ↑ LH (no surge), ↑ GnRH.
Menopause causes **HAVOC:**
Hot flashes, Atrophy of the Vagina, Osteoporosis, Coronary artery disease.

Androgens

Testosterone, dihydrotestosterone (DHT), androstenedione.

Source

DHT (prostate, peripheral conversion), testosterone (testis, adrenal), androstenedione (adrenal).

Potency—DHT > testosterone > androstenedione.

Targets

Skin, prostate, seminal vesicles, epididymis, liver, muscle, brain.

Testosterone is converted to DHT by the enzyme 5α-reductase, which is inhibited by finasteride.

Function

1. Differentiation of wolffian duct system into internal gonadal structures
2. 2° sexual characteristics and growth spurt during puberty
3. Required for normal spermatogenesis
4. Anabolic effects—↑ muscle size, ↑ RBC production
5. ↑ libido

Testosterone and androstenedione are converted to estrogen in adipose tissue by enzyme aromatase.

Male spermatogenesis

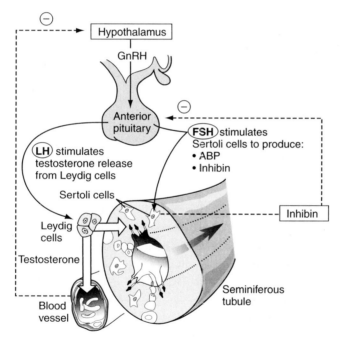

PRODUCTS	FUNCTIONS OF PRODUCTS
Androgen-binding protein (ABP)	Ensures that testosterone in seminiferous tubule is high
Inhibin	Inhibits FSH
Testosterone	Differentiates male genitalia, has anabolic effects on protein metabolism, maintains gametogenesis, maintains libido, inhibits GnRH, and fuses epiphyseal plates in bone.

FSH → **S**ertoli cells → **S**perm production
LH → **L**eydig cell

Response to high altitude

1. Acute ↑ in ventilation
2. Chronic ↑ in ventilation
3. ↑ erythropoietin → ↑ hematocrit and hemoglobin (chronic hypoxia)
4. ↑ 2,3-DPG (binds to Hb so that Hb releases more O_2)
5. Cellular changes (↑ mitochondria)
6. ↑ renal excretion of bicarbonate (e.g., use of acetazolamide) to compensate for the respiratory alkalosis
7. Chronic hypoxic pulmonary vasoconstriction results in right ventricular hypertrophy

---

Important lung products

1. Surfactant—produced by type II pneumocytes, ↓ alveolar surface tension, ↑ compliance
2. Prostaglandins
3. Histamine
4. Angiotensin-converting enzyme (ACE)—AI → AII; inactivates bradykinin (ACE inhibitors ↑ bradykinin and cause cough, angioedema)
5. Kallikrein—activates bradykinin

Surfactant—dipalmitoyl phosphatidylcholine (lecithin) deficient in neonatal RDS.

Collapsing pressure =
$$\frac{2 \text{ (tension)}}{\text{radius}}$$

Lung volumes

1. Residual volume (RV)—air in lung at maximal expiration
2. Expiratory reserve volume (ERV)—air that can still be breathed out after normal expiration
3. Tidal volume (TV)—air that moves into lung with each quiet inspiration, typically 500 mL
4. Inspiratory reserve volume (IRV)—air in excess of tidal volume that moves into lung on maximum inspiration
5. Vital capacity (VC)—TV + IRV + ERV
6. Functional reserve capacity (FRC)—RV + ERV (volume in lungs after a normal respiration)
7. Inspiratory capacity (IC)—IRV + TV
8. Total lung capacity—TLC = IRV + TV + ERV + RV

Vital capacity is everything but the residual volume.

A capacity is a sum of ≥ 2 volumes.

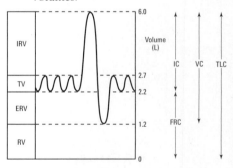

Oxygen-hemoglobin dissociation curve

When curve shifts to the right, ↓ affinity of hemoglobin for O_2 (facilitates unloading of O_2 to tissue).

An ↑ in all factors (except pH) causes a shift of the curve to the right.

A ↓ in all factors (except pH) causes a shift of the curve to the left.

Increased O_2 affinity, decreased P_{50}

Decreased metabolic needs (Decreased Pco_2, decreased temp, decreased H^+/ increased pH)
Decreased 2,3-DPG
Fetal Hb

Decreased O_2 affinity, increased P_{50}

Increased metabolic needs (Increased Pco_2, increased temp, increased H^+/decreased pH)
High altitude (increased 2,3-DPG)

(Graph: O_2 saturation (%) vs Po_2 (mmHg), showing Normal, Hypoxemia, Cyanosis curves)

Pulmonary circulation

Normally a low-resistance, high-compliance system. Pco_2 exert opposite effects on pulmonary and systemic circulation. A ↓ in Pao_2 causes a hypoxic vasoconstriction that shifts blood away from poorly ventilated regions of lung to well-ventilated regions of lung.

1. Perfusion limited—O_2 (normal health), CO_2, N_2O
2. Diffusion limited—O_2 (exercise, emphysema, fibrosis), CO

A consequence of pulmonary hypertension is cor pulmonale and subsequent right ventricular failure (jugular venous distention, edema, hepatomegaly).

Determination of physiologic dead space

$$V_D = V_T \times \frac{(Paco_2 - Peco_2)}{Paco_2}$$

$Paco_2$ = Arterial Pco_2, $Peco_2$ = expired air Pco_2

V/Q mismatch

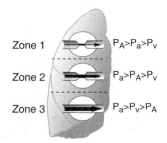

Zone 1 — $P_A > P_a > P_v$
Zone 2 — $P_a > P_A > P_v$
Zone 3 — $P_a > P_v > P_A$

Ideally, ventilation is matched to perfusion (i.e., V/Q = 1) in order for adequate oxygenation to occur efficiently.

Lung zones:
1. Apex of the lung—V/Q = 3 (wasted ventilation)
2. Base of the lung—V/Q = 0.6 (wasted perfusion)

Both ventilation and perfusion are greater at the base of the lung than at the apex of the lung.

With exercise (↑ cardiac output), there is vasodilation of apical capillaries, resulting in a V/Q ratio that approaches 1.

Certain organisms that thrive in high O_2 (e.g., TB) flourish in the apex.

V/Q → 0 = airway obstruction.
V/Q → ∞ = blood flow obstruction.

CO_2 transport

Carbon dioxide is transported from tissues to the lungs in 3 forms:

1. **Bicarbonate (90%)**

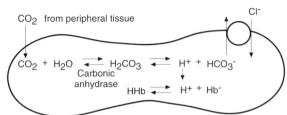

2. Bound to hemoglobin as carbaminohemoglobin (5%)
3. Dissolved CO_2 (5%)

(Adapted, with permission, from Ganong WF. *Review of Medical Physiology*, 20th ed. New York: McGraw-Hill, 2001.)

In lungs, oxygenation of Hb promotes dissociation of CO_2 from Hb (Haldane effect).

In peripheral tissue, ↑ H^+ shifts curve to right, unloading O_2 (Bohr effect).

PHYSIOLOGY — GASTROINTESTINAL

Salivary secretion

Source	Parotid, submandibular, and sublingual glands.	Salivary secretion is stimulated by both sympathetic and parasympathetic activity.
Function	1. α-amylase (ptyalin) begins starch digestion	
	2. Neutralizes oral bacterial acids, maintains dental health	
	3. Mucins (glycoproteins) lubricate food	

Stomach secretions

	Function	Source
Mucus	Lubricant, protects surface from H^+	Mucous cell
Intrinsic factor	Vitamin B_{12} absorption (in small intestine)	Parietal cell
H^+	Kills bacteria, breaks down food, activates pepsinogen to pepsin	Parietal cell
Pepsinogen	Broken down to pepsin (a protease)	Chief cell
Gastrin	Stimulates acid secretion	G cell

GI secretory products

Product	Source	Function	Regulation	Notes
Intrinsic factor	Parietal cells (stomach)	Vitamin B_{12} binding protein required for vitamin's uptake in terminal ileum		Autoimmune destruction of parietal cells → chronic gastritis → pernicious anemia
Gastric acid	Parietal cells	Lowers pH to optimal range for pepsin function; sterilizes chyme	Stimulated by histamine, ACh, gastrin; inhibited by prostaglandin, somatostatin, and GIP	Not essential for digestion; inadequate acid → ↑ risk of *Salmonella* infections
Pepsin	Chief cells (stomach)	Begins protein digestion; optimal function at pH 1.0–3.0	Stimulated by vagal input, local acid	Inactive pepsinogen converted to pepsin by H^+
Gastrin	G cells of antrum and duodenum	1. Stimulates secretion of HCl, IF, and pepsinogen 2. Stimulates gastric motility	Stimulated by stomach distention, amino acids, peptides, vagus (via GRP); inhibited by secretin and stomach acid pH < 1.5	Hypersecreted in Zollinger-Ellison syndrome → peptic ulcers; phenylalanine and tryptophan are potent stimulators
Bicarbonate	Surface mucosal cells of stomach and duodenum	Neutralizes acid; present in unstirred layer with mucus on luminal surface, preventing autodigestion	Stimulated by secretin (potentiated by vagal input, CCK)	
Cholecystokinin (CCK)	I cells of duodenum and jejunum	1. Stimulates gallbladder contraction 2. Stimulates pancreatic enzyme secretion 3. Inhibits gastric emptying	Stimulated by fatty acids, amino acids	In cholelithiasis, pain worsens after eating fatty foods due to CCK release
Secretin	S cells of duodenum	Nature's antacid: 1. Stimulates pancreatic HCO_3^- secretion 2. Inhibits gastric acid secretion	Stimulated by acid and fatty acids in lumen of duodenum	Alkaline pancreatic juice in duodenum neutralizes gastric acid, allowing pancreatic enzymes to function
Somatostatin	D cells in pancreatic islets, gastrointestinal mucosa	Inhibits: 1. Gastric acid and pepsinogen secretion 2. Pancreatic and small intestine fluid secretion 3. Gallbladder contraction 4. Release of both insulin and glucagon	Stimulated by acid; inhibited by vagus	Highly inhibitory hormone; anti–growth hormone effects (↓ digestion and ↓ absorption of substances needed for growth)

GI secretory products (continued)

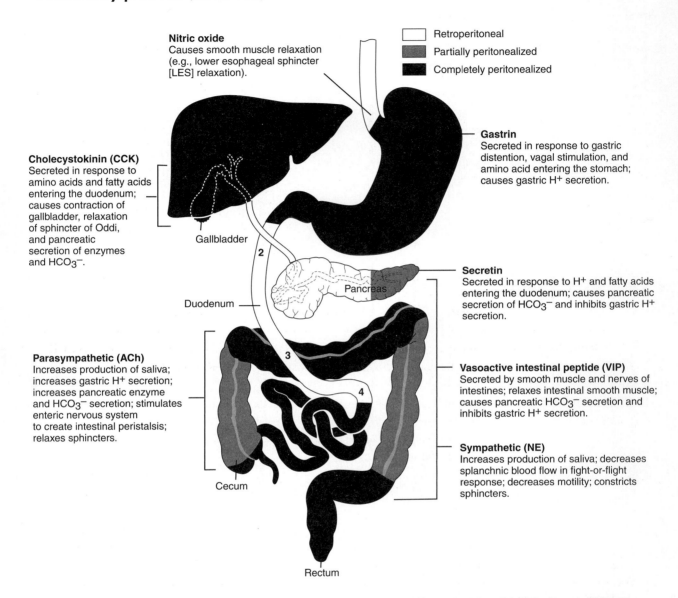

Nitric oxide
Causes smooth muscle relaxation (e.g., lower esophageal sphincter [LES] relaxation).

Retroperitoneal
Partially peritonealized
Completely peritonealized

Cholecystokinin (CCK)
Secreted in response to amino acids and fatty acids entering the duodenum; causes contraction of gallbladder, relaxation of sphincter of Oddi, and pancreatic secretion of enzymes and HCO_3^-.

Gallbladder

Duodenum

Parasympathetic (ACh)
Increases production of saliva; increases gastric H^+ secretion; increases pancreatic enzyme and HCO_3^- secretion; stimulates enteric nervous system to create intestinal peristalsis; relaxes sphincters.

Cecum

Pancreas

Rectum

Gastrin
Secreted in response to gastric distention, vagal stimulation, and amino acid entering the stomach; causes gastric H^+ secretion.

Secretin
Secreted in response to H^+ and fatty acids entering the duodenum; causes pancreatic secretion of HCO_3^- and inhibits gastric H^+ secretion.

Vasoactive intestinal peptide (VIP)
Secreted by smooth muscle and nerves of intestines; relaxes intestinal smooth muscle; causes pancreatic HCO_3^- secretion and inhibits gastric H^+ secretion.

Sympathetic (NE)
Increases production of saliva; decreases splanchnic blood flow in fight-or-flight response; decreases motility; constricts sphincters.

(Adapted, with permission, from Mehta S et al. *Step-Up: A High-Yield, Systems-Based Review for the USMLE Step I Examination.* Philadelphia: Lippincott Williams & Wilkins, 2000: 83.)

Regulation of gastric acid secretion

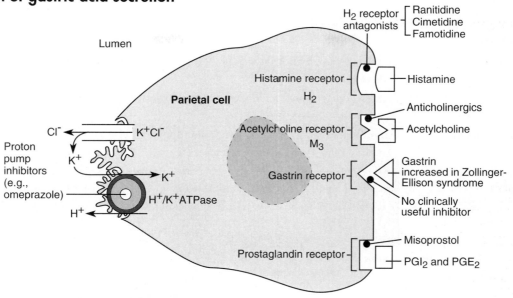

Glucose absorption	Occurs at duodenum and proximal jejunum.
	Absorbed across cell membrane by sodium-glucose cotransporter.

Pancreatic exocrine secretion	Secretory acini synthesize and secrete zymogens, stimulated by acetylcholine and CCK.
	Pancreatic ducts secrete mucus and alkaline fluid when stimulated by secretin.

Pancreatic enzymes	α-amylase—starch digestion, secreted in active form.
	Lipase, phospholipase A, colipase—fat digestion.
	Proteases (trypsin, chymotrypsin, elastase, carboxypeptidases)—protein digestion, secreted as proenzymes.
	Trypsinogen is converted to active enzyme trypsin by enterokinase, a duodenal brush-border enzyme. Trypsin then activates the other proenzymes and can also activate trypsinogen (positive feedback loop).
	Pancreatic insufficiency is seen in CF and other conditions. Patients present with malabsorption, steatorrhea (greasy, malodorous stool). Limit fat intake, monitor for signs of fat-soluble vitamin (A, D, E, K) deficiency.

Stimulation of pancreatic functions

Secretin	Stimulates ductal cells to secrete bicarbonate-rich fluid.
Cholecystokinin	Major stimulus for secretion of enzyme-rich fluid by pancreatic acinar cells.
Acetylcholine	Major stimulus for zymogen release, poor stimulus for bicarbonate secretion.
Somatostatin	Inhibits the release of gastrin and secretin.

Carbohydrate digestion

Only monosaccharides are absorbed.

Salivary amylase

Starts digestion, hydrolyzes α-1,4 linkages to give maltose, maltotriose, and α-limit dextrans.

Pancreatic amylase

Highest concentration in duodenal lumen, hydrolyzes starch to oligosaccharides, maltose, and maltotriose.

Oligosaccharide hydrolases

At brush border of intestine, the rate-limiting step in carbohydrate digestion, produce monosaccharides (glucose, galactose, fructose).

Bilirubin

Product of heme metabolism, actively taken up by hepatocytes. Conjugated version is water soluble. Jaundice (yellow skin, sclerae) results from elevated bilirubin levels.

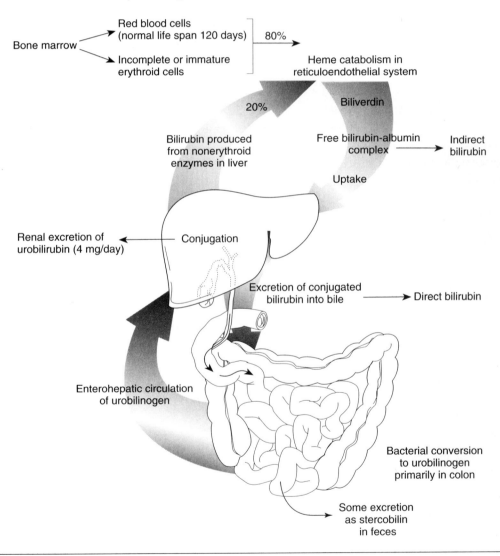

Bile

Secreted by hepatocytes. Composed of bile salts, phospholipids, cholesterol, bilirubin, water (97%). Bile salts are amphipathic (hydrophilic and hydrophobic domains) and solubilize lipids in micelles for absorption.

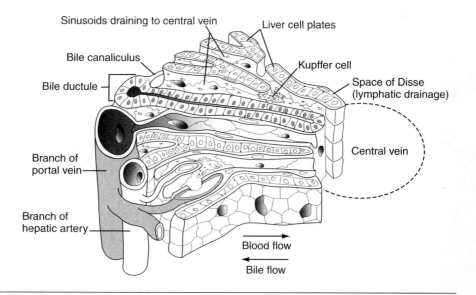

Rapid Review

The following tables represent a collection of high-yield associations of diseases, "buzzwords," findings, and associated pathologies that may be useful for quick review right before the exam.

Classic Findings

Most Common Associations

Disease/Finding	Association
Actinic keratosis	Often precedes squamous cell carcinoma
Addison's disease	1° adrenocortical deficiency
Albright's syndrome	Polyostotic fibrous dysplasia, precocious puberty, café-au-lait spots, short stature, young girls
Albuminocytologic dissociation	Guillain-Barré (↑ protein in CSF with only modest ↑ in cell count)
Alport's syndrome	Hereditary nephritis with nerve deafness
Anti–basement membrane	Goodpasture's syndrome
Anticentromere antibodies	Scleroderma (CREST)
Anti-double-stranded DNA antibodies (ANA antibodies)	SLE (type III hypersensitivity)
Anti–epithelial cell	Pemphigus vulgaris
Antigliadin antibodies	Celiac disease
Antihistone antibodies	Drug-induced SLE
Anti-IgG antibodies	Rheumatoid arthritis
Antimitochondrial antibodies	1° biliary cirrhosis
Antineutrophil antibodies	Vasculitis
Antiplatelet antibodies	Idiopathic thrombocytopenic purpura
Arachnodactyly	Marfan's syndrome
Argyll Robertson pupil	Neurosyphilis
Arnold-Chiari malformation	Cerebellar tonsillar herniation
Aschoff bodies	Rheumatic fever
Atrophy of the mammillary bodies	Wernicke's encephalopathy
Auer rods	Acute myelogenous leukemia (especially the promyelocytic type)
Autosplenectomy	Sickle cell anemia
Babinski's sign	Upper motor neuron lesion
Baker's cyst in popliteal fossa	Rheumatoid arthritis
"Bamboo spine" on x-ray	Ankylosing spondylitis
Bartter's syndrome	Hyperreninemia
Basophilic stippling of RBCs	Lead poisoning
Becker's muscular dystrophy	Defective dystrophin; less severe than Duchenne's
Bell's palsy	CN VII palsy
Bence Jones proteins	Multiple myeloma (kappa or lambda Ig light chains in urine), Waldenström's macroglobulinemia (IgM)

Berger's disease	IgA nephropathy
Bernard-Soulier disease	Defect in platelet adhesion
Bilateral hilar adenopathy, uveitis	Sarcoidosis
Birbeck granules on EM	Histiocytosis X (eosinophilic granuloma)
Bloody tap on LP	Subarachnoid hemorrhage
"Blue bloater"	Chronic bronchitis
Blue-domed cysts	Fibrocystic change of the breast
Blue sclera	Osteogenesis imperfecta
Boot-shaped heart on x-ray	Tetralogy of Fallot; RV hypertrophy
Bouchard's nodes	Osteoarthritis (PIP swelling 2° to osteophytes)
Boutonnière deformity	Rheumatoid arthritis
Branching rods in oral infection	*Actinomyces israelii*
"Brown tumor" of bone	Hemorrhage causes brown color of osteolytic cysts: 　1.　Hyperparathyroidism 　2.　Osteitis fibrosa cystica (von Recklinghausen's disease)
Brushfield's spots	Down syndrome
Bruton's disease	X-linked agammaglobulinemia
Budd-Chiari syndrome	Posthepatic venous thrombosis
Buerger's disease	Small/medium artery vasculitis
Burkitt's lymphoma	8:14 translocation; associated with EBV
Burton's lines	Lead poisoning
C-ANCA, P-ANCA	Wegener's granulomatosis, polyarteritis nodosa
Café-au-lait spots on skin	Neurofibromatosis
Caisson disease	Gas emboli
Calf pseudohypertrophy	Duchenne's muscular dystrophy
Call-Exner bodies	Granulosa/theca cell tumor of the ovary
Cardiomegaly with apical atrophy	Chagas' disease
Cerebriform nuclei	Mycosis fungoides (cutaneous T-cell lymphoma)
Chagas' disease	Trypanosome infection
Chancre	1° syphilis (not painful)
Chancroid	*Haemophilus ducreyi* (painful)
Charcot's triad	Multiple sclerosis (nystagmus, intention tremor, scanning speech), cholangitis (jaundice, RUQ pain, fever)
Charcot-Leyden crystals	Bronchial asthma (eosinophil membranes)
Chédiak-Higashi disease	Phagocyte deficiency

Cherry-red spot on macula	Tay-Sachs, Niemann-Pick disease, central retinal artery occlusion
Cheyne-Stokes respirations	Central apnea in CHF and ↑ ICP
"Chocolate cysts"	Endometriosis (frequently involve both ovaries)
Chronic atrophic gastritis	Predisposition to gastric carcinoma
Chvostek's sign	Hypocalcemia (facial muscle spasm upon tapping)
Clear cell adenocarcinoma of the vagina	Diethylstilbestrol exposure in utero
Clue cells	*Gardnerella* vaginitis
Codman's triangle on x-ray	Osteosarcoma
Cold agglutinins	*Mycoplasma pneumoniae,* infectious mononucleosis
Cold intolerance	Hypothyroidism
Condylomata lata	2° syphilis
Continuous machinery murmur	Patent ductus arteriosus
Cori's disease	Debranching enzyme deficiency
Cotton-wool spots	Chronic hypertension
Cough, conjunctivitis, coryza + fever	Measles
Councilman bodies	Toxic or viral hepatitis
Cowdry type A bodies	Herpesvirus
Crescents in Bowman's capsule	Rapidly progressive crescentic glomerulonephritis
Crigler-Najjar syndrome	Congenital unconjugated hyperbilirubinemia
Curling's ulcer	Acute gastric ulcer associated with severe burns
Currant-jelly sputum	*Klebsiella*
Curschmann's spirals	Bronchial asthma (whorled mucous plugs)
Cushing's ulcer	Acute gastric ulcer associated with CNS injury
D dimers	DIC
Depigmentation of neurons in substantia nigra	Parkinson's disease (basal ganglia disorder—rigidity, resting tremor, bradykinesia)
Dermatitis, dementia, diarrhea	Pellagra (niacin, vitamin B_3 deficiency)
Diabetes insipidus + exophthalmos + lesions of skull	Hand-Schüller-Christian disease
Dog or cat bite	*Pasteurella multocida*
Donovan bodies	Granuloma inguinale
Dressler's syndrome	Post-MI fibrinous pericarditis

Dubin-Johnson syndrome	Congenital conjugated hyperbilirubinemia (black liver)
Duchenne's muscular dystrophy	Deleted dystrophin gene (X-linked recessive)
Eburnation	Osteoarthritis (polished, ivory-like appearance of bone)
Edwards' syndrome	Trisomy 18 associated with rocker-bottom feet, low-set ears, heart disease
Eisenmenger's complex	Late cyanosis shunt (uncorrected L → R shunt becomes R → L shunt)
Elastic skin	Ehlers-Danlos syndrome
Erb-Duchenne palsy	Superior trunk brachial plexus injury ("waiter's tip")
Erythema chronicum migrans	Lyme disease
Fanconi's syndrome	Proximal tubular reabsorption defect
"Fat, female, forty, and fertile"	Acute cholecystitis
Fatty liver	Alcoholism
Ferruginous bodies	Asbestosis
Gardner's syndrome	Colon polyps with osteomas and soft tissue tumors
Gaucher's disease	Glucocerebrosidase deficiency
Ghon focus	Primary TB
Gilbert's syndrome	Benign congenital unconjugated hyperbilirubinemia
Glanzmann's thrombasthenia	Defect in platelet aggregation
Goodpasture's syndrome	Autoantibodies against alveolar and glomerular BM proteins
Gowers' maneuver	Duchenne's (use of patient's arms to help legs pick self off the floor)
Guillain-Barré syndrome	Idiopathic polyneuritis
"Hair-on-end" appearance on x-ray	β-thalassemia, sickle cell anemia (extramedullary hematopoiesis)
Hampton's hump on x-ray	Pulmonary embolism
Hand-Schüller-Christian disease	Chronic progressive histiocytosis
HbS	Sickle cell anemia
hCG elevated	Choriocarcinoma, hyadatidiform mole (occurs with and without embryo)
Heberden's nodes	Osteoarthritis (DIP swelling 2° to osteophytes)
Heinz bodies	G6PD deficiency
Henoch-Schönlein purpura	Hypersensitivity vasculitis associated with hemorrhagic urticaria and URIs
Heterophil antibodies	Infectious mononucleosis (EBV)
Hgb F	Thalassemia major
High-output cardiac failure (dilated cardiomyopathy)	Wet beriberi (thiamine, vitamin B_1 deficiency)
HLA-B27	Reiter's syndrome, ankylosing spondylitis
HLA-DR3 or -DR4	DM type 1 (caused by autoimmune destruction of β cells)
Homer Wright rosettes	Neuroblastoma

HIGH-YIELD FACTS

Rapid Review

Honeycomb lung on x-ray	Interstitial fibrosis
Horner's syndrome	Ptosis, miosis, and anhidrosis
Howell-Jolly bodies	Splenectomy (or nonfunctional spleen)
Huntington's disease	Caudate degeneration (autosomal dominant)
Hyperphagia + hypersexuality + hyperorality + hyperdocility	Klüver-Bucy syndrome (amygdala)
Hyperpigmentation of skin	1° adrenal insufficiency (Addison's disease)
Hypersegmented neutrophils	Macrocytic anemia
Hypertension + hypokalemia	Conn's syndrome
Hypochromic microcytosis	Iron deficiency anemia, lead poisoning
Increased α-fetoprotein in amniotic fluid/maternal serum	Anencephaly, spina bifida (neural tube defects)
Increased uric acid levels	Gout, Lesch-Nyhan syndrome, myeloproliferative disorders, loop and thiazide diuretics
Intussusception	Adenovirus (causes hyperplasia of Peyer's patches)
Janeway lesions	Endocarditis
Jarisch-Herxheimer reaction	Syphilis—overaggressive treatment of an asymptomatic patient that causes symptoms due to rapid lysis
Job's syndrome	Neutrophil chemotaxis abnormality
Kaposi's sarcoma	AIDS in MSM (men who have sex with men)
Kartagener's syndrome	Dynein defect
Kayser-Fleischer rings	Wilson's disease
Keratin pearls	Squamous cell carcinoma
Kimmelstiel-Wilson nodules	Diabetic nephropathy
Klüver-Bucy syndrome	Bilateral amygdala lesions
Koilocytes	HPV
Koplik spots	Measles
Krukenberg tumor	Gastric adenocarcinoma with ovarian metastases
Kussmaul hyperpnea	Diabetic ketoacidosis
Lens dislocation + aortic dissection + joint hyperflexibility	Marfan's syndrome (fibrillin deficit)
Lesch-Nyhan syndrome	HGPRT deficiency
Letterer-Siwe disease	Langerhans cell histiocytosis
Lewy bodies	Parkinson's disease
Libman-Sacks disease	Endocarditis associated with SLE

388

Lines of Zahn	Arterial thrombus
Lisch nodules	Neurofibromatosis (von Recklinghausen's disease)
Low serum ceruloplasmin	Wilson's disease
Lucid interval	Epidural hematoma
"Lumpy-bumpy" appearance of glomeruli on immunofluorescence	Poststreptococcal glomerulonephritis
Lytic bone lesions on x-ray	Multiple myeloma
Mallory bodies	Alcoholic liver disease
Mallory-Weiss syndrome	Esophagogastric lacerations
McArdle's disease	Muscle phosphorylase deficiency
McBurney's sign	Appendicitis
MLF syndrome (INO)	Multiple sclerosis
Monoclonal antibody spike	Multiple myeloma (called the M protein; usually IgG or IgA), MGUS (monoclonal gammopathy of undetermined significance), Waldenström's (M protein = IgM) macroglobulinemia
Myxedema	Hypothyroidism
Necrotizing vasculitis (lungs) and necrotizing glomerulonephritis	Wegener's and Goodpasture's (hemoptysis and glomerular disease)
Needle-shaped, negatively bifringent crystals	Gout
Negri bodies	Rabies
Nephritis + cataracts + hearing loss	Alport's syndrome
Neurofibrillary tangles	Alzheimer's disease
Niemann-Pick disease	Sphingomyelinase deficiency
No lactation postpartum	Sheehan's syndrome (pituitary infarction)
Nutmeg liver	Congestive heart failure
Occupational exposure to asbestos	Malignant mesothelioma
"Orphan Annie" nuclei	Papillary carcinoma of the thyroid
Osler's nodes	Endocarditis
Owl's eye	CMV
Painless jaundice	Pancreatic cancer (head)
Palpable purpura on legs and buttocks	Henoch-Schönlein purpura
Pancoast's tumor	Bronchogenic apical tumor associated with Horner's syndrome
Pannus	Rheumatoid arthritis
Parkinson's disease	Nigrostriatal dopamine depletion
Periosteal elevation on x-ray	Pyogenic osteomyelitis

Peutz-Jeghers syndrome	Benign polyposis
Peyronie's disease	Penile fibrosis
Philadelphia chromosome (*bcr:abl*)	CML (may sometimes be associated with AML)
Pick bodies	Pick's disease
Pick's disease	Progressive dementia, similar to Alzheimer's
"Pink puffer"	Emphysema (centroacinar [smoking], panacinar [α_1-antitrypsin deficiency])
Plummer-Vinson syndrome	Esophageal webs with iron deficiency anemia
Podagra	Gout (MP joint of hallux)
Podocyte fusion	Minimal change disease
Polyneuropathy, cardiac pathology, and edema	Dry beriberi (thiamine, vitamin B_1 deficiency)
Polyneuropathy preceded by GI or respiratory infection	Guillain-Barré syndrome
Pompe's disease	Lysosomal glucosidase deficiency associated with cardiomegaly
Port-wine stain	Hemangioma
Positive anterior "drawer sign"	Anterior cruciate ligament injury
Pott's disease	Vertebral tuberculosis
Pseudopalisade tumor cell arrangement	Glioblastoma multiforme
Pseudorosettes	Ewing's sarcoma
Ptosis, miosis, anhidrosis	Horner's syndrome (Pancoast's tumor)
Rash on palms and soles	2° syphilis, Rocky Mountain spotted fever
Raynaud's syndrome	Recurrent vasospasm in extremities
RBC casts in urine	Acute glomerulonephritis
Recurrent pulmonary *Pseudomonas* and *Staphylococcus aureus* infections	Cystic fibrosis
Red urine in the morning	Paroxysmal nocturnal hemoglobinuria
Reed-Sternberg cells	Hodgkin's lymphoma
Reid index (increased)	Chronic bronchitis
Reinke crystals	Leydig cell tumor
Reiter's syndrome	Urethritis, conjunctivitis, arthritis
Renal cell carcinoma + cavernous hemangiomas + adenomas	Von Hippel–Lindau disease

Renal epithelial casts in urine	Acute toxic/viral nephrosis
Rhomboid crystals, positively bifringent	Pseudogout
Rib notching	Coarctation of aorta
Roth's spots in retina	Endocarditis
Rotor's syndrome	Congenital conjugated hyperbilirubinemia
Rouleaux formation (RBCs)	Multiple myeloma
Russell bodies	Multiple myeloma
S3	Left-to-right shunt (VSD, PDA, ASD), mitral regurgitation, LV failure (CHF)
S4	Aortic stenosis, hypertrophic subaortic stenosis
Schiller-Duval bodies	Yolk sac tumor
Senile plaques	Alzheimer's disease
Sézary syndrome	Cutaneous T-cell lymphoma
Sheehan's syndrome	Postpartum pituitary necrosis
Shwartzman reaction	*Neisseria meningitidis*
Signet-ring cells	Gastric carcinoma
Simian crease	Down syndrome
Sipple's syndrome	MEN type IIa
Sjögren's syndrome	Dry eyes, dry mouth, arthritis
Skip lesions	Crohn's
Slapped cheeks	Erythema infectiosum (fifth disease)
Smith antigen	SLE
"Smudge cell"	CLL
Soap bubble on x-ray	Giant cell tumor of bone
Spike and dome on EM	Membranous glomerulonephritis
Spitz nevus	Benign juvenile melanoma
Splinter hemorrhages in fingernails	Endocarditis
Starry-sky pattern	Burkitt's lymphoma
"Strawberry tongue"	Scarlet fever
Streaky ovaries	Turner's syndrome
String sign on x-ray	Crohn's disease
Subepithelial humps on EM	Poststreptococcal glomerulonephritis
Suboccipital lymphadenopathy	Rubella
Sulfur granules	*Actinomyces israelii*

Swollen gums, bruising, poor wound healing, anemia	Scurvy (ascorbic acid, vitamin C deficiency)—vitamin C is necessary for hydroxylation of proline and lysine in collagen synthesis
Systolic ejection murmur (crescendo-decrescendo)	Aortic valve stenosis
t(8;14)	Burkitt's lymphoma (c-*myc* activation)
t(9;22)	Philadelphia chromosome, CML (*bcr-abl* hybrid)
t(14;18)	Follicular lymphomas (*bcl*-2 activation)
Tabes dorsalis	3° syphilis
Tendon xanthomas (classically Achilles)	Familial hypercholesterolemia
Thumb sign on lateral x-ray	Epiglottitis (*Haemophilus influenzae*)
Thyroidization of kidney	Chronic bacterial pyelonephritis
Tophi	Gout
"Tram-track" appearance on LM	Membranoproliferative glomerulonephritis
Trousseau's sign	Visceral cancer, pancreatic adenocarcinoma (migratory thrombophlebitis), hypocalcemia (carpal spasm)
Virchow's node	Left supraclavicular node enlargement from metastatic carcinoma of the stomach
Virchow's triad	Pulmonary embolism (triad = blood stasis, endothelial damage, hypercoagulation)
von Recklinghausen's disease	Neurofibromatosis with café-au-lait spots
von Recklinghausen's disease of bone	Osteitis fibrosa cystica ("brown tumor")
Wallenberg's syndrome	PICA thrombosis
Waterhouse-Friderichsen syndrome	Adrenal hemorrhage associated with meningococcemia
Waxy casts	Chronic end-stage renal disease
WBC casts in urine	Acute pyelonephritis
WBCs in urine	Acute cystitis
Wermer's syndrome	MEN type I
Whipple's disease	Malabsorption syndrome caused by *Tropheryma whippelii*
Wilson's disease	Hepatolenticular degeneration
"Wire loop" appearance on LM	Lupus nephropathy
"Worst headache of my life"	Berry aneurysm—associated with adult polycystic kidney disease
Xanthochromia (CSF)	Subarachnoid hemorrhage
Xerostomia + arthritis + keratoconjunctivitis sicca	Sjögren's syndrome

Zenker's diverticulum	Upper GI diverticulum
Zollinger-Ellison syndrome	Gastrin-secreting tumor associated with ulcers

Most Common ...	
Bacteremia/pneumonia (IVDA)	*Staphylococcus aureus*
Bacteria associated with cancer	*Helicobacter pylori*
Bacteria found in GI tract	*Bacteroides* (second most common is *Escherichia coli*)
Brain tumor (adults)	Mets > astrocytoma (including glioblastoma multiforme) > meningioma > schwannoma
Brain tumor (kids)	Medulloblastoma (cerebellum)
Brain tumor—supratentorial (kids)	Craniopharyngioma
Breast cancer	Infiltrating ductal carcinoma (in the United States, 1 in 9 women will develop breast cancer)
Breast mass	Fibrocystic change (in postmenopausal women, carcinoma is the most common)
Breast tumor (benign)	Fibroadenoma
Bug in debilitated, hospitalized pneumonia patient	*Klebsiella*
Cardiac 1° tumor (adults)	Myxoma (4:1 left to right atrium; "ball and valve")
Cardiac 1° tumor (kids)	Rhabdomyoma
Cardiac tumor (adults)	Mets
Cardiomyopathy	Dilated cardiomyopathy
Chromosomal disorder	Down syndrome (associated with ALL, Alzheimer's dementia, and endocardial cushion defects)
Chronic arrhythmia	Atrial fibrillation (associated with high risk of emboli)
Congenital cardiac anomaly	VSD
Constrictive pericarditis	Tuberculosis
Coronary artery involved in thrombosis	LAD > RCA > LCA
Cyanosis (early; less common)	Tetralogy of Fallot, transposition of great vessels, truncus arteriosus
Cyanosis (late; more common)	VSD, ASD, PDA (close with indomethacin; open with misoprostol)
Demyelinating disease	Multiple sclerosis
Dietary deficit	Iron
Epiglottitis	*Haemophilus influenzae* type B
Esophageal cancer	Squamous cell carcinoma

Gene involved in cancer	p53 tumor suppressor gene
Group affected by cystic fibrosis	Caucasians (fat-soluble vitamin deficiencies, mucous plugs/lung infections)
Gynecologic malignancy	Endometrial carcinoma
Heart murmur	Mitral valve prolapse
Heart valve in bacterial endocarditis	Mitral
Heart valve in bacterial endocarditis in IVDA	Tricuspid
Heart valve (rheumatic fever)	Mitral valve (aortic is 2nd)
Helminth infection (U.S.)	*Enterobius vermicularis* (*Ascaris lumbricoides* is 2nd most common)
Hereditary bleeding disorder	Von Willebrand's
Kidney stones	Calcium = radiopaque (2nd most common is ammonium = radiopaque; formed by urease-positive organisms such as *Proteus vulgaris* or *Staphylococcus*)
Liver disease	Alcoholic liver disease
Location of brain tumors (adults)	Supratentorial
Location of brain tumors (kids)	Infratentorial
Lysosomal storage disease disorder	Gaucher's
Male cancer	Prostatic carcinoma
Malignancy associated with noninfectious fever	Hodgkin's
Malignant skin tumor	Basal cell carcinoma (rarely metastasizes)
Mets to bone	Breast, lung, thyroid, testes, prostate, kidney
Mets to brain	Lung, breast, skin (melanoma), kidney (renal cell carcinoma), GI
Mets to liver	Colon, gastric, pancreatic, breast, and lung carcinomas
Motor neuron disease	ALS
Neoplasm (kids)	ALL (2nd most common is cerebellar medulloblastoma)
Nephrotic syndrome	Membranous glomerulonephritis
Obstruction of male urinary tract	BPH
Opportunistic infection in AIDS	PCP
Organ receiving mets	Adrenal glands (due to rich blood supply)
Organ sending mets	Lung > breast, stomach
Ovarian tumor (benign)	Serous cystadenoma
Ovarian tumor (malignant)	Serous cystadenocarcinoma
Pancreatic tumor	Adenocarcinoma (head of pancreas)
Patient with ALL/CLL/AML/CML	ALL—child, CLL—adult > 60, AML—adult > 60, CML—adult 35–50

Patient with Hodgkin's	Young male (except nodular sclerosis type—female)
Patient with minimal change disease	Young child
Patient with Reiter's	Male
Pituitary tumor	Prolactinoma (2nd—somatotropic "acidophilic" adenoma)
Preventable cancer	Lung cancer
Primary bone tumor (adults)	Multiple myeloma
Primary hyperparathyroidism	Adenomas (followed by hyperplasia, then carcinoma)
Primary liver tumor	Hepatoma
Renal tumor	Renal cell carcinoma—associated with von Hippel–Lindau and acquired polycystic kidney disease; paraneoplastic syndromes (erythropoietin, renin, PTH, ACTH)
Secondary hyperparathyroidism	Hypocalcemia of chronic renal failure
Sexually transmitted disease	*Chlamydia*
Site of diverticula	Sigmoid colon
Site of metastasis	Regional lymph nodes
Site of metastasis (2nd most common)	Liver
Sites of atherosclerosis	Abdominal aorta > coronary > popliteal > carotid
Skin cancer	Basal cell carcinoma
Stomach cancer	Adenocarcinoma
Testicular tumor	Seminoma
Thyroid cancer	Papillary carcinoma
Tracheoesophageal fistula	Lower esophagus joins trachea/upper esophagus—blind pouch
Tumor in men	Prostate carcinoma
Tumor in women	Leiomyoma (estrogen dependent)
Tumor of infancy	Hemangioma
Tumor of the adrenal medulla (adults)	Pheochromocytoma (benign)
Tumor of the adrenal medulla (kids)	Neuroblastoma (malignant)
Type of Hodgkin's	Nodular sclerosis (vs. mixed cellularity, lymphocytic predominance, lymphocytic depletion)
Type of non-Hodgkin's	Follicular, small cleaved
Type of pituitary adenoma	Prolactinoma
Vasculitis	Temporal arteritis (risk of ipsilateral blindness due to thrombosis of ophthalmic artery)
Viral encephalitis	HSV
Vitamin deficiency (U.S.)	Folic acid (pregnant women are at high risk; body stores only 3- to 4-month supply)

Most Frequent Cause of ...	
Addison's	Autoimmune (infection is the 2nd most common cause)
Aneurysm, dissecting	HTN
Aortic aneurysm, abdominal and descending aorta	Atherosclerosis
Aortic aneurysm, ascending	3° syphilis
Bacterial meningitis (adults)	*Neisseria meningitidis*
Bacterial meningitis (elderly)	*Streptococcus pneumoniae*
Bacterial meningitis (kids)	*Haemophilus influenzae* type B
Bacterial meningitis (newborns)	*Escherichia coli*
Cancer associated with AIDS	Kaposi's sarcoma
Congenital adrenal hyperplasia	21-hydroxylase deficiency
Cretinism	Iodine deficit/hypothyroidism
Cushing's syndrome	Corticosteroid therapy (2nd most common cause is excess ACTH secretion by pituitary)
Death in CML	Blast crisis
Death in SLE	Lupus nephropathy
Dementia	Alzheimer's (2nd most common is multi-infarct)
DIC	Gram-negative sepsis, obstetric complications, cancer, burn trauma
Ejection click	Aortic/pulmonic stenosis
Food poisoning	*Staphylococcus aureus*
Glomerulonephritis (adults)	IgA nephropathy (Berger's disease)
Hematoma—epidural	Rupture of middle meningeal artery (arterial bleeding is fast)
Hematoma—subdural	Rupture of bridging veins (trauma; venous bleeding is slow)
Hemochromatosis	Multiple blood transfusions (can result in CHF, and ↑ risk of hepatocellular carcinoma)
Hepatic cirrhosis	EtOH
Hepatocellular carcinoma	Cirrhotic liver (often associated with hepatitis B and C)
Holosystolic murmur	VSD, tricuspid regurgitation, mitral regurgitation
Hypertension, 2°	Renal disease
Hypoparathyroidism	Thyroidectomy
Hypopituitarism	Adenoma
Infection in blood transfusion	Hepatitis C

Infection in burn victims	*Pseudomonas*
Leukemia (adults)	AML
"Machine-like" murmur	PDA
Mental retardation	Down syndrome (fragile X is the second most common cause)
MI	Atherosclerosis
Mitral valve stenosis	Rheumatic heart disease
Myocarditis	Coxsackie B
Nephrotic syndrome (adults)	Membranous glomerulonephritis
Nephrotic syndrome (kids)	Minimal change disease (associated with infections/vaccinations; treat with corticosteroids)
Opening snap	Mitral stenosis
Osteomyelitis	*Staphylococcus aureus*
Osteomyelitis in patients with sickle cell disease	*Salmonella*
Osteomyelitis with IVDA	*Pseudomonas*
Pancreatitis (acute)	EtOH and gallstones
Pancreatitis (chronic)	EtOH (adults), cystic fibrosis (kids)
Peau d'orange	Carcinoma of the breast
Pelvic inflammatory disease	*Neisseria gonorrhoeae* (monoarticular arthritis)
Pneumonia, hospital-acquired	*Klebsiella*
Pneumonia in CF, burn infection	*Pseudomonas aeruginosa*
Preventable blindness	*Chlamydia*
Primary amenorrhea	Turner's (XO)
Primary hyperaldosteronism	Adenoma of adrenal cortex
Primary hyperparathyroidism	Adenoma
Pulmonary hypertension	COPD
Right heart failure due to a pulmonary cause	Cor pulmonale
Right-sided heart failure	Left-sided heart failure
Sheehan's syndrome	Postpartum pituitary infarction 2° to hemorrhage
SIADH	Small cell carcinoma of the lung
UTI	*Escherichia coli*
UTI (young women)	*E. coli* and *Staphylococcus saprophyticus*

HIGH-YIELD FACTS

Rapid Review

Database of Basic Science Review Resources

Books to GET

UCV Bundle
BRS Path Flashcards
Buzzwords For Boards : usmle step 1 recall.
High yield Behavioral science.

World Wide Web Sites
Comprehensive
Anatomy
Behavioral Science
Biochemistry
Microbiology
Pathology
Pharmacology
Physiology

Commercial Review Courses
Publisher Contacts

This section is a database of current basic science review books, sample examination books, software, Web sites, and commercial review courses marketed to medical students studying for the USMLE Step 1. At the end of this section is a list of publishers and independent bookstores with addresses and phone numbers. For each book, we list the Title of the book, the First Author (or editor), the Series Name (where applicable), the Current Publisher, the Copyright Year, the Number of Pages, the ISBN Code, the Approximate List Price, the Format of the book, and the Number of Test Questions. The entries for most books also include Summary Comments that describe their style and overall utility for studying. Finally, each book receives a Rating. The books are sorted into a comprehensive section as well as into sections corresponding to the seven traditional basic medical science disciplines (anatomy, behavioral science, biochemistry, microbiology, pathology, pharmacology, and physiology). Within each section, books are arranged by Rating, and alphabetically by First Author within each Rating group.

For the 2003 edition of *First Aid for the USMLE Step 1*, the database of rated review books has been reorganized and updated with the addition of many new books and software and the removal of some older, outdated items. A letter rating scale with six different grades reflects the detailed student evaluations for **Rated Resources.** They are followed by **New Resources** that have not yet been reviewed, and finally **Other Resources** for your consideration with detailed student reviews where available. Each rated resource receives a rating as follows:

A+	Excellent for boards review.
A A–	Very good for boards review; choose among the group.
B+ B	Good, but use only after exhausting better sources.
B–	Fair, but there are many better books in the discipline; or low-yield subject material.

The Rating is meant to reflect the overall usefulness of the resource in preparing for the USMLE Step 1 examination. This is based on a number of factors, including:

- The cost
- The readability of the text
- The appropriateness and accuracy of the material
- The quality and number of sample questions
- The quality of written answers to sample questions
- The quality and appropriateness of the illustrations (e.g., graphs, diagrams, photographs)
- The length of the text (longer is not necessarily better)
- The quality and number of other resources available in the same discipline
- The importance of the discipline on the USMLE Step 1 examination

Please note that the rating does not reflect the quality of the resources for purposes other than reviewing for the USMLE Step 1 examination. Many books with lower ratings are well written and informative but are not ideal for boards preparation. We have not listed or commented on general textbooks available in the basic sciences.

Evaluations are based on the cumulative results of formal and informal surveys of thousands of medical students at many medical schools across the country. The summary comments and overall ratings represent a consensus opinion, but there may have been a broad range of opinion or limited student feedback on any particular resource.

Please note that the data listed are subject to change in that:

■ Publishers' prices change frequently.
■ Bookstores often charge an additional markup.
■ New editions come out frequently, and the quality of updating varies.
■ The same book may be reissued through another publisher.

We actively encourage medical students and faculty to submit their opinions and ratings of these basic science review materials so that we may update our database. (See p. xv, How to Contribute.) In addition, we ask that publishers and authors submit for evaluation review copies of basic science review books, including new editions and books not included in our database. We also solicit reviews of new books or suggestions for alternate modes of study that may be useful in preparing for the examination, such as flash cards, computer-based tutorials, commercial review courses, and World Wide Web sites.

Disclaimer/Conflict of Interest Statement

No material in this book, including the ratings, reflects the opinion or influence of the publisher. All errors and omissions will gladly be corrected if brought to the attention of the authors through the publisher. Please note that the entire Underground Clinical Vignette series are independent publications by the authors of this book; their ratings are based solely on data from the student survey and feedback forms.

RATED RESOURCES

Kaplan Medical (Qbank)

Test/2000+ q

www.kaplanmedical.com

Internet-based question bank provides tailored CBT-format exams. Test content and performance feedback are provided by organ system and discipline. Questions are representative in style and at times content to those on the actual exam. E-mail help on USMLE topics. There is a free online demonstration; costs vary with subscription period. Requires time commitment.

WebPath: The Internet Pathology Laboratory

Review/290 q

Klatt

www-medlib.med.utah.edu/WebPath/webpath.html

Features a wealth of outstanding gross and microscopic illustrations, clinical vignette questions, and case studies. Contains many classic, high-quality illustrations. Features 21 exams with more than 290 questions that reflect current boards format and difficulty level but are typically shorter. Online exams include illustrations and a timer. A WebPath CD-ROM is available for $60.00 and features the online Web site plan supplemented with 40% more material, including additional topics, tutorials, and radiology. The CD-ROM is ideal for computers with slow or no Internet access. May be ordered directly from Web site.

B+ Digital Anatomist Interactive Atlases

Review

University of Washington

www9.biostr.washington.edu/da.html

Good site containing an interactive neuroanatomy course along with three-dimensional atlas of the brain, thorax, and knee. Atlases have computer-generated images along with cadaver dissections. Each atlas also has a useful quiz in which users identify structures in the slide images.

B The Whole Brain Atlas

Review

Johnson

www.med.harvard.edu/AANLIB/home.html

Collection of high-quality brain MR and CT images with views of normal, aging, and diseased brains (CVA, degenerative, neoplastic, and inflammatory diseases). The interface is technologically impressive but complex. The guided tours and image correlation to cases are especially useful. Although not all of the images are particularly high yield for the boards, this is an excellent introduction to neuroimaging.

B | **Medrevu.com (*irevu*)** | Test/4500+ q

www.medrevu.com

Subscription-based site affiliated with Lippincott Williams & Wilkins with more than 4500 USMLE-style questions. Some questions not in vignette style. Costs vary with subscription period. There is a free 50-question demonstration. Limited student feedback. Compare with Kaplan's Qbank.

B | **Active Learning Centre** | Test/100+ q

Turchin

www.med.jhu.edu/medcenter/quiz/home.cgi

Quiz engine site based on a large database that has an extensive list of bugs, drugs, and vaccines. The questions generated test the basic characteristics of each element in the database in a multiple-choice, matching, or essay format that the user selects. Questions are not boards style but are useful for learning the memory-intensive subjects of microbiology and pharmacology.

B‾ | **Introduction to Clinical Microbiology** | Review

medic.med.uth.tmc.edu/path/00001450.htm

Basic introduction/review of the fundamentals of microbiology. The site has a useful review of the different types of culture media and lab tests. The information on bugs is a shallow but quick read.

RATED RESOURCES

 NMS Review for USMLE Step 1 Examination $42.95 Test/1000+ q
Lazo
Lippincott Williams & Wilkins, 2002, 436 pages (plus CD-ROM), ISBN
0781732921
Good source of practice questions and answers. Newest edition features
clinically based integrated content with increased numbers of patient-
based questions. Some questions are too picky or difficult. Good annotated explanations, but occasionally offers unnecessary detail. Good buy
for the number of questions. Organized as four 200-question booklets;
good for simulating exam conditions, yet clinical vignettes with multiple
questions per case description do not reflect current boards format. Helpful color plates. CD-ROM provides practice with computer-based format.

 Step Up: A High-Yield Systems-Based Review $32.95 Review only
for the USMLE
Mehta
Lippincott Williams & Wilkins, 2001, 394 pages, ISBN 0781738938
Comprehensive and unique organ-system-based review text that is mainly
composed of outlines, charts, tables, and diagrams. Appendix includes 38
clinical cases and an alphabetical section on pharmacology. Revised
reprint edition now available with new edition expected in 2003.

 Pathophysiology for the Boards $28.95 Review only
and Wards—USMLE Step 1
Ayala
Blackwell Science, 2000, 288 pages, ISBN 0632044853
System-based outline with a focus on pathology. Excellent organization
with color glossy photos. Clinical scenarios and a few questions at the end
of each chapter. Appendix has a helpful overview of neurology, immunology, "zebras," syndromes, and pearls.

B+ Blackwell's Underground Clinical Vignettes $151.00 Review
Step 1 Bundle
Bhushan
Blackwell Science, 2002, 9 volumes, ISBN 0632045590
All nine volumes of the *UCV Step 1* books bundled with a free, 50-plus-
page *Basic Science Color Atlas* containing over 250 full-color photographs
linked to the vignette cases. Designed for easy quizzing. Atlas includes histology, gross pathology, hematology, and microbiology images. Case-based
vignettes provide a good review supplement.

REVIEW RESOURCES

Comprehensive

B+   Board Simulator Series

$25.95 (each)   Test/770 q

Gruber

Lippincott Williams & Wilkins
Body Systems Reviews I: 1997, 338 pages, ISBN 0683302981
Body Systems Reviews II: 1997, 350 pages, ISBN 068330299X
Body Systems Reviews III: 1997, 298 pages, ISBN 0683303007
General Principles in the Basic Sciences: 1997, 306 pages, ISBN 0683302965
Normal and Abnormal Processes in the Basic Sciences: 1997, 304 pages, ISBN 0683302973
USMLE Step 1 Board Simulator on CD-ROM for Windows (includes all volumes), 2000, ISBN 0781792657, $99.95
Four exams per book with approximately 160 questions each. Follows USMLE content outline. Numerous vignettes reflect the clinical slant of the exam. Good black-and-white photographs. Comprehensive systems-based approach that is most effective if all three "Reviews" books are used. For the motivated student. Questions tend to be more picky than those of the actual USMLE exam. Needs updating. Explanations discuss important concepts. *General Principles* has some overlap with *Normal and Abnormal Processes*. *Normal and Abnormal Processes* can be used independently, as it covers all seven major subject areas. The CD-ROM for Windows allows customized testing and performance feedback.

B+   Appleton & Lange's Review for the USMLE Step 1

$39.95   Test/1200 q

King

McGraw-Hill, 2003, 496 pages, ISBN 0071377425
Features seven subject-based tests and three 100-question comprehensive exams. Good buy for the number of questions. Thorough explanations of right and wrong answers. Reasonable, straightforward, question-based review to assess your strengths and weaknesses. Testing includes references to diagrams, images, and a few color plates. Revised and updated to current USMLE format.

B+   NMS USMLE Step 1

$44.95   Software/1000+ q

Lazo

Lippincott Williams & Wilkins, 1998, ISBN 0683300954
Windows/Mac-based testing software. Features questions from Lazo's *NMS Review for USMLE Step 1*. Organized as four comprehensive tests. Flexible test modes. Well-written questions with frequent clinical vignettes. Illustrations are poorly reproduced. Does not accurately reflect CBT format.

B+ | **Clinical Vignettes for the USMLE Step 1: PreTest** | **$24.95** | Test/400 q

McGraw-Hill

McGraw-Hill, 2002, 332 pages, ISBN 0071373764

Clinical vignette-style questions with detailed explanations. Covers all the basic sciences. Good self-evaluation tool, although questions may not mirror like those on actual USMLE exam.

B+ | **Crashing the Boards: USMLE Step 1** | **$19.95** | Review only

Yeh

Lippincott Williams & Wilkins, 1999, 184 pages, ISBN 0781719771

Brief coverage of high-yield topics. Great diagrams and a good sense of humor. No photos. Good organization (bulleted facts and highlighted boxing). Useful for supplementary, last-minute review. Incomplete book reviews in the back. New edition retains outdated strategies for paper-and-pencil exam. Compare with Carl's *Medical Boards—Step 1 Made Ridiculously Simple*.

B | **Integrated Basic Sciences: PreTest** | **$29.95** | Review/453 q

Brown

McGraw-Hill, 1999, 304 pages, ISBN 007052551X

Great clinical review questions. Each of the 151 vignettes is followed by a group of three questions testing anatomy and normal and abnormal function. Answers are discussed in detail. Covers many core diseases, organized by system. Time-consuming; for the motivated student.

B | **Medical Boards—Step 1 Made Ridiculously Simple** | **$24.95** | Review only

Carl

MedMaster, 2002, 353 pages, ISBN 0940780526

Quick and easy reading. Table and chart format is organized by subject. Mixed reviews. Some charts are poorly labeled. Consider as an adjunct. Compare with Yeh's *Crashing the Boards: USMLE Step 1*.

B | **Rapid Preparation for the USMLE Step 1** | **$36.00** | Test/926 q

Johnson

J&S Publishing, 1997, 406 pages, ISBN 1888308028

A "best of J&S" compendium. Questions are organized by subject and are drawn as exact duplicates from other books in the series. Thorough explanations with key concepts in boldface; however, some are incomplete or inaccurate. High-quality black-and-white MRIs, CTs, line drawings, histology, and gross photo illustrations. Clinical vignette–based questions.

B **Kaplan's Organ-Based Review Books** $499.00 Review/1200 q
Kaplan
Kaplan, 2001, Item 634101, ISBN 0X63410101
Includes seven organ-system-based review books, a test-taking and strategy guide, a Qbook of 850 questions, and two CD-ROMs (one with 350 questions divided by organ system and one with a full-length simulation). The software is also available separately. Books and CD-ROMs can be purchased by calling 1-800-KAP-ITEM. Limited student feedback.

B **Gold Standard Prep Set for USMLE Step 1** $265.00 Audio tapes
Knouse
Gold Standard, 2001
Set of 48 approximately 90-minute audio tapes covering USMLE Step 1 material. Limited but positive feedback on updated and expanded set of audiotapes. Popular among some students as a way to review while driving, while working out, and during down time. Has some inaccuracies. Available only by mail order at (740) 592-4124, fax: (740) 592-4045, or www.boardprep.net.

B **Cracking the Boards: USMLE Step 1** $34.95 Review/400 q
The Princeton Review
Random House, 2000, 832 pages, ISBN 0375761632
Comprehensive text review based on the USMLE content outline, written by past and present medical students. Wordy and broad spectrum but few details. Many labeled illustrations, chart, and photos. Student opinion varies widely.

B **Buzzwords for the Boards:** $29.00 Review only
USMLE Step 1 Recall
Reinheimer
Lippincott Williams & Wilkins, 1999, 400 pages, ISBN 0683306391
Quizzes on main topics and key points in a two-column question-and-answer format. Good for self-testing and quick review. Use as a change of pace; hits many important clinical features but is not comprehensive or tightly organized. Questions lack the level of integration found on the exam. Contains several errors.

B **Preparation for USMLE Step 1 Basic** $15.00 Test/315 q
Medical Sciences, Volumes A, B, C **(each)**
Waintrub
Maval Publishing, 1999, 78 pages, ISBN 1884083137 (Vol. A), 1884083143 (Vol. B), 1884083153 (Vol. C)
Three tests with appropriate-format, straightforward questions, and explanatory answers. Suggested time frame for test simulation. Moderate clinical orientation. Good color photographs. Moderately expensive for the number of questions.

B **Preparation for the USMLE Step 1 Basic Medical Sciences, Volumes D, E**   **$15.00**   Test/210 q
                                                                                                  (each)

Waintrub

Maval Publishing, 1995, 57 pages, ISBN 1884083161

Same format and comments as for Volumes A, B, and C, but even more expensive for the number of questions.

B **Preparation for the USMLE Step 1 Basic Medical Sciences, Volume F**   **$18.00**   Test/540 q

Waintrub

Maval Publishing, 1997, 120 pages, ISBN 1884083080

Six practice tests and answers; otherwise same comments as for Volumes A through E. Free with the purchase of the *USMLE Review Book* (listed separately) from the Maval Publishing Web site.

B **USMLE Step 1 Simulated Test 1 & 2**   **$18.00**   Test/180 q
                                                               (each)

Walling

Maval Publishing, 1999, 87 pages, ISBN 1884083188, ISBN 1884083196

Two 90-question simulated exams in each booklet covering all the basic science topics. Clinically oriented, but simplistic questions. Good images. Moderately expensive for the amount of material.

B **USMLE Success**   **$20.00**   How-to/360 q

Zaslau

FMSG, 1999, 150 pages, ISBN 1886468303

Broad overview of all three Steps. Has a useful "what to study" section with a list of classic slides, x-rays, and gross specimens that have appeared on previous USMLE exams; however, no pictures or diagrams. The mnemonic section is helpful. Includes a 180-question mock Step 1 exam with explanations. Appropriate for the IMG student preparing to take all three Step exams in a short time period.

B⁻ **Exam Master Step 1**   **$149.00**   Software/8000 q

Exam Master

Exam Master Corporation, 2001, ISBN 1581290683

Windows/Mac-based testing software with access to up to 8000 Step 1 questions. Questions are relatively simple. Ability to hide multiple-choice options. New version eliminates K-type, nonclinical questions and provides compatibility with Windows 98.

Rypins' Basic Sciences Review, Vol. I $39.95 Review/1000+ q
Frohlich
Lippincott Williams & Wilkins, 2001, 810 pages, ISBN 0781725186
Multitopic textbook with few figures and tables. A good general reference,
but should be used with other subject-specific sources. Well priced for the
number of pages and questions. Requires extensive time commitment.

 Rypins' Questions and Answers $34.95 Test/1600+ q
for Basic Science Review
Frohlich
Lippincott Williams & Wilkins, 2001, 288 pages, ISBN 0781725208
Questions with detailed answers to supplement Rypins' *Basic Sciences Re-*
view. Decent overall question-based review of all subjects. Requires time
commitment. Limited and mixed reviews. Includes CD-ROM.

 USMLE Step 1: The Stanford Solutions $18.95 Answers
to the NBME Computer-Based Sample Test Questions
Kush
J&S Publishing, 1999, 120 pages, ISBN 1893730077
Explanations, with references, for the NBME practice CD-ROM. Expen-
sive for the amount of material.

 USMLE Step 1 Crosswords That Won't $19.95 Review only
Leave You Crosseyed, Volume 1: Basic Sciences
Silverstein
MedHumor Publications, 2000, 200 pages, ISBN 0970028733
USMLE review-oriented crossword puzzle book containing over 750 fre-
quently tested facts, concepts, and key disease associations that are pre-
sented in a way that facilitates learning. Organized by the traditional basic
sciences. Style may not work for most students. Limited student feedback.
Also available at www.passtheboards.com.

 USMLE Review Book, Step 1 $18.00 Review only
Basic Medical Sciences
Walling
Maval Publishing, 1999, 290 pages, ISBN 1884083218
Detailed summaries of important information, organized by USMLE con-
tent outline. Mostly text, with some tables, photos, and diagrams. Re-
quires time commitment; not for quick review. Limited student feedback.

REVIEW RESOURCES

Comprehensive

Basic Science Question Bank　　　　　　　　**$19.00**　Test/500 q
Zaslau
FMSG, 1997, 141 pages, ISBN 1886468176
Three sections designed to simulate the three-hour time periods of the exam. Includes letter answers with explanations and some clinical vignettes. Questions adequately reflect the clinical slant of the USMLE. Includes 90 poor-quality pictures and diagrams. Repeated questions from other books in the series. Limited student feedback.

 Step 1 Success　　　　　　　　　　　　**$38.00**　Test/720 q
Zaslau
FMSG, 1996, 198 pages, ISBN 1886468079
Full-length practice examination with four 180-question booklets with explanations. Features many clinically focused questions similar to the USMLE format. Offers a small number of black-and-white photographs of moderate quality but no color pictures. Limited student feedback. Also available on CD-ROM.

 "Virtual Reality" Step 1　　　　　　　　**$19.00**　Test/370 q
Zaslau
FMSG, 1998, 163 pages, ISBN 1886468230
Includes two "virtual" practice tests. Simple, straightforward questions; few images but in poor-quality black-and-white photocopy. Explanations of both correct and incorrect answers.

 "Virtual Reality" Step 1 Update 1998　　**$10.00**　Test/130 q
Zaslau
FMSG, 1998, 69 pages, ISBN 1886468265
Includes updated questions following the administration of the 1997 USMLE.

USMLE Step 1 (REA)   **$39.95**   Review/1080 q
Cargan
REA, 2001, 558 pages, ISBN 0878910743
Not yet reviewed.

 Rapid Review for the USMLE Step 1   **$32.95**   Review/1400 q
Goljan
Mosby, 2002, 314 pages, ISBN 0323008410
Outline format with high-yield margin notes, figures, and tables that high-
light key content. Narrative clinical boxes illustrate clinical relevance.
Practice exams provide clinically oriented questions. Includes a CD-ROM
of questions. New series.

 USMLE Step1 CD-ROM Version 2.0   **$49.95**   Software/1000+ q
Lazo
Lippincott Williams & Wilkins, 2002, ISBN 0683300954
Not yet reviewed.

 High-Yield Basic Science: PreTest   **$14.95**   Review only
McGraw-Hill
McGraw-Hill, 2002, 172 pages, ISBN 0071386300
Outline format of basic science facts with diagrams and tables. Organized
by subject.

Buzzwords for the Boards: **$29.95**   Software/1000+ q
USMLE Step 1 Recall PDA
Reinheimer
Lippincott Williams & Wilkins, 2001, ISBN 078173343X
Derived from the book of the same name. Not yet reviewed.

REVIEW RESOURCES

Comprehensive

USMLE Step 1 Review: The Study Guide

$32.95   Review only

Goldberg

Sage, 1996, 473 pages, ISBN 0803972849

A comprehensive review that often reads like a textbook. Does not organize ideas in a way that is useful for review purposes. No mnemonics, no questions, and very few diagrams or pictures. Requires a large time commitment and is low yield.

Basic Science Review Success

$18.00   Review only

Zaslau

FMSG, 1997, 138 pages, ISBN 1886468184

A cursory presentation of high-yield facts in all seven basic science topics. However, much more knowledge is required for actual success on the USMLE. No pictures or diagrams. Includes sections on test-taking pointers and a bonus section on the Match, internship, and residency. Limited student feedback.

RATED RESOURCES

A− **Underground Clinical Vignettes: Anatomy** **$17.95** Review only
Bhushan
Blackwell Science, 2002, 100 pages, ISBN 0632045418
Concise clinical cases illustrating approximately 100 frequently tested diseases with an anatomic basis. Cardinal signs, symptoms, and buzzwords are highlighted. Use as a supplement to other sources of review.

A− **High-Yield Embryology** **$17.95** Review only
Dudek
Lippincott Williams & Wilkins, 2002, 192 pages, ISBN 0781730430
Excellent, concise review of embryology for the USMLE. Excellent organization with clinical correlations. High-yield list of embryologic origins of tissues. Expensive for the amount of material. No index.

A− **High-Yield Gross Anatomy** **$19.95** Review only
Dudek
Lippincott Williams & Wilkins, 2001, 144 pages, ISBN 0781730430
Excellent, concise review with clinical correlations. Contains well-labeled, high-yield radiologic images, yet may be useful to supplement with an atlas. No index.

A− **High-Yield Neuroanatomy** **$19.95** Review only
Fix
Lippincott Williams & Wilkins, 2000, 128 pages, ISBN 0683307215
Clean, easy-to-read outline format. Straightforward text with excellent diagrams and illustrations. Compare with Goldberg's *Clinical Neuroanatomy Made Ridiculously Simple*. No index.

B+ **Liebman's Neuroanatomy Made Easy & Understandable** **$31.00** Review/Few q
Gertz
Aspen, 1999, 210 pages, ISBN 0834216329
Easy to read. Contains excellent diagrams. Fast, straightforward, high-yield review. Some humor and interesting facts to help the student remember pathways. Expensive. Incomplete, but more thorough than Goldberg's *Clinical Neuroanatomy Made Ridiculously Simple*.

B+ Clinical Anatomy Made Ridiculously Simple

$19.95   Review only

Goldberg

MedMaster, 2002, 187 pages, ISBN 0940780534

Easy reading, simple diagrams, and lots of mnemonics and amusing associations. Incomplete. Style has variable appeal to students, so browse before buying. Good coverage of selected topics. Best if used during the course.

B+ Clinical Neuroanatomy Made Ridiculously Simple

$13.95   Review/Few q

Goldberg

MedMaster, 2000, 97 pages, ISBN 0940780461

Easy to read, memorable, and simplified, with clever hand-drawn diagrams. Quick, high-yield review of clinical neuroanatomy. Good emphasis on clinically relevant pathways, cranial nerves, and neurologic diseases. Spotty coverage of some key boards topics. No CT or MRI images. Compare with Fix's *High-Yield Neuroanatomy*.

B+ Anatomy: Review for USMLE Step 1

$25.00   Test/560 q

Johnson

J&S Publishing, 1998, 275 pages, ISBN 1888308036

Easy reading. Clinical case-based questions with detailed explanations. Good superficial overview of cell biology, histology, gross anatomy, embryology, and neuroanatomy. Discusses clinically relevant anatomic science with good explanations, illustrations, and pictures; also covers many clinically relevant genetic diseases. Some key topics are not covered. Includes good photomicrographs, cross-sectional imaging-based questions, and patient photos.

B Cell Biology: Review for New National Boards

$25.00   Review/524 q

Adelman

J&S Publishing, 1995, 203 pages, ISBN 0963287389

Question-based review format like other J&S books. Covers classic topics in cell biology. Contains some high-quality micrographs. Recycles some questions and illustrations from J&S's *Anatomy*. Not as useful as other books in series.

B Color Atlas of Embryology

$36.00   Review only

Drews

Thieme, 1995, 421 pages, ISBN 0865775443

Embryology is presented with 176 color plates. Topics range from the basics of reproductive biology to general embryology and topics related to cellular and molecular biology.

B BRS Embryology

Dudek

$29.95   Review/500 q

Lippincott Williams & Wilkins, 199, 293 pages, ISBN 0683302728
Outline-based review of embryology that is typical for books in this series.
Good review of important embryology, but too detailed. Good discussion
of congenital malformations at the end of each chapter. Comprehensive
exam at the end of the book is the most high yield part of the book.

B High-Yield Histology

Dudek

$19.95   Review only

Lippincott Williams & Wilkins, 2000, 120 pages, ISBN 0781721342
Quick and easy review of a relatively low yield subject. Tables with some
high-yield information. Good pictures. Appendix contains classic EMs.

B BRS Neuroanatomy

Fix

$29.95   Review/500 q

Lippincott Williams & Wilkins, 2001, 416 pages, ISBN 0781728290
Updated text. Covers anatomy and embryology of the nervous system.
Complete but lengthy; requires time commitment. Compare with *High-Yield Neuroanatomy* by the same author.

B Clinical Anatomy

Monkhouse

$29.95   Review/264 q

Churchill Livingstone, 2001, 336 pages, ISBN 0443063958
Reviews core concepts in human clinical anatomy, integrating systemic
and regional anatomical description with text boxes highlighting clinical
applications. Self-assessment questions at end of each section. Nicely illustrated and well written. Limited student feedback.

B Review Questions for Neuroanatomy: Structural and Functional

Mosenthal

$19.95   Test/965 q

CRC Press-Parthenon, 1996, 126 pages, ISBN 1850706530
Good, non-boards-style questions with explanations. Some diagrams with
questions on lesions included throughout. Includes embryology of nervous
system. Best of series. Some clinical vignettes.

B Clinical Neuroanatomy: A Review with Questions and Explanations

Snell

$32.00   Review/440 q

Lippincott Williams & Wilkins, 2001, 336 pages, ISBN 0781729890
Comprehensive review book requiring time commitment. Frequent clinical correlations. Many clear diagrams. Reorganized to integrate structure
with function in a systems format.

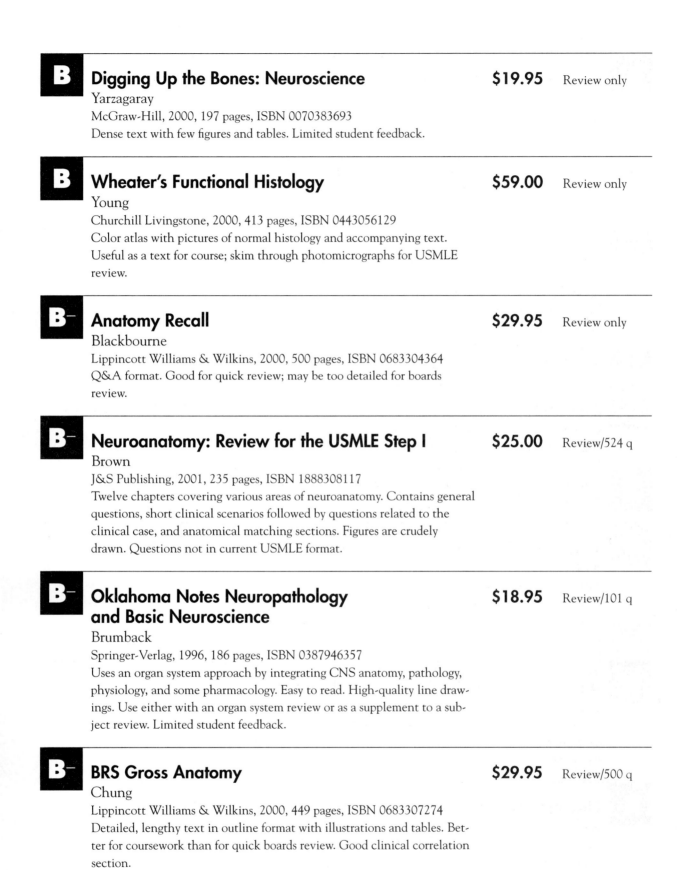

B **Digging Up the Bones: Neuroscience** $19.95   Review only
Yarzagaray
McGraw-Hill, 2000, 197 pages, ISBN 0070383693
Dense text with few figures and tables. Limited student feedback.

B **Wheater's Functional Histology** $59.00   Review only
Young
Churchill Livingstone, 2000, 413 pages, ISBN 0443056129
Color atlas with pictures of normal histology and accompanying text.
Useful as a text for course; skim through photomicrographs for USMLE
review.

B⁻ **Anatomy Recall** $29.95   Review only
Blackbourne
Lippincott Williams & Wilkins, 2000, 500 pages, ISBN 0683304364
Q&A format. Good for quick review; may be too detailed for boards
review.

B⁻ **Neuroanatomy: Review for the USMLE Step I** $25.00   Review/524 q
Brown
J&S Publishing, 2001, 235 pages, ISBN 1888308117
Twelve chapters covering various areas of neuroanatomy. Contains general
questions, short clinical scenarios followed by questions related to the
clinical case, and anatomical matching sections. Figures are crudely
drawn. Questions not in current USMLE format.

B⁻ **Oklahoma Notes Neuropathology** $18.95   Review/101 q
and Basic Neuroscience
Brumback
Springer-Verlag, 1996, 186 pages, ISBN 0387946357
Uses an organ system approach by integrating CNS anatomy, pathology,
physiology, and some pharmacology. Easy to read. High-quality line drawings. Use either with an organ system review or as a supplement to a subject review. Limited student feedback.

B⁻ **BRS Gross Anatomy** $29.95   Review/500 q
Chung
Lippincott Williams & Wilkins, 2000, 449 pages, ISBN 0683307274
Detailed, lengthy text in outline format with illustrations and tables. Bet-
ter for coursework than for quick boards review. Good clinical correlation
section.

Neuroanatomy: Illustrated $39.95

Crossman

Churchill Livingstone, 2000, 172 pages, ISBN 0443062161

Illustrations of neuroanatomical structures using colored line drawings, scanning electron micrographs, confocal micrographs, photographs of cadaveric specimens, MRI, cross sections of brain and spinal cord, and angiograms to highlight the descriptive text. Significant content may have been sacrificed for brevity.

Embryology: Review for New National Boards $25.00   Test/569 q

Gasser

J&S Publishing, 1997, 221 pages, ISBN 188830801X

Typical format for this series. Occasional vignettes reflect the clinical slant of the USMLE. Question format does not reflect the format of the USMLE; however, pictures are of high quality. Too long for boards review for such a low-yield topic. Limited student feedback.

Color Atlas of Neuroscience $34.00   Review only

Greenstein

Thieme, 2000, 448 pages, ISBN 0865777101

Visual approach to the anatomy, physiology, and pharmacology of neuroscience with 193 color plates and concise text. Requires considerable time commitment. Use to supplement larger texts.

Anatomy, Histology & Cell Biology: PreTest $24.95   Test/500 q

Klein

McGraw-Hill, 2002, 497 pages, ISBN 0071370870

Difficult questions with detailed answers. Some illustrations. Requires extensive time commitment. Includes a high-yield section that highlights clinically relevant relationships and lessons.

Basic Concepts in Cell Biology and Histology $29.95   Review only

McKenzie

McGraw-Hill, 2000, 427 pages, ISBN 0070369305

Divided by tissue type and organ system. Lots of diagrams. Overly detailed for boards review.

Neuroscience: PreTest $24.95   Test/500 q

Siegel

McGraw-Hill, 2002, 283 pages, ISBN 0071373500

Detailed questions and answers. Includes photographs of CT/MRIs and drawings of brain sections. Useful after studying from other sources. For the motivated student. Picky questions. High-yield section summarizes pathways and functions. Few helpful diagrams.

Basic Concepts in Neuroscience　　　　　　　　$29.95　　Review only

Slaughter

McGraw-Hill, 2002, 277 pages, ISBN 0071360468

Detailed description of many aspects of neuroscience. More suitable for course than quick review.

 Clinical Anatomy: An Illustrated Review　　　$32.00　　Review/500+ q
with Questions and Explanations

Snell

Lippincott Williams & Wilkins, 2001, 272 pages, ISBN 0781729890

Well-organized summary of Snell's major book. Great diagrams and tables. Questions incorporate radiographs, CT scans, and MRIs. Does not cover neuroanatomy or embryology. Neither text nor questions are as clinical as the title implies. Only some of the answers have explanations, most of which are too short.

 Basic Concepts in Embryology　　　　　　$29.95　　Review only

Sweeney

McGraw-Hill, 1998, 480 pages, ISBN 0070633088

Thorough examination of low-yield topic. Use as a reference and not for boards review.

Anatomy Recall PDA   **$29.95**   Software/Review
Blackbourne
Lippincott Williams & Wilkins, 2000, ISBN 0781733413
Derived from the book of the same name. Not yet reviewed.

 Rapid Review: Histology and Cell Biology   **$32.95**   Review/600 q
Burns
Mosby, 2002, 324 pages, ISBN 0323008348
Outline format with high-yield margin notes, figures, and tables that high-
light key content. Narrative clinical boxes illustrate clinical relevance.
Practice exams provide clinically oriented questions. Includes a CD-ROM
of questions. New series.

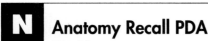 **Neuroscience: An Outline Approach**   **$29.95**   Review/Few q
Castro
Mosby, 2002, 542 pages, ISBN 0323008364
Information nicely organized in combination with tables and margin
notes. Well-illustrated diagrams and figures. Case-based problems at the
end serve to integrate material. May be too detailed for boards review. For
the motivated student.

 Essential Histology   **$42.00**   Review only
Cormack
Lippincott Williams & Wilkins, 2001, 463 pages, ISBN 0781716683
Not yet reviewed.

Essentials of Clinical Neuroanatomy
and Neurophysiology   **$29.95**   Review only
Crossman
F. A. Davis, 2003, 281 pages, ISBN 0803607725
Discussions of neuroanatomy, neurophysiology, and neuropharmacology
with illustrations and images. Well organized but too dense for boards
review.

Netter's Atlas of Embryology   **$39.95**   Review only
George
Icon Learning Systems, 2002, 250 pages, ISBN 0914168991
Not yet reviewed.

REVIEW RESOURCES

Anatomy

N | **Clinical Neuroanatomy Made Ridiculously Simple—Interactive Edition** | $19.95 | Review only

Goldberg

MedMaster, 2003, 96 pages plus CD-ROM, ISBN 0940780577

New interactive edition of classic text with a "Neurologic Localization" CD-ROM of tutorials on localization of neurologic injuries.

N | **Review of Neuroscience** | $34.95 | Review/845 q

Haines

Churchill Livingstone, 2003, 224 pages, ISBN 0443066256

Not yet reviewed.

N | **Netter's Anatomy Flash Cards** | $29.95 | Cards

Hansen

Icon Learning Systems, 2002, ISBN 1929007086

Not yet reviewed.

N | **Netter's Atlas of Human Physiology** | $39.95 | Review only

Hansen

Icon Learning Systems, 2002, ISBN 1929007019

Not yet reviewed.

N | **Histology and Cell Biology** | $46.95 | Review only

Kierszenbaum

Mosby, 2002, 640 pages, ISBN 0323016391

Relies primarily on illustrations to help students master key concepts in histology and cell biology. Great illustrations. May be more suitable as a reference for coursework. For the motivated student.

N | **Picture Tests in Histology** | $26.95 | Review/90 q

Young

Churchill Livingstone, 2001, 246 pages, ISBN 0443060207

Provides five "papers" of 24 questions each on the full range of human histology with full explanatory answers. For the motivated student.

NMS Clinical Anatomy

$32.00 Review/500 q

April

Lippincott Williams & Wilkins, 1997, 670 pages, ISBN 0683061992
Organized in outline form. Questions with detailed answers. Text is too
detailed and low yield. Limited student feedback. However, contains some
good clinical correlations and boards-style questions.

NMS Neuroanatomy

$32.00 Review/300 q

DeMyer

Lippincott Williams & Wilkins, 1998, 480 pages, ISBN 068330075X
Outline form. Nice diagrams, but low yield. Good for coursework, but too
detailed for boards review. Short, comprehensive exam at the end.

Histology Series

$99.95 Software/800+ q

Downing

MedTech Publishing, 1998, ISBN 1889185108
Database of boards-style questions arranged by subject area. Explanations
on demand. Questions cross-referenced to Junqueira's *Histology TextStack*
(sold separately). Expensive for a limited-yield topic; discounts available
directly through the publisher (800-260-2600 or www.medtech.com).
Available for either Macintosh or Windows.

BRS Cell Biology & Histology

$29.95 Review/500 q

Gartner

Lippincott Williams & Wilkins, 1997, 377 pages, ISBN 0683301039
Nice format with mixed-quality reproductions, but too detailed. Nineteen
chapters with detailed answers. For the motivated student.

NMS Histology

$32.00 Review/312 q

Henrickson

Lippincott Williams & Wilkins, 1997, 425 pages, ISBN 0683062255
Good black-and-white images. No color plates. Outline format is easy to
read for main points; however, too dense for boards review. Best used with
course.

Digging Up the Bones: Anatomy

$19.95 Review only

Linardakis

McGraw-Hill, 2000, 117 pages, ISBN 0070384150
Hits the high points of gross anatomy. Not very detailed. Clear diagrams.
Clinical tie-ins throughout, but no vignettes.

Appleton & Lange's Review of Anatomy

$39.95 Test/1400+ q

Montgomery

McGraw-Hill, 1995, 160 pages, ISBN 0838502466

High volume of questions with brief explanations, no text, and few diagrams. New edition expected in 2003. Limited student feedback.

Concepts in Gross Anatomy

$26.95 Review/160 q

Mosenthal

Parthenon, 1997, 250 pages, ISBN 1850709289

Long, detailed narrative format with review questions may be more appropriate for coursework. In-depth coverage of a relatively low yield subject. Clinical correlations hidden in dense text. Some line drawings and fill-in-the-blank drawings are of questionable value for review. Limited student feedback.

Oklahoma Notes Anatomy

$17.95 Review/70 q

Papka

Springer-Verlag, 1995, 231 pages, ISBN 0387943951

Covers embryology, gross anatomy, neuroanatomy, and histology. Broad coverage, but dense text is somewhat difficult to read. Few illustrations. The student is "encouraged to thoughtfully engage the narrative and incorporate mental images of structures."

Histology and Cell Biology: Examination and Board Review

$44.95 Test/1000- q

Paulsen

McGraw-Hill, 2000, 376 pages, ISBN 0838505937

Dense, thorough review, but low yield for boards. Good format with many questions. Designed to complement Junqueira's *Basic Histology* textbook. Requires extensive time commitment. May be useful for course.

IMS Medical Neuroscience

$25.95 Review/150 q

Prichard

Fence Creek, 1998, 448 pages, ISBN 1889325295

Similar to others in the series. Readable but lengthy and detailed text. Many excellent diagrams. Simple questions with good explanations.

Clinical Neuroanatomy: A Review with Questions and Explanations

$32.00 Review/400+ q

Snell

Lippincott Williams & Wilkins, 2001, 256 pages, ISBN 0781729890

Reasonably easy to read; contains some clinical correlations. Too long in relation to the portion of the exam devoted to neuroanatomy.

Review Questions for Human Anatomy

$21.95 Test/1000 q

Tank

Parthenon, 1996, 150 pages, ISBN 1850707952

Highly detailed questions may be more appropriate for coursework. Extensive coverage of very low yield subject with two comprehensive exams at the end. Some clinical correlations are scattered throughout. May be too time-consuming for boards exam. Limited student feedback.

Blond's Anatomy

$17.99 Review only

Tesoriero

Sulzburger & Graham, 1994, 282 pages, ISBN 094581920X

Concise review of gross anatomy. Easy read. Good tables and illustrations. More appropriate for coursework than for boards review.

RATED RESOURCES

A⁻ **BRS Behavioral Science** $29.95 Review/500 q
Fadem
Lippincott Williams & Wilkins, 1999, 352 pages, ISBN 0683306812
Easy-to-read outline format with boldfacing of key terms. Good, detailed
coverage of high-yield topics. Lengthy; gives more information than may
be needed for USMLE. Great tables and charts. Short but complete statis-
tics chapter. Great coverage of ethics and patient communications topics.
Good review questions.

A⁻ **High-Yield Behavioral Science** $19.95 Review only
Fadem
Lippincott Williams & Wilkins, 2001, 144 pages, ISBN 0781730848
Clear, concise, quick review of behavioral science. Logical presentation
with crammable charts, graphs, and tables. Short but adequate statistics
chapter. No index.

B⁺ **Underground Clinical Vignettes:** $17.95 Review only
Behavioral Science
Bhushan
Blackwell Science, 2002, 100 pages, ISBN 0632045434
Concise clinical cases illustrating commonly tested diseases in behavioral
science. Cardinal signs, symptoms, and buzzwords are highlighted. Use as a
supplement to other sources of review. Some cases lack details.

B⁺ **USMLE Behavioral Science** $16.95 Review only
Made Ridiculously Simple
Sierles
MedMaster, 1998, 171 pages, ISBN 0940780348
Easy reading; reasonable yield for the amount of text. Includes medical so-
ciology; strong on psychopathology with illustrative examples. No biosta-
tistics. At times too much detail on low-yield topics.

B **Behavioral Science/Psychiatry: Review** $25.00 Test/500+ q
for New National Boards
Frank
J&S Publishing, 1998, 248 pages, ISBN 1888308001
Answers given in text format with additional information to help teach
and expand on concepts.

B **High-Yield Biostatistics** $18.95   Review only
Glaser
Lippincott Williams & Wilkins, 2001, 96 pages, ISBN 078172242X
Well-written book with extensive coverage of biostatistics. Good review
exercises and tables. Still, low-yield topic. For the motivated student; not
for last-minute cramming. Suitable as a course companion.

B **Appleton & Lange's Review of Epidemiology** $24.95   Review/100 q
and Biostatistics
Hanrahan
McGraw-Hill, 1994, 109 pages, ISBN 083850244X
Excellent, concise overview of epidemiology with complete explanations
and diagrams. Does not include other behavioral science subtopics. Expensive and limited yield. Good for the motivated student.

B **Digging Up the Bones: Biostatistics** $19.95   Review only
and Epidemiology
Linardakis
McGraw-Hill, 1998, 111 pages, ISBN 0070382220
Fairly concise review with clinical applications. Most effective as a quick
refresher. Heavy on low-yield equations. No self-testing opportunities.

B⁻ **Behavioral Science: PreTest Self-Assessment** $24.95   Test/500 q
and Review
Ebert
McGraw-Hill, 2002, 358 pages, ISBN 0071374701
Detailed answers cross-referenced with other resources. Good test ques-
tions. Requires time commitment. Brief high-yield section.

B⁻ **Oklahoma Notes Behavioral Sciences** $19.95   Review/169 q
Krug
Springer-Verlag, 1995, 311 pages, ISBN 0387943935
Typewritten; easy reading. Outline format. Questions of mixed quality.
Good tables. For the motivated student.

B⁻ **Digging Up the Bones: Behavioral Sciences** $19.95   Review only
Linardakis
McGraw-Hill, 1998, 88 pages, ISBN 0070382182
Concise narrative review of behavioral sciences; disorganized format cov-
ers some high-yield topics. Choppy style.

Behavioral Sciences and Outpatient Medicine for the Boards & Wards $15.95   Review
Ayala
Blackwell Science, 2001, 98 pages, ISBN 0632045787
Not yet reviewed. Outline format with a few tables.

 STARS Epidemiology, Biostatistics, and Preventative Medicine Review $39.95   Review/380 q
Jekel
W. B. Saunders, 2001, 430 pages, ISBN 0721690793
Detailed and dense review that is excessive for USMLE Step 1. May be useful for an in-depth biostatistics course.

Medical Biostatistics and Epidemiology: Examination and Board Review

$37.95   Review/100 q

Essex-Sorlie

McGraw-Hill, 1995, 336 pages, ISBN 0838562191

Too in-depth for USMLE biostatistics. Requires time commitment. Consider using with a course. Sample questions may not be representative of the USMLE Step 1.

RATED RESOURCES

 Lippincott's Illustrated Reviews: Biochemistry   **$38.00**   Review/250+ q
Champe
Lippincott Williams & Wilkins, 1994, 443 pages, ISBN 0397510918
Excellent book, but requires time commitment, so an early start is necessary. Best used while taking the course. Excellent diagrams. Emphasizes
"big picture" concepts. Good clinical correlations. Comprehensive review
of biochemistry, including low-yield topics. Skim high-yield diagrams to
maximize USMLE review. New edition expected in 2003.

 BRS Biochemistry   **$29.95**   Review/500 q
Marks
Lippincott Williams & Wilkins, 1998, 350 pages, ISBN 0683304917
Easy-to-read outline with very good boldfaced chapter summaries. Very
thorough; at times too detailed. Mixed-quality diagrams. High-yield clinical correlations are given at the end of each chapter. Questions with short
answers.

B+ **High-Yield Biochemistry**   **$19.95**   Review only
Wilcox
Lippincott Williams & Wilkins, 1999, 106 pages, ISBN 0683304593
Concise and crammable. Outline format with good clinical correlations
at the end of each chapter. Lots of diagrams and tables. Good as a study
supplement.

B **Underground Clinical Vignettes: Biochemistry**   **$17.95**   Review only
Bhushan
Blackwell Science, 2002, 101 pages, ISBN 0632045450
Concise clinical cases illustrating approximately 100 frequently tested dis-
eases with a biochemical basis. Cardinal signs, symptoms, and buzzwords
are highlighted. Useful supplement to other sources of review.

B **Biochemistry Illustrated**   **$39.95**   Review only
Campbell
Churchill Livingstone, 2000, 240 pages, ISBN 044306217X
Excellent diagrams with explanations but no questions. Good for students
who prefer learning by diagrams. Readable but expensive; requires time
commitment.

B | **IMS Metabolism** | $25.95 | Review/170+ q

Coffee

Fence Creek, 1998, 434 pages, ISBN 1889325260

Detailed coverage of general metabolic functions. Good diagrams, tables, and clinical correlations. Most chapters begin with a relevant clinical case and end with its resolution. Review questions after every chapter. Very readable. Compare with *Lippincott's Illustrated Reviews: Biochemistry*.

B | **High-Yield Cell & Molecular Biology** | $19.95 | Review only

Dudek

Lippincott Williams & Wilkins, 1999, 110 pages, ISBN 0683303597

Cellular and molecular biology presented in outline format, with good diagrams and clinical correlations. Brief but complete. Includes description of laboratory techniques and genetic disorders. No questions or vignettes.

B | **Clinical Biochemistry** | $31.00 | Review only

Gaw

Churchill Livingstone, 1999, 176 pages, ISBN 0443061831

Biochemistry and physiology presented in a clinical framework. Visually pleasing. Focuses on adult medicine; skimpy on inherited disorders, genetics, and molecular biochemistry. Case studies throughout, but no standard question-answer exercises. May be more wards than boards oriented.

B | **Clinical Biochemistry Made Ridiculously Simple** | $22.95 | Review only

Goldberg

MedMaster, 1999, 95 pages, ISBN 0940780305

Conceptual approach to clinical biochemistry, with humor. Casual style does not appeal to all students. Mnemonics tend to be somewhat complicated. Good overview and integration for all metabolic pathways. Includes a 23-page clinical review that is very high yield and crammable. Also contains a unique foldout "road map" of metabolism. For students with a firm biochemistry background.

B | **Medical Genetics** | $45.00 | Review

Jorde

Mosby-Year Book, 1999, 352 pages, ISBN 0323012531

Intended as an up-to-date introductory text on medical genetics. Contains numerous well-integrated photographs, diagrams, and drawings. "Clinical commentaries" on specific diseases are used to further illustrate or reinforce the text. Includes study questions. Great for use during course and as a reference for boards review.

B Biochemistry: Review for USMLE Step 1

$25.00 Test/533 q

Kumar

J&S Publishing, 2001, 265 pages, ISBN 1888308109

Quick question-based review of biochemistry. Includes clinical vignettes and extended matching questions but few diagrams. Use in conjunction with other resources.

B Molecular Biology Series

$99.95 Software/500+ q

MedTech Publishing, 1995, ISBN 1889185019

Many good questions with clear explanations. Expensive for student purchase; discount available directly through publisher (800-260-2600 or www.medtech.com). Limited student feedback. Available for either Windows or Macintosh.

B STARS Biochemistry Review

$27.50 Review/600 q

Roskoski

W. B. Saunders, 1996, 242 pages, ISBN 0721651755

Content review in dense outline format with small type. Chapters are short and include only relevant pathways. Good for students who prefer an outline-based review. Parallels a core text by the same authors. Comprehensive exam at the end of the book has some questions with a clinical slant.

B Biochemistry and Genetics: PreTest

$24.95 Test/500 q

Wilson

McGraw-Hill, 2002, 300 pages, ISBN 0071375783

Difficult questions with detailed, referenced explanations. Best for the motivated student who uses this together with a review book. Contains some questions on biochemical disorders but no clinical vignettes. Six pages of high-yield facts focusing on genetically based diseases.

B− Oklahoma Notes Biochemistry

$24.95 Review/549+ q

Briggs

Springer-Verlag, 1995, 287 pages, ISBN 0387943986

Dense text with many hand-drawn diagrams. Good chapter on medical genetics. Non–clinically oriented questions with brief explanations in the margin. Multiple authors; inconsistent style. Easy reading, but not thorough.

B⁻ IMS Medical Molecular Genetics   **$27.95**   Review/150+ q

Hoffee

Fence Creek, 1998, 384 pages, ISBN 1889325287

Detailed coverage of molecular biology and medical genetics. Includes photographs. Easy reading with good explanations and diagrams. Chapters begin and end with clinical cases. Highly clinical, but very lengthy for boards review; focus on chapter outline and review questions.

B⁻ Basic Concepts in Medical Genetics   **$29.95**   Review only

Horwitz

McGraw-Hill, 2000, 149 pages, ISBN 0071345000

Presents concise summaries of medical genetic concepts with clinical applications and anecdotes. Better suited for a specialized genetics course than for boards review.

B⁻ Digging Up the Bones: Biochemistry   **$19.95**   Review only

Linardakis

McGraw-Hill, 1998, 115 pages, ISBN 0070382174

Collection of high-yield biochemistry facts. Use for last-minute review or in conjunction with another review book. Some lists are helpful. Few clinical correlations. Limited student feedback.

Brain Chip for Biochemistry $14.95
Lee
Blackwell Science, 2002, 100 pages, ISBN 0632046368
Not yet reviewed.

1) Secretin
2) ~~Choletsy~~ Cholecystokinin
3) why doesn't the pancreas self digest

Basic Concepts in Biochemistry

$29.95   Review only

Gilbert

McGraw-Hill, 2000, 312 pages, ISBN 0071356576

Presents concise summaries of difficult biochemical concepts and principles. Ignores much high-yield material and thus not very useful for boards
review. Oriented toward undergraduate courses.

Blond's Biochemistry

$19.99   Review only

Guttenplan

Sulzburger & Graham, 1994, 269 pages, ISBN 0945819498

Easy reading. Requires moderate time commitment. Some topics are covered only superficially. Lacks clinical correlations. Not boards oriented;
may be more appropriate with coursework.

Color Atlas of Biochemistry

$34.00   Review only

Koolman

Thieme, 1996, 435 pages, ISBN 0865775842

Excellent four-color diagrams with accompanying explanatory text. Very
little clinical information. Not designed for boards review. Limited student feedback.

REVIEW RESOURCES

Biochemistry

RATED RESOURCES

Clinical Microbiology Made Ridiculously Simple

$25.95 Review only

Gladwin

MedMaster, 2001, 281 pages, ISBN 0940780496

Very good chart-based review of microbiology. Clever and humorous mnemonics. Best of this series. Text easy to read. Excellent antibiotic review helps for pharmacology as well. "Ridiculous" style does not appeal to everyone. Requires supplemental source for immunology. Excellent if you have limited time or are "burning out."

Underground Clinical Vignettes: Microbiology

$17.95 Review only
(each)

Bhushan

Blackwell Science

Microbiology, Vol. I: 2002, 109 pages, ISBN 0632045477

Microbiology, Vol. II: 2002, 105 pages, ISBN 0632045493

Concise clinical cases illustrating approximately 100 frequently tested diseases in microbiology and immunology. Cardinal signs, symptoms, and buzzwords are highlighted. Use as a supplement to other sources of review.

Medical Microbiology & Immunology: Examination and Board Review

$39.95 Review/654 q

Levinson

McGraw-Hill, 2002, 614 pages, ISBN 0071382178

Clear, concise writing with excellent diagrams and tables. Excellent immunology section. Forty-three-page "Summary of Medically Important Organisms" is highly crammable. Requires time commitment. Can be detailed and dense. Best if started early with the course. Covers all topics, including low-yield ones. Good practice questions and comprehensive exam, but questions have letter answers only. Compare with the new Lippincott book.

Microbiology Companion

$27.95 Review/Cards

Topf

Alert and Oriented, 1997, 243 pages, ISBN 0964012413

Chart format is well organized; spiral binding makes it easy to read and carry. Most relevant to microbiology topics. Ties in relevant drugs. Very little immunology. High-yield flash cards (180) are a plus.

B+ **Cases in Medical Microbiology** $39.95   Review/200 q
and Infectious Disease

Gilligan

ASM Press, 1997, 350 pages, ISBN 155581106X

Seventy cases are presented and discussed in detail. Cases test pathogenesis and lab diagnosis of organisms, clinical presentations, epidemiology, and treatment. More than 100 full-color images demonstrate laboratory and clinical diagnosis of disease. Excellent for integrating basic and clinical concepts.

B+ **Case Studies in Immunology:** $33.95   Review/100 q
A Clinical Companion

Rosen

Garland, 2001, 250 pages, ISBN 0815340508

Originally designed as a clinical companion to *Janeway's Immunobiology*, this text provides an excellent synopsis of the major disorders of immunity in a clinical vignette format. Integrates basic and clinical science. Wonderful images, illustrations, questions, and discussion.

B+ **STARS Microbiology Review** $21.95   Review/600 q

Walker

W. B. Saunders, 1998, 255 pages, ISBN 0721646425

Parallels core text by same authors. Learning objectives are clearly defined. Includes numerous questions throughout as well as a 160-question comprehensive exam with answers and a detailed discussion. Immunology not included.

B+ **Clinical Microbiology Review** $36.95   Review only

Warinner

Wysteria, 2001, 152 pages, ISBN 0967783933

Concise yet comprehensive review in chart form with some clinical correlations. Each page is devoted to a single organism with ample space for adding notes during class. No immunology. Spatial organization, color coding, and bulleting of facts facilitate review of subject. Great cross-reference section groups organisms by general characteristics. New edition includes color plates of significant microbes. Limited but positive student feedback. Compare with Topf's *Microbiology Companion*.

B+ Appleton & Lange's Review of Microbiology and Immunology

$34.95 Test/995 q

Yotis

McGraw-Hill, 2001, 288 pages, ISBN 0071362657

Large number of questions with detailed answers. Well referenced. Inadequate as a primary source, but a very good supplement. For the motivated student.

B IMS Immunology

$27.95 Review/170 q

Anderson

Fence Creek, 1999, 194 pages, ISBN 1889325341

Integrates clinical cases and questions into each chapter. Answers and explanations provided. Some chapters contain more detail than necessary for boards preparation.

B Diagnostic Picture Tests in Clinical Infectious Disease

$19.75 Test/178 q

Beeching

Mosby-Year Book, 1996, 124 pages, ISBN 0723424519

One hundred seventy-eight infectious disease images (including MRIs, CTs, x-rays, and gross) are presented with a brief clinical description and questions. Includes answers and index.

B Concepts in Microbiology, Immunology, and Infectious Disease

$17.95 Review/100+ q

Gupta

Parthenon, 1997, 150 pages, ISBN 1850707979

Brief paragraphs in outline form on each disease cover most of the important points. Good clinical questions at the end of each section. Good section on immunologic disorders. No illustrations. Format may not appeal to all students; best for the well-prepared student. For quick review. Many answers not sufficiently explained.

B Buzzwords in Microbiology

$19.95 Review only

Hurst

Bryan Edwards, 1997, 240 pages, ISBN 1878576089

Spiral-bound flash cards contain important facts about the most medically relevant bacteria and fungi. Directed toward boards review. Bullet presentation of information affords easy and quick review. Good pictures and buzzwords. Does not cover virology, parasitology, or immunology.

B **Oklahoma Notes Microbiology and Immunology** $19.95 Review/312+ q

Hyde

Springer-Verlag, 1995, 229 pages, ISBN 0387943927

Easy to read, but not adequate as a sole study source. Good summary statements are given at the end of each chapter. Extended matching questions. Poor typeface and diagrams. Unequal coverage.

B **High-Yield Immunology** $19.95 Review only

Johnson

Lippincott Williams & Wilkins, 1999, 68 pages, ISBN 0683306146

Format typical of high-yield series. Accurately covers high-yield details within the topic in proportion to boards coverage of immunology. Some illustrations and diagrams could improve. Some sections may not be detailed enough.

B **BUGCARDS: The Complete Microbiology Review for Class, the Boards, and the Wards** $26.50 Cards

Levine

BL Publishing, 1998, 154 flash cards, ISBN 0967165504

High-quality flash cards (similar to "Pharm Cards") designed for rapid class and USMLE microbiology review. Cover all medically relevant bacteria, viruses, fungi, and parasites. Include important buzzwords, mnemonics, and clinical vignettes to aid in recall. Unique "disease process cards" summarize all organisms for a particular disease (e.g., UTI or pneumonia). Useful for quick review of facts, but not recommended as a comprehensive primary review source.

B **Digging Up the Bones: Microbiology and Immunology** $19.95 Review

Linardakis

McGraw-Hill, 1998, 107 pages and flash cards, ISBN 0070382158

Easy to read. Brief collection of phrases and associations. A few tables and simple diagrams. Expensive for the amount of material given. Features detachable flash cards. Limited student feedback.

B **Medical MicroCards** $19.95 150 cards

Orlando

Medfiles, 1996, 150 pages, ISBN 0965537307

Concise flash cards cover bacteriology, virology, mycology, and parasitology. Designed for fast review. No extraneous information. Covers disease characteristics, treatment, prevention, and clinical findings. Mixed reviews. Compare with Topf's *Microbiology Companion*.

B Basic Immunology

$32.95 Review/150 q

Sharon

Lippincott Williams & Wilkins, 1998, 300 pages, ISBN 0683077295
Well-organized text with many figures and tables. Unique images of clinical presentations. Includes section on organ transplantation. Comprehensive, but may be better suited to coursework than to boards review. Limited student feedback.

B How the Immune System Works

$22.95 Review only

Sompayrac

Blackwell Science, 1998, 100 pages, ISBN 0632044136
Concise overview of immunology. Attempts to place complicated concepts into a simple but not simplistic "big picture." Good general introduction but use as companion to other more detailed resources. Limited student feedback.

B Microbiology: Review for USMLE Step 1

$19.95 Test/573 q

Stokes

J&S Publishing, 2002, 249 pages, ISBN 1888308125
Easy reading. Covers many high-yield topics and includes case-based questions and extended matching questions. Very good question-and-answer-based review of clinically relevant microbiology and immunology, but lacking somewhat in detailed information. Helpful as a supplement to a review book.

B STARS Microbiology

$32.00 Review

Walker

W. B. Saunders, 1998, 513 pages, ISBN 0721646417
Pathogens are presented in a consistent outline format, from pathogenicity to treatment. Numerous multicolor tables and illustrations. No questions. Requires time commitment. Consider using as a course supplement.

B⁻ Blond's Microbiology

$19.99 Review only

Alcamo

Sulzburger & Graham, 1994, 181 pages, ISBN 0945819412
Text review. Spotty coverage of some key topics. Below average for this series.

B⁻ Basic Concepts in Immunology

$29.95 Review only

Clancy

McGraw-Hill, 1998, 223 pages, ISBN 0070113718
Review book similar to others in the *Student's Survival Guide* series. Not sufficiently high yield for boards review. However, appropriate for coursework. Limited student feedback.

B⁻ Microbiology: PreTest   **$24.95**   Test/500 q

Tilton

McGraw-Hill, 2002, 264 pages, ISBN 0071374957

Mixed-quality questions with detailed, sometimes verbose explanations.
Useful for additional question-based review in bacteriology and virology,
but not high yield. Includes three pages of high-yield facts.

B⁻ Flash Micro   **$27.95**   Cards

Ting

Stanford Ink, 1999, 131 cards, ISBN 0967231809

Concise flash cards designed for boards review. Includes 190 pathogens.
No immunology. Color coded. Compare with Orlando's *Medical Micro-
Cards*. Mixed student feedback.

B⁻ NMS Microbiology and Infectious Disease   **$35.95**   Review/500 q

Virella

Lippincott Williams & Wilkins, 1996, 575 pages, ISBN 0683062352

Outline format. Too detailed in some areas. Insufficient immunology;
NMS has a separate immunology book. Lacks a good explanation of bacterial genetics. Updated material on AIDS. Useful only if previously used
as a textbook. Limited student feedback.

N **Basic Immunology** $39.95
Abbas
W. B. Saunders, 2001, 320 pages, ISBN 0721693164
Not yet reviewed.

N **Immunology for the Boards and Wards** $14.95   Review/19 q
Ayala
Blackwell Science, 2001, 80 pages, ISBN 0632045744
Not yet reviewed. Outline format with a few tables.

N **Microbiology for the Boards and Wards** $14.95   Review/22 q
Ayala
Blackwell Science, 2001, 163 pages, ISBN 0632045760
Not yet reviewed. Focused on quick review of frequently tested pathogens.

N **Color Atlas of Immunology** $36.00   Review only
Burmester
Thieme, 2002, 293 pages, ISBN 0865779643
Not yet reviewed.

N **Medical Microbiology and Infection at a Glance** $19.95   Review only
Gillespie
Blackwell Science, 2000, 120 pages, ISBN 0632050268
Not yet reviewed.

N **Microcards** $26.95   Cards
Harpavat
Lippincott Williams & Wilkins, 2001, 380 pages, ISBN 0781722004
Microbiology flash cards. Coverage of clinically relevant viruses, bacteria,
fungi, protozoa, and helminths with a clinical case and annotated picture
summarizing the laboratory diagnosis on each card.

N **Color Guide: Microbiology** $19.95   Review only
Inglis
Churchill Livingstone, 1997, 141 pages, ISBN 0443057729
Not yet reviewed.

N **BrainChip Microbiology** $18.95   Review only
Lee
Blackwell Science, 2001, 100 pages, ISBN 063204568X
Not yet reviewed.

REVIEW RESOURCES

Microbiology

N **Visual Mnemonics Microbiology**   **$18.95**

Marbas

Blackwell Science, 2001, 100 pages, ISBN 0632045876

For the visual learner. Not yet reviewed.

N **Immunology for Medical Students**   **$34.95**   Review only

Nairn

Mosby, 2002, 326 pages, ISBN 0723431906

Easy reading. Good color illustrations with clinical examples. Best used as
a reference; too detailed for boards review.

N **Immunology at a Glance**   **$25.95**

Playfair

Blackwell Science, 2001, 120 pages, ISBN 0632054069

Not yet reviewed.

N **Really Essential Immunology**   **$34.95**

Roitt

Blackwell Science, 2000, 150 pages, ISBN 0632055065

Not yet reviewed.

N **Rapid Review: Microbiology and Immunology**   **$32.95**   Review/600 q

Rosenthal

Mosby, 2002, 362 pages, ISBN 0323008402

Outline format with high-yield margin notes, figures, and tables that highlight key content. Narrative clinical boxes illustrate clinical relevance.
Practice exams provide clinically oriented questions. Includes a CD-ROM
of questions. New series.

N **Lippincott's Illustrated Reviews: Microbiology**   **$35.95**   Review/few q

Strohl

Lippincott Williams & Wilkins, 2001, 528 pages, ISBN 0397515685

Comprehensive, highly illustrated review of microbiology similar in style
to Champe's *Lippincott's Illustrated Reviews: Biochemistry*. Includes a 50-
page color section with over 150 clinical and laboratory photographs.
Compare with Levinson's *Medical Microbiology*.

Quick Look Medicine: Immunology

$19.95 Review/100+ q

Mamula
Fence Creek, 2000, 130 pages, ISBN 1889325384
Not yet reviewed.

IMS Microbial Pathogenesis

$25.95 Review/150+ q

McClane
Fence Creek, 2000, 350 pages, ISBN 1889325279
Not yet reviewed.

Medical Microbiology Made Memorable

$24.95 Review only

Myint
Churchill Livingstone, 1999, 138 pages, ISBN 0443061351
Presents material in brief two-page summaries. Contains numerous charts,
tables, and illustrations. Seven case studies are presented with brief
discussions.

Review Questions for Microbiology and Immunology

$20.95 Review/625 q

Reese
Parthenon, 2000, 113 pages, ISBN 1850700206
Review of main subtopics in microbiology and immunology through
question-and-answer format. Answers face questions on opposing pages.
Figures, graphs, and line drawings enhance answers.

Essential Immunology Review

$21.95 Test/422 q

Roitt
Blackwell Science, 1995, 319 pages, ISBN 0865424586
Boards-style questions with explanations that also discuss incorrect an-
swers. Required text at some medical schools. Mixed reviews.

RATED RESOURCES

A | BRS Pathology
Schneider

$29.95 Review/500 q

Lippincott Williams & Wilkins, 2001, 470 pages, ISBN 068302655
Excellent, concise review with appropriate content emphasis. Outline-format chapters with boldfacing of key facts. Excellent questions with explanations at the end of each chapter and a comprehensive exam at the end of the book. Well-organized tables and diagrams. Some good black-and-white photographs representative of classic pathology. Correlate with color photographs from an atlas. Latest edition contains a new chapter on laboratory testing and "key associations" with each disease. Short on clinical details for vignette questions. Consistently high student recommendations. Very worthwhile to master this book. Most effective if started early and then reviewed during study period.

A⁻ | Underground Clinical Vignettes: Pathophysiology
Bhushan

$17.95 (each) Review only

Blackwell Science
Pathophysiology, Vol. I: 2002, 103 pages, ISBN 0632045515
Pathophysiology, Vol. II: 2002, 93 pages, ISBN 0632045531
Pathophysiology, Vol. III: 2002, 97 pages, ISBN 0632045558
Concise clinical cases illustrating approximately 100 frequently tested pathology and physiology cases in each book. Cardinal signs, symptoms, and buzzwords are highlighted. Use as a supplement to other sources of review.

A⁻ | Robbins Review of Pathology
Goljan

$34.95 Review/1100+ q

W. B. Saunders, 2000, 310 pages, ISBN 0721682596
Question book of pathology with answer explanations. Questions are almost entirely clinically based and are accompanied by a number of high-quality histologic and gross images as well as references to the *Robbins Pathologic Basis of Disease* and *Basic Pathology* textbooks. Questions can be difficult or picky. Answer explanations are brief but well written. Very good review resource.

REVIEW RESOURCES

Pathology

STARS Pathology Review
Goljan

$24.95   Review/500+ q

W. B. Saunders, 1998, 352 pages, ISBN 0721670245

Companion book to STARS *Pathology*. Uses a concise outline to summarize key concepts. Includes chapter questions with answers and detailed explanations as well as a comprehensive 150-question practice exam. Features more than 100 illustrations and includes photos and histologic images.

 STARS Pathology
Goljan

$34.00   Review only

W. B. Saunders, 1998, 528 pages, ISBN 0721670237

Well-organized, concise, and easy-to-read explanations of pathology. Illustrated with diagrams; lacks photos and imaging. Excellent charts and tables. Some students use this text as a primary source.

B+ **Interactive Case Study Companion to Robbins Pathologic Basis of Disease**
Kumar

$49.95   Software/ Case Studies

W. B. Saunders, 1999, ISBN 0721684629

Ninety-nine clinical cases with 1500 images covering a full range of topics in general and systemic pathology. Great learning supplement. Time-consuming. For the motivated student.

B+ **Pathophysiology of Heart Disease**
Lilly

$34.95   Review only

Lippincott Williams & Wilkins, 2003, 445 pages, ISBN 0781740274

Collaborative project by medical students and faculty at Harvard. Well organized, easy to read, and concise; offers comprehensive coverage of cardiovascular pathophysiology from the medical student's perspective. Provides an excellent bridge between the basic and clinical sciences. Very good for review of this subject, but does not cover other areas of pathology tested on the boards. New edition expected in 2003.

B+ **Digging Up the Bones: Pathology**
Linardakis

$19.95   Review only

McGraw-Hill, 1998, 130 pages, ISBN 0070382166

Easy reading. Brief collection of phrases and associations, often based on answers to assorted multiple-choice questions. Expensive for the amount of material. Features photomicrographs (gross and microscopic).

B+ **Pathophysiology of Disease: An Introduction to Clinical Medicine**   **$44.95**   Review/Few q

McPhee

McGraw-Hill, 2000, 662 pages, ISBN 0838581609

Interdisciplinary course text useful for understanding the pathophysiology of clinical symptoms. Excellent integration of basic sciences with mechanisms of disease. Great graphs, diagrams, and tables. Most helpful if used during coursework owing to length. Few non-boards-style questions. Clinical emphasis nicely complements *BRS Pathology*.

B+ **Pathology: Review for New National Boards**   **$25.00**   Test/509 q

Miller

J&S Publishing, 1993, 222 pages, ISBN 0963287338

Question-and-answer-based review of pathology. Includes many case-based questions. Focuses on high-yield topics. Good black-and-white photographs. Some picky questions with incomplete answers. Inadequate as a sole source of review. Expensive for the number of questions.

B+ **Pathophysiology: PreTest**   **$24.95**   Test/500 q

Mufson

McGraw-Hill, 2002, 253 pages, ISBN 0071375074

Includes 500 questions and answers with detailed explanations. Questions may be more difficult than those on the boards. Includes a very brief section of high-yield topics.

B **Pathology: PreTest**   **$24.95**   Test/500 q

Brown

McGraw-Hill, 2002, 530 pages, ISBN 0071372237

Picky, difficult questions with detailed, complete answers. Questions are often obscure or esoteric. High-quality black-and-white photographs, but no color photographs. Can be used as a supplement to other review books. For the motivated student who desires exposure to a variety of photographs. Thirty-five pages of high-yield facts are useful for concept summaries.

B **Appleton & Lange's Review of General Pathology**   **$34.95**   Test/1300+ q

Catalano

McGraw-Hill, 2003, 352 pages, ISBN 0071389954

Short text sections followed by numerous questions with answers. Some useful high-yield tables at the beginning of each section. Good photomicrographs. Covers only general pathology (i.e., no organ-based pathology). Can be used as a supplement to more detailed texts. Good review when time is short.

B | **Colour Atlas of Anatomical Pathology** | **$55.00** | Review only

Cooke

Churchill Livingstone, 1995, 261 pages, ISBN 0443050627

Beautifully photographed atlas of gross pathology. Easy-to-read, clinically relevant content.

B | **Lange Smart Charts** | **$24.95** | Review only

Groysman

McGraw-Hill, 2001, 356 pages, ISBN 0838581757

Flip chart of tables with information grouped together for ease of recall. Organized by body systems with mnemonics. Best used as a summary reference for fast review.

B | **USMLE Pathology Review: The Study Guide** | **$25.95** | Review/300+ q

Hassanein

Sage, 1998, 398 pages, ISBN 0761905170

Key pathology concepts presented in an outline format. Numerous questions with answers and explanations. Includes a comprehensive 184-question exam. No index.

B | **EBS Essentials of Pathophysiology** | **$39.95** | Review/69 q

Kaufman

Lippincott Williams & Wilkins, 1996, 816 pages, ISBN 0316484059

Review book with few questions. Features clinical descriptions of important diseases, but too detailed for high-yield review. Good diagrams, tables, and black-and-white photographs. More appropriate as a course text and reference. For the highly motivated student. Limited student feedback.

B | **NMS Pathology** | **$32.00** | Review/500 q

LiVolsi

Lippincott Williams & Wilkins, 1994, 525 pages, ISBN 0683062433

Outline form. Comprehensive review of a large amount of material. Sometimes too detailed for boards review. Slow reading. Best if used with course.

B | **Pathology: Examination and Board Review** | **$32.95** | Review/Few q

Newland

McGraw-Hill, 1995, 360 pages, ISBN 0838577199

Concise text review with some high-quality charts and photomicrographs. Non-boards-style questions at the end of each chapter with letter answers only.

B | **Pocket Companion to Robbins Pathologic Basis of Disease** | $29.95 | Review only

Robbins

W. B. Saunders, 1999, 800 pages, ISBN 0721678599

Good for reviewing associations between keywords and specific diseases. Highly condensed and easy to understand. Explains most important diseases and pathologic processes. No photographs or illustrations. Useful as a quick reference.

B | **Renal Pathophysiology: The Essentials** | $29.95 | Review only

Rose

Lippincott Williams & Wilkins, 1994, 351 pages, ISBN 0683073540

Excellent review and explanations of various disease processes of the kidney. Review questions within text for comprehension; not boards style. Good reference during boards review.

B | **Color Atlas of Pathophysiology** | $36.00 | Review only

Silbernagl

Thieme, 380 pages, 2000, ISBN 0865778663

Over 180 high-quality illustrations that demonstrate disturbed physiologic processes that lead to dysfunction. Limited student feedback.

B | **Case Studies in General and Systemic Pathology** | $30.00 | Review/300+ q

Underwood

Churchill-Livingstone, 1996, 172 pages, ISBN 0443050961

Presents 60 cases with excellent images and integrated questions/answers. Full-color images include gross specimens, histology, and MRIs. Closely linked to Underwood's *General and Systemic Pathology*.

B⁻ | **Basic Concepts in Pathology** | $29.95 | Review only

Brown

McGraw-Hill, 1998, 456 pages, ISBN 0070083215

Good review of basic concepts. No images. Not entirely suitable for USMLE review.

B⁻ | **Wheater's Basic Histopathology** | $52.95 | Review only

Burkitt

Churchill-Livingstone, 1996, 252 pages, ISBN 0443050880

Color atlas with text. Contains pictures of pathologic histology. Not directed toward boards-type review. May be more useful for photomicrograph-based questions.

B− **Pathologic Basis of Disease Self-Assessment and Review** **$23.00** Test/1600+ q
Compton
W. B. Saunders, 2000, 239 pages, ISBN 0721678572
Large number of practice questions, some very difficult and detailed. A good buy for the number of questions. Time-consuming. Only for the dedicated student.

B− **Pulmonary Pathophysiology** **$27.95** Review/100+ q
Criner
Fence Creek, 1999, 300 pages, ISBN 1889325058
Typical of this series. Well organized with integrated clinical case presentations. For the motivated student.

B− **Rypins' Intensive Reviews: Pathology** **$21.95** Review/220+ q
Damjanov
Lippincott Williams & Wilkins, 1998, 432 pages, ISBN 0397515553
Typical of this series. Includes a comprehensive exam with answers and explanations. Illustrated with simple diagrams; no photos included.

B− **IMS Renal System** **$24.95** Review/150+ q
Jackson
Fence Creek, 1998, 350 pages, ISBN 1889325317
Well-organized text with integrated clinical cases. Features questions with answers and explanations. Best if used with course.

B− **Review Questions for Human Pathology** **$19.95** Test/1300+ q
Jones
Parthenon, 1999, 322 pages, ISBN 1850705992
Includes more than 1300 questions with answers and discussions. Many questions are in outdated USMLE format. Step 1–level questions are interspersed with questions at the level of Step 2 and Step 3. Good value for the price.

B− **Cardiovascular Pathophysiology** **$27.95** Review/100+ q
Kusomoto
Fence Creek, 1999, 278 pages, ISBN 1889325007
Numerous charts and illustrations. Each chapter offers summary questions. Too detailed for boards review.

B- | **Endocrine Pathophysiology** | **$27.95** | Review/100+ q

Niewoehner

Fence Creek, 1999, 270 pages, ISBN 1889325023

Well organized and easy to read with integrated clinical cases. High-quality content, but too detailed for boards review.

B- | **IMS Cardiopulmonary System** | **$25.95** | Review/150+ q

Richardson

Fence Creek, 1997, 336 pages, ISBN 1889325309

Integrates clinical cases throughout the text. Well organized but lengthy. Best if used with course.

B- | **Gastrointestinal and Hepatobiliary Pathophysiology** | **$27.95** | Review/100+ q

Rose

Fence Creek, 1998, 451 pages, ISBN 1889325015

Well organized but lengthy. For the motivated student. Detailed and comprehensive explanations.

B- | **Hematologic Pathophysiology** | **$25.95** | Review/100+ q

Rubin

Fence Creek, 1998, 129 pages, ISBN 188932504X

Emphasis on clinical aspects of disease and treatment.

N **Churchill Mastery of Medicine: Pathology** $29.00 Review only
Bass
Churchill Livingstone, 1996, 127 pages, ISBN 0443050031
Limited coverage of topics.

N **Pathology Recall** $29.95 Review only
Chhabra
Lippincott Williams & Wilkins, 2002, 624 pages, ISBN 0781734061
Similar in format to rest of Recall series. "Power reviews" at end of each
chapter to reinforce concepts.

N **Pathology Recall PDA** $29.95 Software
Chhabra
Lippincott Williams & Wilkins, 2002, ISBN 0781733413
Derived from the book of the same name. Not yet reviewed.

N **BrainChip Pathology** $18.95
Garcia
Blackwell Science, 2002, 100 pages, ISBN 0632046392
Not yet reviewed.

N **Pocket Brain for Clinical Pathophysiology** $17.95
Griffin
Blackwell Science, 2001, 90 pages, ISBN 0632046341
Not yet reviewed.

N **BRS Pathology Flash Cards** $27.95 Cards
Swanson
Lippincott Williams & Wilkins, 2002, ISBN 0781737109
Companion to BRS Pathology. Intended for quick review. No diagrams.

N **Pulmonary Physiology and Pathophysiology:** $31.95 Review/100 q
An Integrated, Case-Based Approach
West
Lippincott Williams & Wilkins, 2001, 162 pages, ISBN 0781729106
Not yet reviewed.

Oklahoma Notes Pathology
$19.95 Review/140 q

Holliman

Springer-Verlag, 1994, 279 pages, ISBN 0387943900

Dense text. Few diagrams and tables. No illustrations. Questions with letter answers only. Good when you have no time for comprehensive review books.

Pathology Illustrated
$62.00 Review only

MacFarlane

Churchill Livingstone, 2000, 696 pages, ISBN 044305956X

Lengthy, but fast reading. Well illustrated with many line drawings. User-friendly format. Some errors. Worth considering despite price.

Essential Pathology
$59.95 Review only

Rubin

Lippincott Williams & Wilkins, 2001, 786 pages, ISBN 0781723957

Thin book with excellent color illustrations and pictures that are useful for the second year and beyond. Use as a text for coursework; too detailed for boards review. Limited student feedback.

RATED RESOURCES

B+ **Underground Clinical Vignettes: Pharmacology** $17.95 Review only
Bhushan
Blackwell Science, 2002, 102 pages, ISBN 0632045574
Concise clinical cases illustrating approximately 100 frequently tested
pharmacology concepts. Cardinal signs, symptoms, and buzzwords are
highlighted. Clinical vignette style less effective for pharmacology. Use as
a supplement to other sources of review.

B+ **Pharmacology: Review for New National Boards** $25.00 Test/539 q
Billingsley
J&S Publishing, 1995, 186 pages, ISBN 0963287370
Question-and-answer book typical for this series. Includes clinical vi-
gnettes. Good explanations cover many high-yield pharmacology topics.
Easy, fast reading. Questions about drug structures probably low yield. Use-
ful adjunct to a review book. Limited student feedback.

B+ **Lippincott's Illustrated Reviews: Pharmacology** $35.95 Review/230+ q
Harvey
Lippincott Williams & Wilkins, 2000, 514 pages, ISBN 0781724139
Outline format with practice questions and many excellent and memorable illustrations and tables. Cross-referenced to *Lippincott's Illustrated Reviews: Biochemistry.* Good for the "big picture." Good pathophysiologic approach. Detailed, so use with course and review for USMLE. For the
motivated student. Ten illustrated case studies with questions and answers
in the appendix. Revised printing edition includes a "special millennium
update" that covers all new drugs introduced since 1996.

B+ **Pharm Cards: A Review for Medical Students** $29.95 Cards
Johannsen
Lippincott Williams & Wilkins, 2002, 228 cards, ISBN 0781734010
Updated edition highlights important features of major drugs/drug classes.
Good for class review; also offers a quick, focused review for the USMLE.
Lacks pharmacokinetics. Good charts and diagrams. Highly rated by stu-
dents who enjoy flash-card-based review. Bulky to carry around.

Digging Up the Bones: Pharmacology　　　　**$19.95**　Review/Cards
Linardakis
McGraw-Hill, 1998, 99 pages and 100+ flash cards, ISBN 007038214X
Easy reading. Brief collection of phrases and drug associations. Contains
more than 100 flash cards of top drugs with clinical use, mechanisms, and
side effects. Use as a supplement.

 Pharm Recall　　　　**$25.00**　Test
Ramachandran
Lippincott Williams & Wilkins, 1999, 528 pages, ISBN 068330285X
Approach to pharmacology review in question-and-answer "recall" format.
High-yield drug summary included.

 Basic Concepts in Pharmacology　　　　**$29.95**　Review only
Stringer
McGraw-Hill, 2001, 285 pages, ISBN 0071356991
Presents summaries of "elusive" concepts in pharmacology, from simple to
complex. No questions. Limited student feedback.

Katzung and Trevor's Pharmacology: Examination and Board Review　　　　**$39.95**　Review/1000 q
Trevor
McGraw-Hill, 2002, 662 pages, ISBN 0838581471
Text is well organized in a narrative format with concise explanations.
Good charts and tables. Good for drug interactions and toxicities. Fea-
tures two practice exams and 17 case studies with questions and detailed
answers. Includes some low-yield/obscure drugs. The 40-page crammable
list of "top boards drugs" is especially high yield. Compare closely with
Lippincott's Illustrated Reviews: Pharmacology.

STARS Pharmacology Review　　　　**$22.95**　Review/Some q
Brenner
W. B. Saunders, 2000, 271 pages, ISBN 0721677584
Focuses on prototypical drugs and their mechanisms and clinical uses. Em-
phasizes application of basic science concepts to everyday clinical problem
solving. Includes section examinations and a comprehensive exam of
USMLE-style questions based on clinical vignettes. Answers and detailed
rationales for each question are provided.

B Pharmacology Companion

$27.95   Review/Cards

Gallia

Alert and Oriented, 1997, 339 pages, ISBN 096401243X

Spiral bound with high-yield flash cards. Chart format illustrates mechanisms, uses, and side effects of each drug or class of drugs. However, few diagrams, and format does not seem to work as well as it does in Topf's *Microbiology Companion*. Limited student feedback.

B NMS Pharmacology

$32.00   Review/450+ q

Jacob

Lippincott Williams & Wilkins, 1995, 385 pages, ISBN 0683062514

Outline format. More tables and diagrams in the new edition. Often too detailed. Lacks emphasis on high-yield material. Has a lengthy USMLE-type exam. Requires time commitment. Typical for this series.

B Blond's Pharmacology

$19.99   Review only

Kostrzewa

Sulzburger & Graham, 1995, 398 pages, ISBN 094581948X

Concise review of pharmacology. Many good diagrams. Some key topics are inadequately covered.

B Color Atlas of Pharmacology

$36.00   Review only

Luellmann

Thieme, 386 pages, 2000, ISBN 0865778434

Highly visual approach to pharmacology. No questions. One hundred forty-nine color plates are accompanied by brief descriptions.

B Clinical Pharmacology Made Ridiculously Simple

$20.95   Review only

Olson

MedMaster, 2001, 164 pages, ISBN 094078050X

Includes general principles and many drug summary charts. Particularly strong in cardiovascular drugs and antimicrobials; incomplete in other areas. Mostly tables; lacks the humorous illustrations and mnemonics typical of this series. Well organized, but occasionally too detailed. Effective as a chart-based review book but not as a sole study source. Must supplement with a more detailed text.

B Quick Look Medicine: Pharmacology

$21.95   Review/100+ q

Raffa

Fence Creek, 1999, 204 pages, ISBN 1889325384

Covers essential facts and concepts using diagrams. Includes numerous questions, answers, and explanations. Limited student feedback.

B **Instant Pharmacology** $39.99   Review/130 q
Saeb-Parsy
John Wiley & Sons, Inc., 1999, 349 pages, ISBN 0471976393
This text is divided into several parts. The first addresses basic mechanisms found in pharmacology. Drugs encountered in this section are summarized in the "Dictionary of Drugs." The text ends with a comprehensive
exam. Answers, but not explanations, are included.

B **Pharmacology: PreTest** $24.95   Test/500 q
Stern
McGraw-Hill, 2002, 294 pages, ISBN 0071367047
Picky, difficult questions with detailed answers. New high-yield chapter is
a comparison chart intended only as a sample learning tool.

B⁻ **High-Yield Pharmacology** $19.95   Review only
Christ
Lippincott Williams & Wilkins, 1999, 122 pages, ISBN 0683307134
Pharmacology review in an easy-to-follow outline format. No questions;
no index.

B⁻ **EBS Essentials of Pharmacology** $29.95   Review/250+ q
Theoharides
Lippincott Williams & Wilkins, 1996, 479 pages, ISBN 0316839361
Review text with some boards-style questions and letter answers. May be
more appropriate as a course text than as a review book. New edition has
many good tables that summarize important drug mechanisms and toxicities. Good text, but not focused enough for boards.

Visual Mnemonics Pharmacology $18.95

Marbas

Blackwell Science, 2001, 112 pages, ISBN 063204585X

Not yet reviewed. For the visual learner.

 Rapid Review: Pharmacology $32.95   Review/600 q

Pazdernik

Mosby, 2003, 316 pages, ISBN 0323008380

Outline format with high-yield margin notes, figures, and tables that high-light key content. Narrative clinical boxes illustrate clinical relevance. Practice exams provide clinically oriented questions. Includes a CD-ROM of questions. New series.

 Recall Pharmacology PDA $29.95   Software

Ramachandran

Lippincott Williams & Wilkins, 2001, ISBN 078173343X

Derived from the book of the same name. Not yet reviewed.

REVIEW RESOURCES

Pharmacology

Medical PharmFile

$22.95   Cards

Feinstein

Medfiles, 1998, ISBN 0965537315

High-yield pharmacology in flash-card format similar to *Medical Micro-Cards*. Cards have printing on one side only. Not conducive to self-testing.

Oklahoma Notes Pharmacology

$19.95   Review/560+ q

Moore

Springer-Verlag, 1995, 235 pages, ISBN 0387943943

Conceptual approach. Features USMLE-type questions with brief explanations. Readable but outdated review book.

BRS Pharmacology

$29.95   Review/450 q

Rosenfeld

Lippincott Williams & Wilkins, 1997, 455 pages, ISBN 0683180509

Outline format. Good use of boldface, but few tables. Questions are of moderate difficulty with short answers. Worse than average for this series.

RATED RESOURCES

BRS Physiology
Costanzo

$29.95 Review/400 q

Lippincott Williams & Wilkins, 1998, 326 pages, ISBN 0683303961
Clear, concise review of physiology. Fast, easy reading. Comprehensive
and efficient. Great charts and tables. Good practice questions with explanations and a clinically oriented final exam. Excellent review book, but
may not be enough for in-depth coursework. Comparatively weak respiratory and acid-base sections.

Physiology
Costanzo

$36.95 Review only

W. B. Saunders, 2002, 395 pages, ISBN 0721695493
Comprehensive coverage of concepts outlined in *BRS Physiology*. Excellent diagrams and charts. Each systems-based chapter includes a detailed
summary of objectives and a boards-relevant clinical case. Requires time.

Appleton & Lange's Review of Physiology
Penney

$32.95 Test/700+ q

McGraw-Hill, 1998, 227 pages, ISBN 0838502741
Boards-style questions with letter answers and explanations. No vignettes.
Questions somewhat picky. Limited review.

NMS Physiology
Bullock

$32.00 Review/300 q

Lippincott Williams & Wilkins, 2000, 853 pages, ISBN 0683306030
Very complete text in outline form. Often too detailed, but some good diagrams. Moderately difficult questions with detailed answers. Provides
some pathophysiology and clinical correlations. More useful if used as a
course text and reference; too long as a review text. Inexpensive for the
amount of material. For the motivated student.

Color Atlas of Physiology
Despopoulos

$35.00 Review only

Thieme, 1991, 369 pages, ISBN 0865773823
Compact, with more than 150 colorful but complicated diagrams on the
right and dense explanatory text on the left. Some translation problems.
A unique, highly visual approach worthy of consideration. Useful as an
adjunct to other review books.

REVIEW RESOURCES

Physiology

B | **Clinical Physiology Made Ridiculously Simple** | $19.95 | Review only

Goldberg

MedMaster, 2001, 152 pages, ISBN 0940780216

Easy reading with many amusing associations. Style does not work for everyone. Not as well illustrated as the rest of the series. Use as a supplement to other review books.

B | **Blond's Physiology** | $20.00 | Review only

Grossman

Sulzburger & Graham, 1995, 439 pages, ISBN 0945819420

Comprehensive but easy-to-read review text of physiology. Clear and simple classic diagrams and charts. Better than average for this series. Strong endocrine chapter. Good hormone list.

B | **Concepts in Physiology** | $17.95 | Review/100+ q

Gupta

Parthenon, 1996, 135 pages, ISBN 1850707308

System-based review in paragraph form. Some sections have clinical questions at the end of the chapter with explanations. Format may not appeal to all students. Limited student feedback.

B | **Physiology: Review for New National Boards** | $25.00 | Test/506 q

Jakoi

J&S Publishing, 1994, 214 pages, ISBN 0963287346

Good review book, but inadequate as a sole source of review. Quick reading. Below-average question quality for this series. Answer discussions cover many important topics.

B | **High-Yield Acid Base** | $18.95 | Review only

Longnecker

Lippincott Williams & Wilkins, 1998, 100 pages, ISBN 0683303937

Concise and well-written description of acid-base disorders. Includes chapters discussing differential diagnosis and 12 clinical cases. Introduces a multistep approach to the material. Bookmark with useful factoids included with text. No index or questions.

B | **Quick Look Medicine: Cardiopulmonary System** | $19.95 | Review/117 q

Richardson

Fence Creek, 1999, 164 pages, ISBN 1889325422

Presents concepts in diagram format. Includes questions, answers, and detailed explanations for self-assessment. Discussion covers cardiovascular and pulmonary physiology as well as cardiopulmonary pathophysiology.

B ## Physiology: PreTest $24.95 Test/500 q
Ryan
McGraw-Hill, 2002, 322 pages, ISBN 0071371990
Questions with detailed, well-written explanations. Some questions too difficult or picky. May be useful for the motivated student following extensive review from other sources. Includes 34 pages of high-yield facts.

B ## Memorix Physiology $35.25 Review
Schmidt
Chapman & Hall, 1997, 281 pages, ISBN 041271440X
Systems-based coverage of key concepts in an easy-to-carry handbook. Similar in format to the *Color Atlas of Physiology*. Contains more than 200 color illustrations and tables. Expensive for the amount of material.

B ## Respiratory Physiology: The Essentials $31.00 Review/100+ q
West
Lippincott Williams & Wilkins, 2000, 171 pages, ISBN 0683307347
Comprehensive coverage of respiratory physiology. Limited student feedback. New edition includes appendices with more than 100 questions and answers with explanations. Best used as a course supplement.

B– ## Digging Up the Bones: Physiology $19.95 Review only
Linardakis
McGraw-Hill, 1998, 146 pages, ISBN 0070382212
Organ-based collection of facts. Text includes tables, graphs, and some illustrations. Clinical vignettes accompany each topic.

B– ## Linardakis' Illustrated Review of Physiology $37.95 Review/200 q
Linardakis
Michaelis Medical, 1998, 340 pages, ISBN 1884084176
Comprehensive, illustration-based review of medical physiology. Color illustrations integrated into text.

B– ## Review Questions for Physiology $19.95 Test/700 q
Pasley
CRC Press-Parthenon, 1998, 136 pages, ISBN 1850706018
Few clinical vignette–type questions. Answers are on the same page as questions, making it easy to move through questions and check answers at the same time.

N | **Cardiovascular System at a Glance** | $26.95
Aaronson
Blackwell Science, 2000, 120 pages, ISBN 0632049715
Not yet reviewed.

N | **Physiology Cases and Problems (Board Review Series)** | $22.00 | Review/Many q
Costanzo
Lippincott Williams & Wilkins, 2001, 338 pages, ISBN 0781724821
About 50 cases in vignette format with several questions per case. Detailed explanatory answers. For the motivated student.

N | **Pocket Companion to Guyton's Textbook of Physiology** | $26.95 | Handbook
Guyton
W. B. Saunders, 2001, 730 pages, ISBN 0721687296
At-a-glance reference to facts and concepts in Guyton's *Textbook of Medical Physiology*. No diagrams.

N | **How the Circulatory System Works** | $19.95
Mehler
Blackwell Science, 2000, 100 pages, ISBN 0865425485
Not yet reviewed.

N | **Hematology at a Glance** | $19.95
Mehta
Blackwell Science, 2000, 120 pages, ISBN 0632047933
Not yet reviewed.

N | **How the Endocrine System Works** | $19.95
Neal
Blackwell Science, 2001, 100 pages, ISBN 0632045566
Not yet reviewed.

Oklahoma Notes Physiology

$19.95 Review/345 q

Thies

Springer-Verlag, 1995, 280 pages, ISBN 0387943978

Dense text. Inconsistent quality of sections. Emphasizes general concepts, but incomplete. Boards-type questions with short answers. Some errors.

Commercial Review Courses

Kaplan Medical
Northwestern Learning
  Center
Postgraduate Medical
  Review Education
The Princeton Review
Youel's Prep, Inc.

Commercial preparation courses can be helpful for some students, but these courses are expensive and require significant time commitment. They are usually effective in organizing study material for students who feel overwhelmed by the volume of material. Note that the multiweek courses may be quite intense and may thus leave limited time for independent study. Also note that some commercial courses are designed for first-time test takers while others focus on students who are repeating the examination. Some courses focus on international medical graduates who want to take all three Steps in a limited amount of time. Student experience and satisfaction with review courses are highly variable. We suggest that you discuss options with recent graduates of review courses you are considering. Course content and structure can evolve rapidly. Some student opinions can be found in discussion groups on the World Wide Web.

Kaplan Medical

Kaplan Educational Centers, National Medical School Review (NMSR), and Compass Medical Education Network have merged to form Kaplan Medical. All program offerings are designed around the new computer-based USMLE.

Live Lectures

Kaplan Medical offers the IntensePrep™ live-lecture program created by Compass. This 15-day live course is designed specifically for second-year students and is offered on more than 20 U.S. medical school campuses across the nation. The fast pace and high-yield structure of the course make it suitable for (and restricted to) first-time takers of the exam. Many of the lecturers have authored USMLE review books, and all are experienced instructors. The course includes a full set of lecture notes, hundreds of practice questions, an organ-system-based CD-ROM, and a full-length simulated exam on CD-ROM. The course lecture notes are available before the start of the actual lectures for advance preparation. Tuition for this course is $999.

Longer live-lecture program options include a Prep version (approximately seven weeks) and an ExtendedPrep version (approximately 13 weeks) for repeaters of the exam or for students or physicians seeking more time to prepare. Call 1-800-533-8850 for more information about these courses.

Kaplan Center Study

Center-based review gives students access to more than 170 hours of lectures on video. At more than 120 Kaplan Educational Centers nationwide, students can use the video library as well as access the Kaplan library of medical texts. There are two center-based course options, both of which include access to the videos, lecture notes, an 850-question book with complete explanations, a simulated exam on CD-ROM, and an in-center exam simulation. Tuition for this course is $799. Call 1-800-533-8850 for more information on these courses.

Qreview

Reviewing USMLE-style questions is a popular method of preparing for the boards. Kaplan offers a questions-only Qreview program that features 3500 unique, exam-style questions with complete explanations. Qreview includes six months of access to Kaplan Medical's Step 1 Qbank and new Integrated Vignette Qbank. Qreview provides students with collective reporting of their results across both

Qbanks. A simulated full-length exam in the local center is also included. Tuition is $429. Qbank and IVQbank are also offered separately in either one-month or three-month increments. A demo is available online at www.kaplanmedical.com.

Northwestern Learning Center

Northwestern Learning Center offers live-lecture review courses for both the USMLE Step 1 and the COMLEX Level 1 examinations. Two types of courses are available for each exam: NBI 100—Primary Care for the Boards and NBI 300—Intensive Care for the Boards. NBI 100 is an on-site, 15-hour live-lecture review offered in two- and three-day formats that uses Northwestern Learning Center's TALLP techniques in conjunction with a systematic review of high-yield USMLE facts and concepts. This course is designed to organize students and to help them focus on the most essential aspects of their boards preparation. NBI 300 is a comprehensive, live boards preparation review conducted by a team of university faculty and authors of review notes. It also includes organized lecture notes, a large pool of practice questions, and simulated exams. NBI 300 is offered each year in two-, three-, and four-week formats both across the country and overseas. NBI 300 is also available in a customized, on-site format for groups of second-year students from individual U.S. medical schools. Sites are East Lansing, Ann Arbor, and Detroit, Michigan; Philadelphia; Los Angeles; and Long Island, New York. International sites in 2001 were in India, Saudi Arabia, the West Indies, and Tehran.

Tuition for NBI 100 ranges from $130 to $250 and for NBI 300 from $500 to $950 per student, depending on group size and early-enrollment discounts. NBI 100 home-study materials are available for $110. The Center also offers a retake option and a liberal cancellation policy. For more information, call 517-332-0777, or write to:

Northwestern Medical Review
2501 Coolidge
P.O. Box 22174
Lansing, MI 48909-2174
E-mail should be sent to testbuster@aol.com

The Center may also be found online at www.northwesternlearningcenter.com.

Postgraduate Medical Review Education

Postgraduate Medical Review Education (PMRE) has 24 years of experience with medical licensing exam preparation.

PMRE offers a complete home-study course for the USMLE Step 1 in the form of audio cassettes and concise books beginning at $300. PMRE has packages of 4200 questions and answers for both basic and clinical sciences for $220.

Every month, PMRE offers video reviews for $300 and live reviews for $990. PMRE guarantees that if a student does not pass the USMLE, he or she will receive a free additional live, video, or audio three-week review. The home-study course also comes with study materials totaling over $900.

PMRE uses professors who write questions for USMLE exams and professionally recorded materials.

For more information, call 1-800-ECFMG-30, or write to:

PMRE
407 Lincoln Road, Suite 12E
Miami Beach, FL 33139

E-mail should be sent to PMRE@aol.com

PMRE can also be found online at www.PMRE.com.

The Princeton Review

Several preparation options are available from The Princeton Review for the USMLE Steps 1 and 2. Medical students and graduates who thrive in a structured, classroom environment are likely to be more interested in The Princeton Review's Total Prep and Premium Prep courses, while its Exam Review and Self-Study options are more likely to appeal to those who wish to augment their own study plans with the benefits that review courses offer.

Total Prep ($1499) provides complete USMLE Step 1 preparation, including online diagnostic testing, a complete set of review manuals and workbooks, and more than 100 hours of class time devoted to reviewing high-yield Step 1 topics and practice exam results. Exam Review ($449), designed for students who will be doing the majority of their preparation on their own, includes full access to online diagnostic testing (more than 1000 practice items) and 28 hours of class time devoted to reviewing test results. No review manuals or workbooks are provided. Self-Study ($299) includes a complete set of review manuals and workbooks (over 2000 pages) and live test-taking strategy and wrap-up workshops. Exam Review Plus ($649) offers a combination of the Exam Review and Self-Study programs. A complete set of review materials and online diagnostic testing are included in addition to 28 hours of class time reviewing test results. No time in class will be provided to go over material from the manuals and workbooks.

The Princeton Review recruits and trains medical students and physicians who have achieved high USMLE scores to teach its preparation courses and contribute to its materials and tests. Classes are small, with no more than 30 students in each Exam Review section or 20 in each Total or Premium Prep course section.

You may request more information from The Princeton Review about its USMLE preparation options by calling 1-800-USMLE84 or by sending an e-mail message to gustavoj@review.com. Information is also available at www.review.com.

Youel's Prep, Inc.

Youel's Prep, Inc. has specialized in medical board preparation for 25 years. Youel's Prep provides web casts (*Youel's WebPrep*™), videotapes (*VideoPrep*™), audiotapes (*AudioPrep*™), books (*BookPrep*™), live lectures (*Youel's LivePrep*™), and tutorials for small groups and for individuals (*TutorialPrep*™). All web casts, videotapes, audiotapes, live lectures, and tutorials are correlated with the 3 book set, *Prep Notes©*: 2 textbooks, *Youel's Jewels I©* and *Youel's Jewels II©* (984 pages) and question and answer book, *Case Studies*.

FastTrac for the Basic Sciences©, available in audiotapes and books, 984 questions, answers, and explanations, is designed for both a HeadStart and FastFinish for the boards. *ClinicalSkillsAssesmentPrep*™ (*C-SAPPrep*™), available in videotape (24 hours) or audiotape (24 hours) and book, provides a concise summary of the symptoms, signs, and syndromes essential to taking a focused history and physical and preparing proper patient notes. *ClerkPrep*©, available in videotape, audiotape, and books, provides a HeadStart for clinical clerkships. *ClerkPrep*™ is offered in 24-hour and 40-hour programs. Q-Prep consists of 2 books with 1,854 questions, answers, and explanations.

All Youel's Prep are physician taught and written, reflecting the clinical slant of the boards. All programs are updated continuously, not just annually or every other year. Reflecting this, books are not printed until the order is received. Delivery in the United States is usually within 1 week. Optional express delivery is available.

Youel's Prep Home Study Program™—*Youel's Web Prep*™, *VideoPrep*™, *AudioPrep*™, *BookPrep*™— means the student owns the materials and can use them for repetitive study in the convenience of their homes.

Purchasers of any of the Youel's Prep programs are enrolled as members of the *Youel's Prep Family of Students*™. This provides free telephone tutoring by Youel.

Youel's Prep live lectures are held at select medical schools, at the invitation of the school and students. These programs are customized to meet individual and school needs. They can be custom-designed for 16–56 hours. First year students are urged to call early to arrange live lecture programs at their schools for next year. Youel's Prep-India & Nepal offers on-site programs in selected cities.

For more information contact:

Youel's Prep, Inc.
P.O. Box 4605
West Palm Beach, FL 33402
Phone: 1-800-645-3985
Fax: 1-561-366-8628
E-mail: youelsprep@bellsouth.net
Web site: www.youelsprep.com

Publisher Contacts

If you do not have convenient access to a medical bookstore, consider ordering directly from the publisher.

Alert & Oriented
13025 Candela Place
San Diego, CA 92130-1866
(888) 253-7844
joel@alertandonline.com
www.alertandonline.com

Appleton & Lange
(see McGraw-Hill)

BL Publishing
3614 North Raven Wash Drive
Tucson, Arizona 85745
(520) 743-1711
blpublishing@hotmail.com

Blackwell Science
Commerce Place
350 Main Street
Malden, MA 02148
(800) 759-6102
(781) 388-8255
Fax: (781) 388-8250
www.blackwellscience.com

Churchill Livingstone
300 Lighting Way
Secaucus, NJ 07094
(800) 553-5426
(973) 319-9800
Fax: (201) 319-9659

FMSG Publishing Co.
35 Hollow Pine Drive
DeBary, FL 32713
(904) 774-5277
Fax: (904) 774-5563
fmsgco@n-jcenter.com

Gold Standard Board Prep.
6374 Long Run Road
Athens, OH 45701
(740) 592-4124
Fax: (740) 592-4045
www.boardprep.net

J&S Publishing
1300 Bishop Lane
Alexandria, VA 22302
(703) 823-9833
Fax: (703) 823-9834
Jandspub@ix.netcom.com
www.jandspub.com

Lippincott Williams & Wilkins
P.O. Box 1580
Hagerstown, MD 21741
(800) 777-2295
Fax: (301) 824-7390
www.lww.com

Maval Publishing, Inc.
567 Harrison Street
Denver, CO 80206

McGraw-Hill/Appleton & Lange Customer Service
P.O. Box 545
Blacklick, OH 43004-0545
(800) 722-4726
Fax: (614) 755-5645
www.mghmedical.com

MedMaster, Inc.
P.O. Box 640028
Miami, FL 33164
(800) 335-3480
(305) 653-3480
Fax: (954) 962-4508
mmbks@aol.com

MedTech USA
6310 San Vicente Boulevard
Suite #425
Los Angeles, CA 90048
(800) 260-2600
Fax: (301) 824-7390
mail@medtech.com
www.medtech.com

Mosby-Year Book
11830 Westline Industrial Drive
St. Louis, MO 63146
(800) 325-4177 ext. 5017
Fax: (800) 535-9935
www.mosby.com

National Learning Corporation
212 Michael Drive
Syosset, NY 11791
(800) 645-6337
Fax: (516) 921-8743

Parthenon Publishing
One Blue Hill Plaza
P.O. Box 1564
Pearl River, NY 10965
(914) 735-9363
(800) 735-4744
usa@parthpub.com
www.parthpub.com

Springer-Verlag, NY Inc.
P.O. Box 2485
Secaucus, NJ 07096
(800) 777-4643
Fax: (201) 348-5405
orders@Springer-NY.com
www.Springer-NY.com

W. B. Saunders
6277 Sea Harbor Drive
Orlando, FL 32887
(800) 545-2522
Fax: (800) 874-6418

Sulzburger & Graham
165 West 91st Street
New York, NY 10024
(212) 947-0100

Abbreviations and Symbols

Abbreviation	Meaning
1°	primary
2°	secondary
3°	tertiary
AA	amino acid
AAV	adeno-associated virus
Ab	antibody
ABP	androgen-binding protein
Ac-CoA	acetylcoenzyme A
ACE	angiotensin-converting enzyme
ACh	acetylcholine
AChE	acetylcholinesterase
ACL	anterior cruciate ligament
ACTH	adrenocorticotropic hormone
AD	autosomal dominant
ADA	adenosine deaminase, Americans with Disabilities Act
ADH	antidiuretic hormone
ADHD	attention deficit hyperactivity disorder
ADP	adenosine diphosphate
AFP	α-fetoprotein
Ag	antigen
AICA	anterior inferior cerebellar artery
AIDS	acquired immunodeficiency syndrome
AII	angiotensin II
ALA	aminolevulinic acid
ALL	acute lymphocytic leukemia
ALS	amyotrophic lateral sclerosis
ALT	alanine transaminase
AML	acute myelocytic leukemia
AMP	adenosine monophosphate
ANA	antinuclear antibody
ANOVA	analysis of variance
ANP	atrial natriuretic peptide
ANS	autonomic nervous system
AOA	American Osteopathic Association
AP	action potential
APC	antigen-presenting cell
APKD	adult polycystic kidney disease
APSAC	anistreplase
aPTT	activated partial thromboplastin time
ARC	Appalachian Regional Commission
ARDS	acute respiratory distress syndrome
ARF	acute renal failure
Arg	arginine
ASD	atrial septal defect
ASO	antistreptolysin O
Asp	aspartic acid
AST	aspartate transaminase
ATP	adenosine triphosphate
ATPase	adenosine triphosphatase
AV	atrioventricular
AVM	arteriovenous malformation
AZT	azidothymidine [zidovudine]
BAL	British anti-Lewisite [dimercaprol]
BM	basement membrane

Abbreviation	Meaning
BP	blood pressure
BPG	bis-phosphoglycerate
BPH	benign prostatic hyperplasia
BS	Bowman's space
BUN	blood urea nitrogen
CAD	coronary artery disease
cAMP	cyclic adenosine monophosphate
C-ANCA	cytoplasmic antineutrophil cytoplasmic antibody
CBT	computer-based testing
CCK	cholecystokinin
CCl₄	carbon tetrachloride
CCT	cortical collecting tubule
CD	cluster of differentiation
CDP	cytidine diphosphate
CE	cholesterol ester
CEA	carcinoembryonic antigen
CETP	cholesterol-ester transfer protein
CF	cystic fibrosis
CFTR	cystic fibrosis transmembrane regulator
CFX	circumflex [artery]
cGMP	cyclic guanosine monophosphate
ChAT	choline acetyltransferase
CHF	congestive heart failure
CIN	candidate identification number, cervical intraepithelial neoplasia
CJD	Creutzfeldt-Jakob disease
CK-MB	creatine kinase, MB fraction
CL	clearance
CLL	chronic lymphocytic leukemia
CM	chylomicron
CML	chronic myeloid leukemia
CMT	Computerized Mastery Test
CMV	cytomegalovirus
CN	cranial nerve
CNS	central nervous system
CO	cardiac output
CoA	coenzyme A
COGME	Council on Graduate Medical Education
COM	communications [score]
COMLEX	Comprehensive Osteopathic Medical Licensing Examination
COPD	chronic obstructive pulmonary disease
COX	cyclooxygenase
CPAP	continuous positive airway pressure
CPK	creatine phosphokinase
Cr	creatinine
CRF	chronic renal failure
CRH	corticotropin-releasing hormone
CSA	Clinical Skills Assessment
CSF	cerebrospinal fluid, colony-stimulating factor
CT	computed tomography
CV	cardiovascular
CVA	costovertebral angle

Abbreviation	Meaning	Abbreviation	Meaning
Cx	complication	5f-dUMP	5-fluorodeoxyuridine monophosphate
CXR	chest x-ray	FE_{Na}	excreted fraction of filtered sodium
Cys	cysteine	FEV_1	forced expiratory volume in 1 second
D	dopamine	FF	filtration fraction
d4T	didehydrodeoxythymidine [stavudine]	FFA	free fatty acid
DAF	decay-accelerating factor	FLEX	Federation Licensing Examination
DAG	diacylglycerol	f-met	formylmethionine
dATP	deoxyadenosine triphosphate	FMG	foreign medical graduate
DCT	distal convoluted tubule	FMN	flavin mononucleotide
ddC	dideoxycytidine	FRC	functional residual capacity
ddI	didanosine	FSH	follicle-stimulating hormone
DES	diethylstilbestrol	FSMB	Federation of State Medical Boards
DG	data-gathering [score]	FTA-ABS	fluorescent treponemal antibody—
DHPG	dihydroxy-2-propoxymethyl guanine		absorbed
DHT	dihydrotestosterone	5-FU	5-fluorouracil
DI	diabetes insipidus	FVC	forced vital capacity
DIC	disseminated intravascular coagulation	G3P	glucose-3-phosphate
DIP	distal interphalangeal [joint]	G6P	glucose-6-phosphate
DKA	diabetic ketoacidosis	G6PD	glucose-6-phospate dehydrogenase
DM	diabetes mellitus	GABA	γ-aminobutyric acid
DMD	Duchenne's muscular dystrophy	GBM	glomerular basement membrane
DNA	deoxyribonucleic acid	GC	glomerular capillary
2,4-DNP	2,4-dinitrophenol	G-CSF	granulocyte colony-stimulating factor
DO	doctor of osteopathy	GFR	glomerular filtration rate
DOPA	dihydroxyphenylalanine [methyldopa]	GGT	γ-glutamyl transpeptidase
2,3-DPG	2,3-diphosphoglycerate	GH	growth hormone
DPM	doctor of podiatric medicine	GI	gastrointestinal
DPPC	dipalmitoyl phosphatidylcholine	γ-IFN	γ interferon
D/S	duration of status	GIP	gastric inhibitory peptide
dsDNA	double-stranded deoxyribonucleic acid	Glu	glutamic acid
dsRNA	double-stranded ribonucleic acid	GM-CSF	granulocyte-macrophage colony-
dTMP	deoxythymidine monophosphate		stimulating factor
DTR	deep tendon reflex	GMP	guanosine monophosphate
DTs	delirium tremens	GN	glomerulonephritis
DVT	deep venous thrombosis	GnRH	gonadotropin-releasing hormone
EBV	Epstein-Barr virus	GRP	gastrin-releasing peptide
EC_{50}	median effective concentration	GS	glomerulosclerosis
ECF	extracellular fluid	GSH	reduced glutathione
ECFMG	Educational Commission for Foreign	GSSG	oxidized glutathione
	Medical Graduates	GTP	guanosine triphosphate
ECG	electrocardiogram	GU	genitourinary
ECT	electroconvulsive therapy	H&E	hematoxylin and eosin
EDTA	ethylenediamine tetra-acetic acid	HAV	hepatitis A virus
EDV	end-diastolic volume	Hb	hemoglobin
EEG	electroencephalogram	HBcAb	hepatitis B core antibody
EF	ejection fraction	HBcAg	hepatitis B core antigen
EF-2	elongation factor 2	HBeAb	hepatitis B early antibody
ELISA	enzyme-linked immunosorbent assay	HBeAg	hepatitis B early antigen
EM	electron micrograph, electron	HBsAb	hepatitis B surface antibody
	microscopic, electron microscopy	HBsAg	hepatitis B surface antigen
EMB	eosin–methylene blue	HBV	hepatitis B virus
EOM	extraocular muscle	hCG	human chorionic gonadotropin
epi	epinephrine	HCV	hepatitis C virus
EPO	erythropoietin	HDL	high-density lipoprotein
ER	endoplasmic reticulum	HDV	hepatitis D virus
ERAS	Electronic Residency Application	HEV	hepatitis E virus
	Service	Hgb	hemoglobin
ERP	effective refractory period	HGPRTase	hypoxanthine-guanine
ERV	expiratory reserve volume		phosphoribosyltransferase
ESR	erythrocyte sedimentation rate	HHS	[Department of] Health and Human
ESV	end-systolic volume		Services
EtOH	ethyl alcohol	HHV	human herpesvirus
FAD	oxidized flavin adenine dinucleotide	5-HIAA	5-hydroxyindoleacetic acid
$FADH_2$	reduced flavin adenine dinucleotide	His	histidine
FAP	familial adenomatous polyposis	HIV	human immunodeficiency virus

Abbreviation	Meaning	Abbreviation	Meaning
HLA	human leukocyte antigen	LMN	lower motor neuron
HMG-CoA	hydroxymethylglutaryl-coenzyme A	LP	lymphocyte predominant, lumbar puncture
HMP	hexose monophosphate	LSE	Libman-Sacks endocarditis
HNPCC	hereditary nonpolyposis colorectal cancer	LT	leukotriene
HPSA	Health Professional Shortage Area	LV	left ventricle, left ventricular
HPV	human papillomavirus	Lys	lysine
HR	heart rate	MAC	membrane attack complex
HSV	herpes simplex virus	MAO	monoamine oxidase
HSV-1	herpes simplex virus 1	MAOI	monoamine oxidase inhibitor
HSV-2	herpes simplex virus 2	MAP	mean arterial pressure
5-HT	5-hydroxytryptamine (serotonin)	MC	mixed cellularity
HTLV	human T-cell leukemia virus	MCA	middle cerebral artery
HTN	hypertension	MCHC	mean corpuscular hemoglobin concentration
HUS	hemolytic-uremic syndrome	MCL	medial collateral ligament
IBD	inflammatory bowel disease	MCP	metacarpophalangeal [joint]
IC	inspiratory capacity	MCV	mean corpuscular volume
ICA	internal carotid artery	MD	muscular dystrophy
ICE	Integrated Clinical Encounter	MEN	multiple endocrine neoplasia
ICF	intracellular fluid	MEOS	microsomal ethanol oxidizing system
ICP	intracranial pressure	Met	methionine
ID_{50}	median infectious dose	MGUS	monoclonal gammopathy of undetermined significance
IDDM	insulin-dependent diabetes mellitus	MHC	major histocompatibility complex
IDL	intermediate-density lipoprotein	MI	myocardial infarction
IF	immunofluorescence	MLF	medial longitudinal fasciculus
Ig	immunoglobulin	6-MP	6-mercaptopurine
IHSS	idiopathic hypertrophic subaortic stenosis	MPO	myeloperoxidase
IL	interleukin	MPTP	1-methyl-4-phenyl-1,2,3,6-tetrahydropyridine
Ile	isoleucine	MRI	magnetic resonance imaging
IMA	inferior mesenteric artery	mRNA	messenger ribonucleic acid
IMG	international medical graduate	MS	multiple sclerosis
IMP	inosine monophosphate	MSH	melanocyte-stimulating hormone
INH	isonicotine hydrazine [isoniazid]	MVA	motor vehicle accident
INO	internuclear ophthalmoplegia	MVO_2	myocardial oxygen consumption
INS	Immigration and Naturalization Service	NAD^+	oxidized nicotinamide adenine dinucleotide
IP_3	inositol triphosphate	NADH	reduced nicotinamide adenine dinucleotide
IRV	inspiratory reserve volume	$NADP^+$	oxidized nicotinamide adenine dinucleotide phosphate
ITP	idiopathic thrombocytopenic purpura	NADPH	reduced nicotinamide adenine dinucleotide phosphate
IV	intravenous	NBME	National Board of Medical Examiners
IVC	inferior vena cava	NBOME	National Board of Osteopathic Medicine Examiners
IVDA	intravenous drug abuse	NBPME	National Board of Podiatric Medicine Examiners
JG	juxtaglomerular [cells]	NE	norepinephrine
JGA	juxtaglomerular apparatus	NF2	neurofibromatosis type 2
KOH	potassium hydroxide	NHL	non-Hodgkin's lymphoma
KPV	killed polio vaccine	NIDDM	non-insulin-dependent diabetes mellitus
KSHV	Kaposi's sarcoma–associated herpesvirus	NK	natural killer [cells]
LA	left atrial	NMJ	neuromuscular junction
LAD	left anterior descending [artery]	NPV	negative predictive value
LCA	left coronary artery	NS	nodular sclerosing
LCAT	lecithin-cholesterol acyltransferase	NSAID	nonsteroidal anti-inflammatory drug
LCL	lateral collateral ligament	OAA	oxaloacetic acid
LCME	Liaison Committee on Medical Education	OCD	obsessive-compulsive disorder
LCV	lymphocytic choriomeningitis virus	OCP	oral contraceptive pill
LD	lymphocyte depleted	OMT	osteopathic manipulative technique
LDH	lactate dehydrogenase	OPV	oral polio vaccine
LDL	low-density lipoprotein		
LES	lower esophageal sphincter		
Leu	leucine		
LFA-1	leukocyte function–associated antigen 1		
LFT	liver function test		
LH	luteinizing hormone		
LLQ	left lower quadrant		
LM	light microscopy		

473

Abbreviation	Meaning	Abbreviation	Meaning
OR	odds ratio	SC	subcutaneous
OSCE	objective structured clinical examination	SCID	severe combined immunodeficiency disease
PA	posteroanterior	SD	standard deviation
PABA	para-aminobenzoic acid	SEM	standard error of the mean
PAH	para-aminohippuric acid	SER	smooth endoplasmic reticulum
PALS	periarteriolar lymphoid sheath	SGOT	serum glutamic oxaloacetic transaminase
PAN	polyarteritis nodosa	SGPT	serum glutamic pyruvate transaminase
P-ANCA	perinuclear antineutrophil cytoplasmic antibody	SIADH	syndrome of inappropriate antidiuretic hormone
PCL	posterior cruciate ligament	SLC	Sylvan Learning Center
PCP	phencyclidine hydrochloride, *Pneumocystis carinii* pneumonia	SLE	systemic lupus erythematosus
		SLL	small lymphocytic lymphoma
PCR	polymerase chain reaction	SMA	superior mesenteric artery
PCWP	pulmonary capillary wedge pressure	SMX	sulfamethoxazole
PD	posterior descending [artery]	SOD	superoxide dismutase
PDA	patent ductus arteriosus	SP	standardized patient
PDE	phosphodiesterase	SR	sarcoplasmic reticulum
PEP	phosphoenolpyruvate	SRP	sponsoring residency program
PFK	phosphofructokinase	SRS-A	slow-reacting substance of anaphylaxis
PFT	pulmonary function test	ssDNA	single-stranded deoxyribonucleic acid
PG	prostaglandin	SSRI	selective serotonin reuptake inhibitor
Phe	phenylalanine	ssRNA	single-stranded ribonucleic acid
PICA	posterior inferior cerebellar artery	STC	Sylvan Technology Center
PID	pelvic inflammatory disease	STD	sexually transmitted disease
PIP	proximal interphalangeal [joint]	SV	stroke volume
PIP_2	phosphatidylinositol 4,5-bisphosphate	SVC	superior vena cava
PK	pyruvate kinase	SVT	supraventricular tachycardia
PKD	polycystic kidney disease	$t_{1/2}$	half-life
PKU	phenylketonuria	T_3	triiodothyronine
PML	progressive multifocal leukoencephalopathy	T_4	thyroxine
		TB	tuberculosis
PMN	polymorphonuclear [leukocyte]	TBW	total body water
PN	patient note	3TC	dideoxythiacytidine [lamivudine]
PNH	paroxysmal nocturnal hemoglobinuria	Tc cell	cytotoxic T cell
PNS	peripheral nervous system	TCA	tricyclic antidepressant
PPRF	paramedian pontine reticular formation	TCR	T-cell receptor
PPV	positive predictive value	TFT	thyroid function test
PRPP	phosphoribosylpyrophosphate	TG	triglyceride
PSA	prostate-specific antigen	TGF	transforming growth factor
PSS	progressive systemic sclerosis	Th cell	helper T cell
PT	prothrombin time	THF	tetrahydrofolate
PTH	parathyroid hormone	Thr	threonine
PTHrP	parathyroid hormone–related protein	TIBC	total iron-binding capacity
PTT	partial thromboplastin time	TLC	total lung capacity
PV	plasma volume	TMP-SMX	trimethoprim-sulfamethoxazole
RA	rheumatoid arthritis	TN	trigeminal neuralgia
RBC	red blood cell	TNF	tumor necrosis factor
RBF	renal blood flow	TOEFL	Test of English as a Foreign Language
RCA	right coronary artery	t-PA	tissue plasminogen activator
RDS	respiratory distress syndrome	TPP	thiamine pyrophosphate
REM	rapid eye movement	TRH	thyrotropin-releasing hormone
RER	rough endoplasmic reticulum	tRNA	transfer ribonucleic acid
RNA	ribonucleic acid	Trp	tryptophan
RPF	renal plasma flow	TSH	thyroid-stimulating hormone
RPR	rapid plasma reagin	TSI	thyroid-stimulating immunoglobulin
RR	relative risk	TSS	toxic shock syndrome
rRNA	ribosomal ribonucleic acid	TSST	toxic shock syndrome toxin
RS	Reed-Sternberg [cells]	TTP	thrombotic thrombocytopenic purpura
RSV	respiratory syncytial virus	TV	tidal volume
RUQ	right upper quadrant	TXA	thromboxane
RV	right ventricle, right ventricular, residual volume	UCV	*Underground Clinical Vignettes*
		UDP	uridine diphosphate
RVH	right ventricular hypertrophy	UMN	upper motor neuron
SA	sinoatrial	URI	upper respiratory infection
SAM	*S*-adenosylmethionine		

Abbreviation	Meaning	Abbreviation	Meaning
USDA	United States Department of Agriculture	VF	ventricular fibrillation
USIA	United States Information Agency	VHL	von Hippel–Lindau [disease]
USMLE	United States Medical Licensing Examination	VIPoma	vasoactive intestinal polypeptide-secreting tumor
UTI	urinary tract infection	VLDL	very low density lipoprotein
UV	ultraviolet	V/Q	ratio of ventilation to perfusion
VA	Veterans Administration	VSD	ventricular septal defect
Val	valine	VZV	varicella-zoster virus
VC	vital capacity	WBC	white blood cell
V_d	volume of distribution	ZE	Zollinger-Ellison [syndrome]
VDRL	Venereal Disease Research Laboratory		

Index

A

methotrexate, 333
multiple myeloma, 254
pancreatic enzymes, 379
poliomyelitis, 264
ribosome, 183
rough endoplasmic reticulum, 101
serum sickness, 223
tacrolimus, 346
Proteinuria, 284, 324
Proteoglycan, 101
Proteus, 193, 196
Proteus mirabilis, 214, 215, 302, 303
Prothrombin time (PT), 176, 250
Protozoa, medically important, 201
Proximal jejunum, 379
Psammoma bodies, 291
Pseudocyesis, 136
Pseudocyst formation, 259
Pseudogout, 267
Pseudohermaphroditism, 237
Pseudomembranous colitis, 305
Pseudomonas, 185, 213, 238, 303
Pseudomonas aeruginosa, 189, 194, 213
Psoriasis, 291, 333
Psychiatry, 122
   See also under Behavioral science
Psychology, 122
   See also under Behavioral science
Psychosis, 272, 289, 318, 319, 335
Pterygoid, 90
Ptosis, 262, 265
Ptyalin, 376
Publications, NBME/USMLE, 14
   See also Review resources, database
      of basic science
Public Health, State Departments of, 48
Publisher contacts, 470
Pudendal nerve block, 98
Pulmonary edema, 279, 288, 320
Pulmonary embolus, 281
Pulmonary fibrosis, 330, 333, 334
Pulmonary stenosis, 234
Pulse, 235, 283
Pulsus paradoxus, 260, 282
Pupillary light reflex, 109
Purines, 146, 333
Purine salvage deficiencies, 166
Purkinje fibers, 351
Pyelonephritis, 213, 285, 287, 288
Pyloric stenosis, 234, 254
Pyoderma gangrenosum, 255
Pyrantel pamoate, 202, 311
Pyrazinamide, 307
Pyridostigmine, 313
Pyridoxal phosphate, 174
Pyrimethamine, 201
Pyrimidines, 146, 333
Pyruvate, 160, 170, 171, 173, 174

Q

Questions, exam, 3, 10, 28–29, 57
Quinidine, 327, 329
Quinine, 311
Quinolones, 302
Q waves, 279

R

Rabies, 208
Race
   blood dyscrasias, 249
   celiac sprue, 267
   cystic fibrosis, 238
   gallstones, 259
   glucose-6-phosphate dehydrogenase
      deficiency, 162
   lactase deficiency, 163
   osteoporosis, 273
   sarcoidosis, 267
   systemic lupus erythematosus, 267
   Takayasu's arteritis, 283
   uterine pathology, 275
   See also Genetics
Radial nerve, 117
Radiation, 249
Radiology, 76
   See also X-rays
Raloxifene, 335
Random error, 124
Ranitidine, 339
Rapacuronium, 314
Rapid eye movements (REM), 131
Rapidly progressive
      glomerulonephritis, 284
Rathke's pouch, 246
Rationalization, 140
Raynaud's phenomenon, 267, 283
Reaction formation, 140
Reassortment, 206
Recall bias, 125
Recombination, 206
Red blood cells
   aplastic anemia, 249
   casts, 290
   Cori cycle, 161
   forms, 291
   gallstones, 259
   glucose, 370
   glucose-6-phosphate dehydrogenase
      deficiency, 162
   glycolytic enzyme deficiency, 160
   hereditary spherocytosis, 249
   leukemias, 252
   metabolism, 162
   mononucleosis, 209
   multiple myeloma, 254
   normocytic anemia, 248
   overview, 77
   pathology, 291
   physiologic chloride shift, 77
   plasma membrane composition, 155
   sickle cell anemia, 249
   vitamin E, 176
Red infarcts, 277
Red man syndrome, 304
Reductase deficiency, 237
Reed-Sternberg cells, 291
Reflexes, 115, 117, 266, 270, 288, 323
Registering to take the exam, 7–8
Regression, 129, 140
Reichert's cartilage, 84
Reinforcement schedules, 141

Reiter's syndrome, 214, 268, 291
Rejection, transplant, 225
Reliability, 124
REM sleep, 131
Renal cell carcinoma, 247
Renal failure, 287, 290
Renal insufficiency, 368
Renal tubular necrosis, 307
Renin, 269, 317, 323, 324
Renin-angiotensin system, 97, 269, 365
Reoviruses, 205–207
Replication, DNA/RNA, 147, 206
Reportable diseases, 126
Repression, 140
Reproduction. *See* endocrine/
      reproductive *under* Pathology
      and Physiology; Pregnancy
Reserpine, 323
Residencies and International medical
      graduates, 42–43
Residual volume (RV), 374
Resistance mechanisms for various
      antibiotics, 308
Respiratory acidosis, 285, 286
Respiratory alkalosis, 285, 286
Respiratory distress syndrome, 129
Respiratory system
   antimuscarinic drugs, 314
   atropine, 313
   benzodiazepines, 318, 322
   chemical carcinogens, 243
   cystic fibrosis, 238
   diabetic ketoacidosis, 272
   inhaled anesthetics, 322
   macrolides, 305
   myocardial infarction, 278
   opioids, 320
   oxygen-dependent respiratory burst,
      159
   sympathomimetics, 315
   syndrome of inappropriate
      antidiuretic hormone, 272
   tricyclic antidepressants, 319
   See also Pulmonary *listings*;
      respiratory *under* Pathology
      and Physiology
Restrictive lung disease, 260, 267
Restrictive/obliterative
      cardiomyopathy, 279
Reticular activating system, 107
Reticulocyte, 77
Reticulocytosis, 248
Retinalis, 169
Retinoblastoma, 242
Retrograde amnesia, 133
Retroperitoneal structures, 95
Retroviruses, 205, 206
Reverse transcriptase inhibitors, 310
Review resources, database of basic
      science
   anatomy (new resources)
      Anatomy Recall PDA
         (Blackbourne), 421
      *Clinical Neuroanatomy Made
         Ridiculously Simple-Interactive
         Edition* (Goldberg), 422

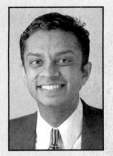 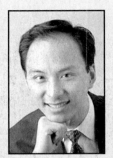 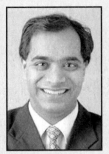 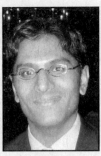 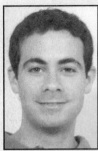

Vikas Bhushan, MD   Tao Le, MD   Chirag Amin, MD   Anil Shivaram   Joshua Klein

Vikas Bhushan, MD Dr. Bhushan is a world-renowned author, publisher, entrepreneur, and board-certified diagnostic radiologist who resides in Los Angeles, California. Dr. Bhushan conceived and authored the original *First Aid for the USMLE Step 1* in 1992, which, after eleven consecutive editions, has become the most popular medical review book in the world. Following this, he co-authored three additional *First Aid* books as well as developed the highly acclaimed 17-title *Underground Clinical Vignettes* series. He completed his training in diagnostic radiology at the University of California, Los Angeles. Dr. Bhushan has more than 13 years of entrepreneurial experience and started two successful software and publishing companies prior to co-founding Medsn. He has worked directly with dozens of medical school faculty, colleagues, and consultants and corresponded with thousands of medical students from around the world. Dr. Bhushan earned his bachelor's degree in biochemistry from the University of California, Berkeley, and his MD with thesis from the University of California, San Francisco.

Tao Le, MD Dr. Le has led multiple medical education projects over the past seven years. As a medical student, he was editor-in-chief of the University of California, San Francisco Synapse, a university newspaper with a weekly circulation of 9,000. Subsequently, he authored *First Aid for the Wards* and *First Aid for the Match* and led the most recent revision of *First Aid for the USMLE Step 2*. At Yale, he was a regular guest lecturer on the USMLE review courses and an adviser to the Yale University School of Medicine curriculum committee. Dr. Le earned his medical degree from the University of California, San Francisco in 1996 and completed his residency training and board certification in internal medicine at Yale-New Haven Hospital. Dr. Le subsequently went on to co-found Medsn and currently serves as its Chief Medical Officer.

Chirag Amin, MD Dr. Amin has extensive experience in the field of medical education and has served as a co-author with Drs. Bhushan and Le on the entire *First Aid* series. He also led the completion of *The Insider's Guide to the MCAT,* published by Lippincott Williams & Wilkins. Dr. Amin has an extensive background in Internet-related enterprises; he actively follows a number of development-stage Internet companies. Dr. Amin earned his BS in biology at the University of Illinois in 1992. He then went on to get his MD with Research Distinction from the University of Miami School of Medicine in 1996 and completed three years of residency training in orthopedic surgery at Orlando Regional Medical Center.

Anil Shivaram Anil is a senior medical student at Yale University School of Medicine. As an undergraduate at Columbia University (Roar Lions, Roar!), he graduated with a degree in MEALAC (huh?) aka Sanskrit and parlayed his love of extinct languages into graduate studies at Oxford. He served as a Fellow in Ethics at the AMA's Institute for Ethics, where he was re-made into the fine, upstanding, and ethical being he is today. His research interest in eyeballs steered him out to LA where he found a home studying the migration of retinal microglia and a renewed passion to pursue ophthalmology. He can sometimes be found having it out with the likes of Scoopy, Oog, Nk, and Taco (boy), but ultimately they all agree that he does not flail while scuba diving. A level-headed, soon-to-be physician, he can be reached at anil.shivaram@yale.edu, unless he happens to be in one of his "Omni" phases.

Joshua Klein Josh is currently a fifth year student in the MD/PhD program at Yale University School of Medicine. He is originally from Roslyn, NY and went to college at the University of Pennsylvania, where he studied biology and music theory and graduated with a BA in 1997. He is completing his thesis in Dr. Stephen Waxman's neurology lab at Yale and has published several clinical and basic science papers. Josh would like to acknowledge the support of Meredith, Willard and Bradley at the University of Illinois College of Veterinary Medicine. This is Josh's third year working for First Aid for the USMLE Step I. He can be contacted at joshua.p.klein@yale.edu.

About the Authors

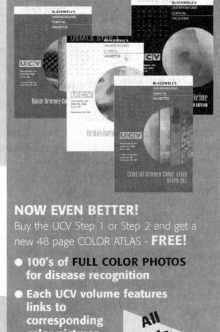

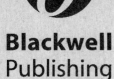

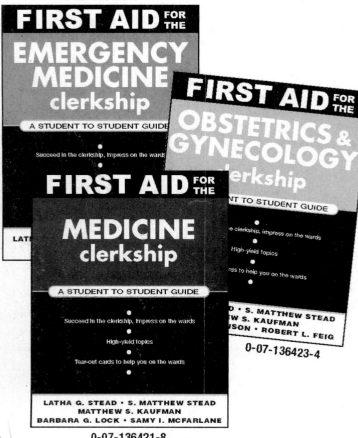
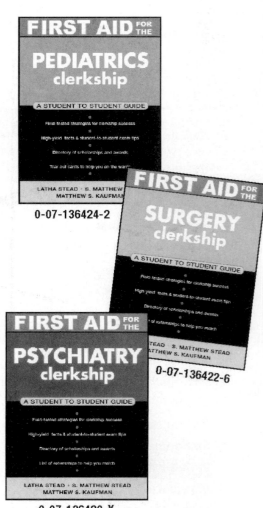